Medical Electronic Records Education Programs

Certificate, Diploma, Degree and Postgraduate Courses

Medical Electronic Records Education Programs

Certificate, Diploma, Degree and Postgraduate Courses

GD Mogli PhD, MBA, FHRIM (UK), FAHIMA (USA)
(Father of Medical Records of India and Middle East)
(Known as Champion of Developing Countries by IFHIMA (World))
Visiting Professor, Medical Informatics
Mahatma Gandhi Institute of Medical Sciences, Sevagram, Maharashtra
Ex WHO Consultant and Senior Consultant, eHealth Management, HEARTCOM (USA)
Dean, Health Information Management (HIM) Program, MOH Oman
Associate Professor, HIM Degree Program, King Faisal University, Saudi Arabia
Head the Department, HIM Diploma Program, Kuwait Institute of Health Sciences, Kuwait
Head of the Department, HIM Program (JIPMER), University of Madras, India
Senior Consultant/Adviser to the Ministries of Health
India, Afghanistan, Iran, Kuwait, Saudi Arabia, Oman, Bahrain, Qatar and UAE
gdmogli@yahoo.com

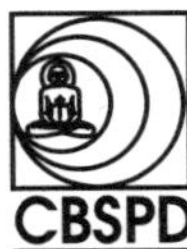

CBS Publishers & Distributors Pvt Ltd

New Delhi • Bengaluru • Chennai • Kochi • Kolkata • Lucknow • Mumbai
Hyderabad • Jharkhand • Nagpur • Patna • Pune • Uttarakhand

Disclaimer

Science and technology are constantly changing fields. New research and experience broaden the scope of information and knowledge. The author has tried his best in giving information available to him while preparing the material for this book. Although, all efforts have been made to ensure optimum accuracy of the material, yet it is quite possible some errors might have been left uncorrected. The publisher, printer and the author will not be held responsible for any inadvertent errors, omissions or inaccuracies.

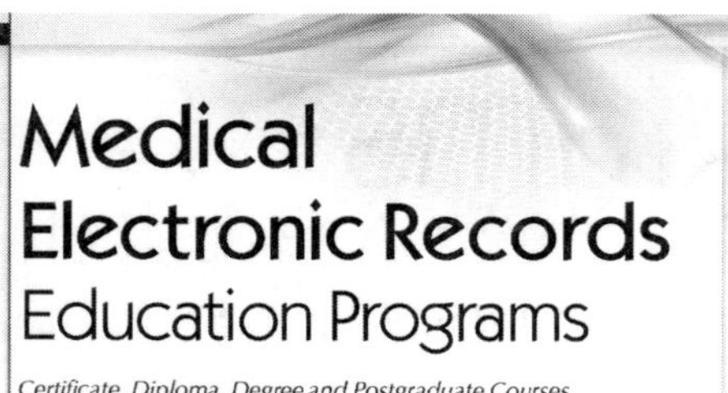

ISBN: 978-93-5466-248-5

First Edition: 2025

Published by Satish Kumar Jain and produced by Varun Jain for

CBS Publishers & Distributors Pvt Ltd
4819/XI Prahlad Street, 24 Ansari Road, Daryaganj, New Delhi 110 002, India
Ph: 011-23289259, 23266838 Website: www.cbspd.com
e-mail: delhi@cbspd.com

Corporate Office: 204 FIE, Industrial Area, Patparganj, Delhi 110 092
Ph: 011-4934 4934 Fax: 011-4934 4935 e-mail: publishing@cbspd.com; publicity@cbspd.com

Branches

- **Bengaluru:** Seema House 2975, 17th Cross, K.R. Road, Banasankari 2nd Stage, Bengaluru 560 070, Karnataka, India
  Ph: +91-80-26771678/79 Fax: +91-80-26771680 e-mail: bangalore@cbspd.com
- **Chennai:** 7, Subbaraya Street, Shenoy Nagar, Chennai 600 030, Tamil Nadu, India
  Ph: +91-44-26680620, 26681266 Fax: +91-44-42032115 e-mail: chennai@cbspd.com
- **Kochi:** 42/1325, 1326, Power House Road, Opp KSEB, Power House, Ernakulam 682 018, Kerala, India
  Ph: +91-484-4059061-65 Fax: +91-484-4059065 e-mail: kochi@cbspd.com
- **Kolkata:** 147, Hind Ceramics Compound, 1st Floor, Nilgunj Road, Belghoria, Kolkata-700056 West Bengal, India
  Ph: 033-25633055, 033-25633056 e-mail: kolkata@cbspd.com
- **Lucknow:** Basement, Khushnuma Complex, 7-Meerabai Marg (Behind Jawahar Bhawan), Lucknow 226001, India
  Ph: 0522-4000032 e-mail: tiwari.lucknow@cbspd.com
- **Mumbai:** PWD Shed. Gala no. 25/26, Ramchandra Bhatt Marg, Next to JJ Hospital Gate no. 2, Opp. Union Bank of India Noorbaug Mumbai-400009, Maharashtra, India
  Ph: 022-66661880/89 e-mail: mumbai@cbspd.com

Representatives

- **Hyderabad** 0-9885175004 • **Jharkhand** 0-9811541605 • **Nagpur** 0-8692091830
- **Patna** 0-9334159340 • **Pune** 0-9664372571 • **Uttarakhand** 0-9716462459

Printed at Glorious Printers, Delhi, India

to

Government of India and Other Nations

for

Standardization of Electronic Medical Health Records and Standardization of HIM Educational Programs

Preface

In the study and practice of medicine and other allied paramedical fields, there is constant need for guiding principles, brief summaries of subjects related to the allied medical sciences, and explanations of techniques and procedures are require to learn. It is evident that students of medical, nursing and paramedic science courses cannot become proficient in their respective field without having continuing education and team work among all the medical, nursing and other allied health science professionals and also to be part of global development in the advancement of medicine.

In the course of my four-decade career as medical record administrator, educator, consultant and adviser, dealing with health professionals in diverse organizations, in nine different countries, felt the need for a comprehensive education book encompassing diploma, degree, masters and specialty certificate program syllabus, course content coupled with practical (directed practice) of latest at par with international standard practice book to meet the global needs. A handbook for the present users, especially the students of medical records which is transformed as health information management (HIM) as popularly known globally, to have the basics of the role and functions of health information management system at their regular professional studies to be well equipped with the hospital electronic record systems and management which are the common place in any modern hospital around the globe. With this objective, a considerable time and efforts have gone in preparing this comprehensive education/training book with various level educational programs to meet the facet of entire health information management field.

This book's objective is to serve the medical and allied educational institutions, faculty members to develop HIM multifarious educational and training programs across the nation in order to benefit extremely the HIM and allied health science students, and medical, nursing and other allied healthcare workers to gain with specialty certificate programs. Now, it is right time the educational programs to be initiated by all the medical colleges and schools of medicine, nursing and other allied health science branches so that the future healthcare providers are well conversant with the modern digital system used in healthcare institutions. This book also absorbs the concept of the healthcare delivery system in comprehensive manner practiced with the use of modern technology and communication to provide swift, safe, quality and cost contained care. Precisely, this is an amalgamation of all ingredients vital to be an efficient health information management professional once he/she qualifies.

This book consists of 24 chapters, 5 annexures, and bibliography; first eight chapters deal with introduction to health information management (HIM) standards, HIM role in efficient management of health information, professional skills to meet future emerging technology, insurance and reimbursement methods. And challenges in implementing electronic health records, elements of EHR functional requirements and tips for evaluating the pre-implementation of EHRs services in selection of software and challenges of hospital IT and network design for EHRS, the need for exchange clinical knowledge and a guide to better physician's practice. Chapter 9 is dedicated to personnel requirements, and job descriptions for medical records (health information) management department, job opportunities, various skills to be acquired to meet the challenges. Most importantly, from Chapters 10 to 12 deal with comprehensively diploma, degree and master's syllabus, course content classified into semester programs with details of course content. Chapter 13 encompasses detailed directed professional practice and internship project assignments at the hospital site. And from chapters 14 to 21 cover EMR specialised certificate/diploma programs in IT and medical and health informatics for clinical pathways; for medical, nursing, operation theatre, ward, MR personnel, and coders.

Chapter 22 is dedicated to provide guidelines for establishing at the national and state level, HIM center for excellence, the national institute for HIM and allied health sciences with building plan with allocation of needed specialized services rooms furnished for the Ministry of Health and Family Welfare of Government of India and also at state level institutions to oversee the entire electronic medical records standards and educational programs to meet those requirements at all levels and in all the institutions. The other chapters include a sample medical record diploma education program in Kuwait, and Government of India's recommendations of electronic medical records standards for Indian hospitals and health institutions. Important annexure-related to glossary terms for medical specialties, software structure for EMR, terms and definition used in healthcare management, standardization of medical abbreviations and concludes with bibliography.

The need for qualified HIM professionals is so huge, there is an acute shortage and dire need of health records/information management professionals across the country, in order to improve healthcare delivery system including primary, secondary and tertiary care at all levels of the nation through improving health record information management system. For which adequate professionals are needed to manage HIM departments in all the health institutions. Without which, the health institutions especially, the hospitals have to function without HIM departments or with non-qualified persons to maintain highly sensitive and most vital records of patients written by highly paid and qualified healthcare providers. Through this stimulus, it is possible for all the institutions to implement the standardized electronic medical/health records and standardized HIM educational programs in all the health and educational centers.

Salient features of this book:

Our country is embarking on medical tourism and a huge number of corporate hospitals is investing heavily on infrastructure and equipping with latest technologies and world class expert specialists to meet the patient care services at par with the international standards. The work of specialist expert healthcare providers is documented either manually or electronically in medical records which reflect the quantitative and qualitative care provided by the health institutions. Hence the maintenance of records is of paramount importance as they not only meet the needs of quality and continuity of patient care, but also required for medical education, research, legal, and insurance, public health information required by national and international authorities. The persons who manage these documents, including manual and electronic, are well educated and trained in the field are called earlier medical records managers or officers, lately, they are known as health information managers or administrators.

The author had the unique advantage of visiting many educational universities, colleges and institutions around the world, he had visited USA as a Dean and envoy of the Ministry of Health, Sultanate of Oman and signed Memorandum of Understanding (MOU) with three renowned universities, e.g. Loma Linda University of California, Duquesne University in Pittsburgh and the State University of Chicago, for two-year Medical Record

Diploma Program with syllabus and course content and got approved so that the two-year diploma qualified student can enter directly into 3rd year of four-year baccalaureate program. The two-year diploma program specified in this book is in line with the internationally practiced program. Similarly, the HIM baccalaureate and Master's programs was developed for King Faisal University, Saudi Arabia.

This type of book is not available, either in India or other parts of the world to generate required professionals. In order to meet this challenge around the globe, most imperative need is to have adequate educated or trained professionals to implement the system efficiently. It is estimated that India needs at least 2,00,000 qualified managerial and supervisory HIM-skilled healthcare technologists to work in about 70,000+ public and private hospitals (2021) to meet the demand as the healthcare field has the responsibility to ensure proper maintenance of medical records in any form and protect the privacy, confidentiality and security of information.

This book will be of immense value to all medical colleges, allied health institutions, faculty members of medical, nursing and allied health sciences. Medical record or HIM professionals, the organizers of medical record or health information departments, health directorates, ministries of health besides medical record educational and paramedical courses and research institutions will also be immensely benefit by this masterpiece.

GD Mogli

Acknowledgements

In the course of experience gained in nine nations by serving in the Ministries of Health at national level as Senior Medical Record Consultant Adviser and WHO Consultant from 1981–2008, in all the six Gulf Cooperative Council (GCC) Countries (Kuwait, Saudi Arabia, Bahrain, Qatar, UAE and Oman). Apart from this, I had also served in India and Afghanistan from 1966 to 1980. With this background, felt the need of hour is to provide a concise but practical educational book that would help in HIM teaching; certificate, diploma, degree, master's with comprehensive syllabus, course content, course objective and directed practice at the hospital site. This book should serve all the medical colleges and allied health science colleges or institutions for establishing HIM programs and to teach to generate excellent professionals to deal with the emerging technologies to provide best possible healthcare to the needy people. The faculty of HIM program will find the book handy in their teaching and learning methods. I owe my respectful gratitude to each and every one with who I had an association.

At the outset, my grateful thanks to CBS Publishers & Distributors Pvt Ltd., New Delhi, for bringing out this invaluable book.

My sincere gratitude to State Health Ministers and Deputy Ministers of Gulf Cooperation Council (GCC) Countries and other administrators, and professional colleagues of India, Afghanistan, Iran, Kuwait, Kingdom of Saudi Arabia, Oman, Bahrain, Qatar, and United Arab Emirates (UAE), for their support, encouragement and cooperation.

My thanks are due to Mr Selvakumar Ramalingam, ACC (UK), AHRIM (UK), BMRSc, MA, MS, PGDHM, Team Leader, Clinical Coding, University College of London Hospital and Moorfields Ophthalmology Hospital, NHS Foundation Trust, London, UK.

My special thanks to Mr Narendar Sampath Kumar, MBA (Hospital Management), Master's of Population Studies, BMRSc, PGDCS, CHRIM (UK), CCS, CCA (AHIMA), Health Information Manager, Mediclinic, Middle East Dubai, and United Arab Emirates.

My special thanks to Mr Vikky (ND Vikram) MBA, DMRS, BMRSc, CHRIM, QMS, Lead Auditor, IRCA, Prince 2, ITIL, Sr IMIT Clinical Business/Systems—Projects Analyst, Cerner, Allscripts, NOVA Scotia Health Authority, Pro Government of NS, Halifax, Novascotia, Canada.

My sincere gratitude to Dr Saadoun Faris Al Azmi, MS, PhD (USA), Associate Professor, College of Health Sciences, The Public Authority for applied Education and Training, Kuwait, for contributing Chapter 23: "Medical Records Diploma Education Program in Kuwait".

My special thanks to Dr Raniya Al Kiyumi, MHIM, BSc, GCertEd. Studs, PhD (Australia), Senior Lecturer, Oman College of Health Sciences, and Associate Deanship for Health Information Management, Ministry of Health, Oman.

Mrs Mary Stella Alexander, BSc, BMRSc, CHRIM (UK), Medical Record Manager, Hamad General Hospital, Doha, Qatar.

And lastly, I owe my sincere gratitude to my family for their unconditional support.

GD Mogli

Contents

Chapter 1

Introduction to Health Information Management

Electronic Medical Records (EMR) Management is also known as Health Record Management. In India and some developing countries use the term Electronic Medical Records while most of Western countries especially USA and Canada use the term Electronic Health Records (EHR). There is slight difference; electronic medical records are mostly used for ambulatory and most hospital-based records for curative; mostly for secondary and tertiary care purpose, while electronic health records are comprehensive longitudinal records encompass primary, secondary and tertiary information from birth to death.

Health Information Management (HIM) Professionals: HIM professionals may not deal with patient directly, but help patients indirectly by maintaining their records or taking care of medical data and ensure reliability, timeliness, accuracy and completeness. They maintain patient records in the strictest of all confidences making sure these records remain securely protected and ensure the information is readily available to authorized healthcare providers whenever and wherever needed. HIM plans information systems, develops health policy, identifies current and future information needs and applies the science of informatics to the collection, analysis, storage, use and transmission of information to meet legal, professional, ethical and administrative records-keeping requirements of healthcare delivery. Their services are used in clinical, epidemiological, demographic, financial services. The HIM plays a crucial role in the healthcare delivery system of any health institution.

There are three distinct career-oriented areas concerning health information, all professionals seeking careers should inspect that include health information management, health information technology and health informatics.

Health Information Management (HIM): HIM activity focuses mainly on obtaining, analyzing in a systematic order the traditional and digital medical information for continuity of patient care and many other purposes such as medical education, research, legal and public health, etc. With the widespread computerization of health records, traditional (paper-based) records are being replaced with Electronic Health Records (EHRs). The tools of health informatics and health information technology are being increasingly utilized to introduce efficiency in information management practices in the healthcare sector.

Both hospital information systems and health human resources information systems (HRHS) are common implementations of HIM.

Health information management professionals are specialized in this field to maintain efficiently the patient medical records and health information according to the highest standards, and protecting data integrity, the confidentiality and secure data and making available only to authorized personnel.

HIM STANDARDS BEGAN WITH ESTABLISHMENT OF AHIMA

History of HIM standard is dated back to the introduction of American Health Information Management Association, founded in 1928 "when the American College of Surgeons established the Association of Record Librarians of North America (ARLNA) to elevate the standards of clinical records in hospitals and other medical institutions". In 1938, AHIMA was known as American Association of Medical Record Librarians (AAMRL) and its members were known as medical record librarians who studied medical record science. The goal was to raise the standards of record keeping in hospitals and other healthcare facilities. The individuals involved in this profession were promoters for the successful management of clinical records to guarantee accuracy and precision. Over time, the organization's name changed to reflect the evolving field of health information management practices, eventually becoming the American Health Information Management Association (AHIMA). AHIMA members affect the quality of patient information and patient care at every touch point in the healthcare delivery cycle. They often serve in bridge roles, connecting clinical, operational, and administrative functions.

Health Information Technology (HIT): HIT is a vital aspect that deals with management of patient's health data in digital format, safe storage and exchange system. The health information technologists specialized in IT hardware and software employed to manage and store patient health information and focus strictly on technical aspects concerning information management. The HIT professionals possess specific knowledge and skills related to management of computer-based health records and information as well as other systems designed to aid the healthcare providers including other allied health workers in efficient management of healthcare delivery system including patient care.

Health Informatics (HI) describes how patient information is technically received, stored, transmitted and used. The focus is mainly dealing with health information generated by the healthcare providers including medical, nursing and other allied healthcare workers in healthcare institutions, its technology and operating principles involved in daily application process. The HI is a science, engineering principles and is an integrated computer technology discipline. HI by its application and process offers varieties of different options for multifarious activities of health institutions technically in securing, storing, transforming comprehensive data in a secured manner.

OPPORTUNITIES FOR HEATH INFORMATICS (HI)

- *Biomedical informatics*: A physician-based research focus that attracts medical students to HI.
- *Nursing informatics*: Nursing-based clinical research focused on nursing issues related healthcare delivered in primary, secondary and tertiary care for the benefit of nursing professionals and especially nursing graduates.
- *Public health informatics*: The public health related issues, conducting research, reporting and managing with the support of technology dealing with epidemiological data including morbidity and mortality that attract student graduates in public health administration.

- *Application informatics*: This is the endeavor of professionals making use of technology; focus on flow of information in digital environment with policies, and procedures to arrive at information management solutions to the identified problems or other problems which need some sort of remedial actions.

Accredited HM educational program development: The Commission on Accreditation for Health Informatics and Information Management Education (CAHIM) defines standards with higher education health information management and technology programs must meet to qualify for accreditation. Students who graduate from an accredited associate's, bachelor's or certificate program are qualified to sit for their respective exams for certification as a Registered Health Information Technician (RHIT), via graduation from an accreditation associate or certification program or Registered Health Information Administrator (RHIA), which requires education through an accredited bachelor or certification program.

What Makes a Health Information Management Career a Good Choice?

A health information management professional is highly trained person, acquaints with the latest technology applications, policies and procedures affecting healthcare provider workflow. Opportunities are available to work in small medical practices and the large hospital systems with many locations. Health information management professionals perform essential operations needed to be executed in the daily healthcare provider environment. An exciting and challenging career in health information management is possible only if the individual willing to gain the specific education leading to great personal and professional rewards provided the individual committed to the profession to do his/her best.

Methods to Ensure Data Quality

The mother of information is the patient health record, and its well planned and organized maintenance can produce accurate and comprehensive data. The accuracy of data depends on the manual or computer information system design for collecting, recording, storing, processing, accessing and displaying data as well as the ability and follow through the people involved in each phase of these activities. Everyone involved with documenting or using health information is responsible for its quality. According to AHIMA's Data Quality Management Model, there are four key processes for data:

1. Application: The purpose for which the data are collected.
2. Collection: The processes by which data elements are accumulated.
3. Warehousing: The processes and systems used to store and maintain data and data journals.
4. Analysis: The process of translating data into information utilized for an application.

Each aspect is analyzed with 10 different data characteristics:

1. *Accuracy:* Data are the correct values and are valid.
2. *Accessibility:* Data items should be easily obtainable and legal to collect.
3. *Comprehensiveness:* All required data items are included. Ensure that the entire scope of the data is collected and document intentional limitations.
4. *Consistency:* The value of the data should be reliable and the same across applications.
5. *Currency:* The data should be up-to-date. A datum value is up-to-date if it is current for a specific point in time. It is outdate if it was current at some preceding time yet incorrect at a later time.

6. *Definition:* Clear definitions should be provided so that current and future data users will know what the data mean. Each data element should have clear meaning and acceptable values.
7. *Granularity:* The attributes and values of data should be defined at the correct level of detail.
8. *Precision:* Data values should be just large enough to support the application or process.
9. *Relevancy:* The data are meaningful to the performance of the process or application for which they are collected.
10. *Timeliness:* Timeliness is determined by how the data are being used and their context.

Health information professionals: Health information management field is a broad and successful as there are several career opportunities in health information management and many different customary and non-traditional settings for an HIM professional to work within.

- **Customary settings include:** Managing an HIM medical records department, cancer registry, coding, trauma registry, transcription, quality improvement, release of information. Patient admissions, compliance auditor, physician accreditation, utilization review, physician offices and risk management.
- **Non-traditional settings include:** Consulting firms, government agencies, law firms, insurance companies, correctional facilities, extended care facilities, pharmaceutical research, information technology and medical software companies.
- Health information managers

Professional health information managers design and construct health information programs to ensure that they accommodate medical, legal, and ethical standards. They play a crucial role in the maintenance, collection, and analyzing of data that is received by doctors, nurses, and other healthcare providers. In return these healthcare data contributors rely on the information to deliver quality healthcare. Managers must work with a group of HIM technicians to guarantee that the patient's medical records are complete, accurate and are easily retrievable whenever needed.

Health information management: Health information management (HIM) is a vital part of the healthcare delivery system that provides for the maintenance of health records in hospitals, clinics, health departments, insurance companies, governmental agencies, and many other health related settings. HIM professional's responsibilities are becoming increasingly significant as the healthcare industry continues to transition to Electronic Health Records (EHRs). As Health Information Management professional works with hospitals and allied health institutions, insurance, clinical, financial, and software companies are responsible for the management of health information in a scientific way that is not only useful for patient, physician, hospitals, medical education and research, but also for legal, insurance, public health or national health and international health agencies.

One of the roles of the HIM is maintaining complete and accurate record which is a central part of providing medical care to people in any medical settings. Such information is necessary to track health conditions, move records from place to place, get insurance coverage, and receive accurate treatment. With a degree in Bachelor of Science in Health Information Management, one get equipped with the required knowledge, competent skills, and with positive attitude, will be able to provide these services effectively by the institutions where the HIM serves.

Reimbursement process: The prominence of HM department is in addition to initiating and maintaining patient health records, have many important responsibilities to carry out, and to do that effectively and efficiently, emphasis on timely completion of documentation accurate classification of diseases by coding efficiently, the HIM staff can expedite key audits for proper reimbursement and quality is more significant in the present day situation and this entails having right HIM education. HIM professional should conduct chart audits and quality assurance assessments; for content completion, timeliness of documentation that support the healthcare providers in rendering healthcare effectively. There are mainly two types of audits; quantitative and qualitative audits.

- Quantitative audit is focused mainly on the patient record which is properly organized and all the required documents are in chronological order, the information is accurate, complete and timely. The auditor's job is to ensure that all the records and documentation system are carried out systematically so that the records are useful for the purpose they are created and maintained.
- Qualitative audit's objective is to ensure that the quality of documentation by healthcare providers are in-line with the recommended guidelines, standards of practice. The auditor's job is to focus on reason for admission, investigations or tests carried out, diagnosis, treatment, length of stay and end results have been in-line with established criteria by medical staff group. Hence, to do this job efficiently the HIM professional must have right education and experience in the field.

There are different types of audits which are carried out by health institutions, the frequency and type of audit varies from institution to institution. The terminology used for audits are: New admission audit, that is conducted within 24–72 hours of a resident's admission to ensure that the accurate and complete information is documented from the beginning of the admission process. Re-admission audit: This is similar to new admission, as done for new admission, the re-admission episode, need to understand the cause for re-admission and required information to be documented. Discharge audits are carried out for all the discharged patients records, and special emphasis is made for long-term care cases. The main focus is to ensure that all the documents are in place and required information is complete at the earliest but not later than 30 days. Health information manager needs to report or takes measures those records which are delinquency for more than 30 days. In order to control or minimize the delinquency rate, hospital management applies different measures such as taking away the certain hospital privileges from the physicians, or not releasing the monthly salary payment bill till the records are completed, etc. An efficient HIM professional with good cooperation and coordination of physicians can alleviate this situation to a greater extent.

Chapter 2

Health Information Management's Professional Role in Efficient Management of Health Information in USA

INTRODUCTION

Health information management (HIM) is the practice of acquiring, analyzing, and protecting traditional and digital medical information vital to providing quality patient care. HIM professionals are highly trained in the latest information management technology applications and understand the workflow in any healthcare provider organization from large hospital systems to the private physician practice. They are vital to the daily operations management of health information and electronic health records. They are responsible to health insurers, state and federal government and other regulatory agencies.

HIM Work Multi-settings

Health information management professionals work in a variety of different settings and job titles. HIM professionals do not just work in hospitals. They work for accounting firms, insurance companies, information systems vendors, government agencies, pharmaceutical research companies and others. They often serve in bridge roles such as connecting clinical, operational and administrative functions. These professionals affect the quality of patient care at every touch point in the healthcare delivery cycle. Having skilled HIM professionals on staff ensures an organization has the right information on hand when and where it is needed while maintaining the highest standards of data integrity, confidentiality and security.

HIM is an Expert

HIM professional is an expert who possesses comprehensive knowledge of medical, administrative, ethical and legal requirements related to healthcare delivery and privacy of protected patient information. Manages people and operational units like release of information, file room, transcription coding and billing, etc. Participates administrative committees and prepares budgets. HIM interacts with all levels of an organization such as clinical, financial, and administrative and information systems.

HIM's Challenges

Ensuring the privacy, security and confidentiality of personal healthcare information has been a fundamental principle for the Health Information Management (HIM). Today HIM professionals continue to face the challenge of maintaining the privacy and security of patient information becomes more and more distributed in electronic systems. The challenge of this responsibility has been increased due to the constantly changing legislative and regulatory environment.

Regulations which have impacted privacy and security:

1. The Health Insurance Portability and Accountability Act of 1996 (HIPPA)
2. The American Recovery and Reinvestment Act of 2009 (ARRA)
3. Modifications to the HIPPA Privacy, security and Enforcement Rules the Health Information Technology for Economic and Clinical Health Act; Final Rule.

HIM professionals use their expertise to protect health information and ensure the right information is available to the right people at the right time.

While operations still demand continued focus on day-to-day activities like EHR implementation, coding, revenue cycle, privacy and security and Release of Information (RIO) to name a few Health Information Exchange (HIE) and emerging technologies and payment reform initiatives are rapidly changing how healthcare documentation will be.

Health Information Technology (HIT)

Health information technology refers to the framework used to manage health information and the exchange of health information in a digital format. Professionals who work in Health Information technology (HIT) are focused on the technical side of managing health information, working with software and hardware used to manage and store patient data. HIT professionals are usually from information technology backgrounds, and provide support for electronic health records and other systems HIM professionals use to secure health information.

Health Informatics (HI)

It is a science that defines how health information is technically captured, transmitted and utilized. Health informatics focuses on information systems, informatics principles and information technology as it is applied to the continuum of healthcare delivery. It is an integrated discipline with specialty domains that include management science, management engineering principles, healthcare delivery and public health, patient safety, information science and computer technology. Health informatics programs demonstrate uniqueness by offering varied options for practice or research focus.

Health information management (HIM) roles are evolving as the industry moves forward with a variety of initiatives, including implementation of an electronic health records. As the health record evolves into a complete and accurate picture of the patient's treatment, including information from personal health records and health information exchange the need for advanced information management skills are needed.

HIM PROFESSIONAL SKILL SET

Organizations depend on HIM professional skill set. The convergence of clinical, documentation and coding processes is vital to a healthy revenue cycle, and more importantly to a healthy patient. To that end, Clinical Documentation Improvement (CDI) has a direct impact on patient care by providing information to all members of the care team, as well as those downstream who may be treating the patient at a later date.

A CDI program includes a myriad of people processes, and technology that must work together to ensure success. Organizations need a well-rounded individual who can articulate effectively all of the pieces, documentation requirements, code assignment, coding guidelines and quality reporting.

In response to this changing environment, CDI specialist must improve work processes, communicate with clinical providers and redesign clinical documentation improvement practices. CDI specialist must continue to learn and develop new skills and move forward with regulatory changes.

HIM professionals hold diverse roles within the revenue cycle for their organizations and physician practices such as CDI specialists, CDI managers, coding professionals and revenue cycle auditors.

As a retired Health Information Manager, Department of Veterans Affairs Medical Center, I would like to mention that, over 8 million Veterans are currently (ex-servicemen) with Healthcare Administration, 153 active Veterans Administration Hospitals and 773 Community Based Outpatient Clinics (CBOCs).

Veterans Healthcare Administration (VHA) is the largest integrated healthcare system in the United States of America. The VHA has generated a number of accolades in the recent past from outside healthcare systems and HMOs and has received rave reviews from the national press as well as VA providers, administrators and staff. MY HEALTH VET is computer system where a veteran can see her/his own medical records.

One most important and particular contribution to the Veterans Administration commitment to excellence in the healthcare field is its award winning CPRS (computerized patient record system). The CPRS interface has proven to be an efficient model; many non-VA healthcare systems around the country and abroad have adopted the Veterans Administration's lead in complete incorporation of a patient's records within a singular database. For example, if a veteran has had treatment at the Chicago Veterans Administration Medical Center, he/she can get treatment at Long Beach, California Veterans Administration Medical Center and their healthcare provider at Long Beach, California will be able to see the patient's entire treatment records from Chicago VAMC or another VAMC. The Veterans Health Administration has embraced these technologies, thus eliminating the need for patients to retrieve copies of their healthcare records from other VAMC professionals. CPRS really was a godsend to providers who remember the paper- only record days. Now, there is no such thing as a "lost record". Another added benefit of converting to all electronic records has been the amount of paper that is saved each year.

Policy Statement

Patients receiving continuing care in the acute and ambulatory setting are required to have a problem list as part of the Medical Record. The problem list is intended to promote continuity of care over time and among providers for the patient.

Purpose

The purpose of this policy is to provide guidance on initiating the problem list. When used properly and consistently, the problem list serves as a valuable tool in patient care management. The problem list compiles all past and current patient problems, including social, psychological and medical problems in one location. At one glance, providers can determine which problems are active, which are resolved and formulate treatment plans accordingly. Additionally the problem list serves as a communication tool and aides in the evaluation and treatment decision when the patient is referred to a specialty physician for care.

Procedure

1. All clinic patients will have a problem list initiated and maintained by the third visit. For inpatients treated for chronic or critical conditions, problems are entered into the problem list upon discharge.
2. All providers should review the problem list, add problems, and enter updates as appropriate.
3. Primary care providers have ultimate responsibility for maintaining an accurate problem list.
4. To maintain usefulness of the problem list, problems will be entered in a timely manner
5. Only approved staff will enter problems. Medical Directors will identify approved staff within their clinic/department.
6. All problems will be listed as active until a licensed independent practitioner changes the problem to "resolved".
7. If copy/paste functionality is utilized, the entry must be edited to ensure documentation integrity.
8. Problems will include:
   i. Items from organization—defined national standards
   ii. Known significant medical diagnoses and conditions
   iii. Known significant operative and invasive procedures affecting current health
   iv. Known adverse and allergic reactions
9. All entries, when possible will utilize a standard vocabulary to ensure classification of data for rules, alerts, and potential reporting. HIM professionals and clinic users will determine whether a classification or vocabulary system should be used for the entries on the problem list.
10. Only providers will be allowed to enter or edit designated problems or diagnoses onto the patient problem list, this is not within the role or scope of coding or coding audit professionals.
11. Development of system level problem folders requires approval by the HIM committee.
12. Abbreviations will be avoided in the problem list to ensure clear communication among all disciplines.
13. The HIM committee must approve all rules, alerts and system-generated problems at least one month before implementation. System-generated problems will be updated with resolved status by the requesting provider groups.
14. The problem list is considered a permanent part of the medical record and is included in the designated record set.

HIMSS establishment in 1961 increased industry knowledge

The Healthcare Information and Management Systems Society (HIMSS) was organized in 1961 as the Hospital Management Systems Society (HMSS), an independent, unincorporated, nonprofit, voluntary association of individuals. It was preceded by increasing amounts of management engineering activity in healthcare during the 1950s, when teachings of Bunker Gilberth and Frank Bunker Gilberth, Sr. began to attract the attention of health leaders.

The HIMSS grew to include chapters, membership categories, publications, conventions, and continues to grow in different parts of the world via its Europe, Asia Pacific, and Middle Eastern branches.

EDUCATIONAL PROGRAMS

The requisites and accreditation processes for health information management education and professional activity vary across jurisdictions.

In the United States, the CAHIIM requires continued accreditation for accredited programs in health information management. The current standard is that accreditation may be maintained with periodic site visits, submission of an annual report, informing CAHIIM of adverse changes within the program and paying CAHIIM administrative fees. HIM students may opt to participate in a full-time bridge program called the Joint Bachelor of Science/ Masters Program. With this program, students can achieve both the Bachelor of Science in Health Information Management and the Master of Health Services Administration Program (BSHIM/MHSA). The full-time bridge program allows students to achieve both degrees in five years. Students pursuing the BSHIM/MHSA will be prepared to assume management and executive positions in health-related organizations such as: Hospitals, managed care organizations, health information system developers and vendors, and pharmaceutical companies, and bring their knowledge in HIM to these positions.

Records

- The patient health record is the primary legal record documenting the health care services provided to a person in any aspect of the health care system. The term includes routine clinical or office records, records of care in any health related setting, preventive care, lifestyle evaluation, research protocols and various clinical databases. This repository of information about a single patient is generated by healthcare professionals as a direct result of interaction with a patient or with individuals who have personal knowledge of the patient.
- The primary patient record is the record that is used by healthcare professionals while providing patient care services to review patient data or document their own observations, actions, or instructions.
- The secondary patient record is a record that is derived from the primary record and contains selected data elements to aid non-clinical persons in supporting, evaluating and advancing patient care. Patient care support refers to administration, regulation, and payment functions.

PRACTICES

Health Information Managers

Professional health information managers manage and construct health information programs to guarantee they accommodate medical, legal, and ethical standards. They play a vital role in the maintenance, collection, and analyzing of data that is received by doctors, nurses, and other healthcare players. In return these healthcare data contributors rely on the information to deliver quality healthcare. Managers must work with a group of information technicians to guarantee that the patient's medical records are accurate and are available when needed.

Medical Records and Health Information Technicians

Medical records (MR) and Health information technicians (HIT) are described as having the following duties according to the US Bureau of Labor Statistics' Occupational Outlook Handbook.

Assemble patients' health information including medical history, symptoms, examination results, diagnostic tests, treatment methods, and all other healthcare provider services. Technicians organize and manage health information data by ensuring its quality, accuracy, accessibility, and security. They regularly communicate with physicians and other healthcare professionals to clarify diagnoses or to obtain additional information.

The International Labor Organization's International Standard Classification of Occupations further notes: "Occupations included in this category require knowledge of medical terminology, legal aspects of health information, health data standards, and computer- or paper-based data management as obtained through formal education and/or prolonged on-the-job training.

MRHITs usually work in hospitals. However, they also work in a variety of other healthcare settings, including office-based physician practices, nursing homes, home health agencies, mental health facilities, and public health agencies. Technicians who specialize in coding are called medical coders or coding specialists.

In the United States, health information technicians are certified as a Registered Health Information Technician (RHIT) after completing an associate's degree in health information technology from a school accredited by the Commission on Accreditation for Health Informatics and Information Management Education (CAHIIM) before they may take their certification exam.

Professional Organizations

- American Society of Health Informatics Managers (ASHIM)
- American Health Information Management Association (AHIMA)
- Commission on Accreditation of Health Informatics and Information Management Education (CHIIM)
- Health Information Management and Systems Society (HIMSS)
- Health Information Management Association of Australia Limited (HIMAA)
- Institute of Health Records and Information Management (HRIM)

Summary

Efficient management of health information is not that simple, it needs besides acquiring professional qualification, e.g. RHIM, etc. one has to and not limited to the following:

- Have good communication skills
- Build up good public relationship
- Pursue continue education in the field by participating in the seminars, workshops, group discussions, and conferences national and international.
- Undertake specialized courses related to HIM to be proficient in the field
- Be a good leader with team building ability and other positive characteristics

With this few tips, any HIM professional can achieve as adage goes "Sky is the limit" *

Chapter 3

Health Information Management Professionals Future Challenges

The health information management (HIM) profession is the heart of the health organization; with each beat it supplies much-needed health information to all users, such as doctors, nurses, allied health professionals, health administrations, insurance companies, software companies and other health related institutions. The principal role of the HIM professional is to maintain organized and accurate data, to accomplish, the health information professionals need to integrate a variety of skills, such as expertise in computer and information technology (IT), a strong knowledge of anatomy and physiology, medical terminology, disease processes and other conditions, experience of clinical classification systems and excellent managerial skills, to enable them to manage the range of health information services. The HIM professional plays a critical role in completing, protecting and ensuring the availability of high-quality clinical information for purposes including patient care, medical education, research, legal, insurance, reimbursement, quality assurance, and management decision making.

Advent of technology has changed the medical records management into health information management. The earlier record management which was dealing with manual records, the introduction of IT has had a great influence in changing the responsibilities of HIM professionals, and due to electronic health records (EHRs) its role is more complex and divergent. The integration of IT in the healthcare system has increased the need for HIMs who understand the use and meaning of the information that forms the health record, and the language used to describe the reality of clinical treatments and allied operations that has created a threat and opportunities. The threat, in the sense, HIM need to equip him/herself with new knowledge and skills that are essential and opportunities can be availed by HIM by playing a vital role in the new environment.

What is HIM? However, many HIM professionals still believe that one of the greatest challenges facing them is having the ability to provide a simple answer to the question, "What is HIM?" in the current electronic world. The HIM can play a vital role only when he/she clearly updates her knowledge in emerging technologies, and needs of implementing electronic health records, and acquiring required ingredients. Otherwise, the professional will take back seat and the information technologists due to compulsion will take driver's place. HIM, if he thinks quietly has tremendous expertise in developing and managing the manual or paper records for years and fulfilled the needs of divergent specialists and administrators, then, due to the technology, the situation has transformed greatly, and in this arena, the HIM has lot to offer, by taking new challenges of learning new techniques and skills instead of considering be hidden profession, if they remain as traditional workforce. Therefore, the HIM professionals unless are able to clearly articulate what it is that they have to do and what it is that makes them unique, otherwise, the profession will find it difficult to convince others of the importance of HIM in the future health sector workforce. The HIM professionals are the ones, who understand how information is used in healthcare institutions, and they play significant roles in managing, analyzing and protecting digital healthcare information; therefore, it is necessary for them to be visible at the forefront of the process.

As such, there is a critical need to define the HIM profession accurately and to determine its key roles in the healthcare system. The HIM has many challenges ahead of him/her as a professional, hence, to get equipped with all necessary ingredients to meet multifarious challenges including diverse responsibilities by becoming a successful professional leader. The main responsibility of the HIM profession lies in collecting, maintaining, analyzing and protecting patients' clinical information in order to facilitate quality patient care. In addition, it is important to ensure that accurate health information is made available to authorized people at the right time for different purposes while, at the same time, maintaining the privacy, security and confidentiality of a patient's clinical information. With the development of EHRs, the roles and responsibilities of the HIM profession have become more crucial to safeguarding the confidentiality and security of patient clinical information despite its importance, there are many challenges influencing the sustainability of the HIM profession within the healthcare system. Therefore, the future of HIM little bit mystifying, needs to work out critically, the HIM profession and where it is taking us what need to be done to remain in the profession to contribute significantly as being done traditionally for decades. What is that new knowledge, skills and attitude to be added to our profession to be an efficient HIM professional to be a key person in the health institution setup.

HIM Profession

The HIM profession takes responsibility for assessing the quality of health information in the health sector, particularly in hospitals. It has been observed that due to insignificant participation in healthcare delivery system to be precise, not effectively, participating with the healthcare provider team in their daily patient care services, or not meeting to their expectation level, have given the least importance of HIM professional existence coupled with low profile of some HIM professionals have contributed for the de-recognition of the professional status. At the same time, some HIM professionals have proved beyond doubt, that their participation and contribution in the healthcare delivery system has enhanced the healthcare quality and brought laurels to the institutions. This is other side of the HIM professional coin. We, HIM professionals, have a problem to be discussed critically and find the problems that are affecting the professional's growth or the progress to be addressed suitably. In addition to this, the disciplines covered in the HIM study field, to attain clear consensus on the scope of practice, roles, job titles, competencies and educational needs have to be carefully planned and executed.

Revolutionized HIM Practice

The implementation of technology in healthcare has revolutionized HIM practice. Many studies have found that the availability of a well-trained and qualified workforce is an important factor affecting the implementation of EHR. However, a conflict exists in determining the appropriate qualified staff member to ensure the success of EHR implementation. Is it the HIM professional, or is it an IT or other professional? Alternatively, is it the responsibility of different bodies, with different roles for each? It is not one particular profession can claim to implement electronic health records; it is the combination of information technologies, and HIM professionals as domain experts in collaboration can execute the job satisfactorily. It is important to understand and clarify the meaning of success in EHR implementation, as it includes factors such as privacy and security issues, the provision of quality data and the provision of data that is fit for purpose. The roles have to be clearly defined in order to avoid any overlap in responsibilities. One thing is sure, what technologist can do, is not possible by HIM and what HIM is equipped with is not entirely possible by an IT person. It is a mutual team work needs to be shared and executed jointly.

It is vital to note that the reality is qualified HIM professional demand is so high, and the supply is very meager, makes a big challenge for the health institutions to have right HIM professionals to be placed in right position. Though the studies have noted the shortage due to various challenges, e.g. unavailability of right educational institutions, and not having proper syllabus, or curriculum content to meet the present requirement, or license or certification to work in the field, the number of the HIM workforce where a staff member with specific credential is doing more than one job, not necessarily based on their title or job description because of the high demand and to make personal financial gains by working overtime.

It is well-known that a skilled HIM workforce is a critical component of a well-functioning healthcare system. Thus, many studies emphasized the need for changes to the future configuration of the HIM workforce to take on new roles and responsibilities and to highlight the importance of capacity development as a means of improving data quality. The HIM workforce need to come out from the traditional education system and the educational institutions which offer the diploma, bachelor or master degree in HIM field are required to modify in view of emerging technologies in the health field. The knowledge, skills and attitude towards to meet the HIM new roles or the past roles with modification to meet new challenges to provide high-quality data for decision-making for patient care management and planning and executing various other responsibilities of HIM efficiently. It is critical to be able to clearly determine the status of the HIM profession and develop a detailed plan for the health information workforce because the relationship between staffing and service quality is irrefutable. It is also necessary to determine a means for entry into the HIM workforce, and to set clear criteria for recruitment into that workforce based on position descriptions, job titles and the qualifications required at each level. In order to meet the demand, it is imperative to encourage more people to become competent HIM professionals by taking required educational programs.

Education is Crucial for HIM Workforce

Education is a cornerstone in supplying the healthcare system with a qualified and trained workforce to provide a quality service and, specifically for the HIM profession, to provide high-quality data. In fact, the US Bureau of Labor Statistics showed that the HIM field is growing; medical records and health information technicians is one of the 20 fastest-growing occupations in the USA, with an expected growth of 22% between 2012 and 2022 (Bureau of Labor Statistics, 2014). In addition, according to an article by US News and World Report, HIM is now considered to be among the top developing study majors in the USA (AHIMA, 2012). Coordination between educational institutions and practicing professionals is crucial in ensuring that education meets the market demand. In addition, modification to Education and Training Skilled Workforce Service Delivery Service

Development and the creation of new materials for an HIM educational program should be based on stakeholders' need. However, there is no clear picture, as to how many graduates are in the field working for the HIM field and how many are really satisfied with the job and how many feel that they are holding the positions that are below in terms of financial remuneration or not getting the esteem which they deserve. Therefore, it is necessary to review and possibly revise the HIM competencies by many educational institutions of different countries which offer these programs.

Therefore, it is necessary to determine the qualifications framework, the allocated job titles and the key competencies. It is also important to determine the certification body for those involved in HIM before they join the workforce. The relationship between education and training in providing a qualified workforce to an organization that must deliver a service. It also clarifies that service development influences the education and training sector; therefore, educators must be involved in supporting the workforce through in-service training and continuing education. Due to rapid developments in the HIM profession, there are many new job titles and responsibilities for HIM professionals due to that development, and AHIMA has created a career map for the HIM profession. Despite, having good career, the HIM strategic planning and workforce planning are done in certain cases without involving HIM professionals and also while decisions are made for creating policies and standards, the HIM professionals are not invited to attend. Previous studies have acknowledged generally that responsibility for ensuring the sustainability and availability of the HIM workforce lies with the government, educational and training institutions, healthcare institutions and HIM professional associations.

In spite of the importance of HIM to the healthcare system in recent years, policymakers and leaders have paid scant attention to the role of HIM professionals. Thus, there is now a specific and crucial need to raise the recognition of the HIM profession by addressing all current challenges and making plans to cope with the ones to come. This will require all loyal HIM professionals to join hands in each of their contexts. In addition, HIM professionals must maintain their own strength and motivation, and that of their subordinates by joining in the national professional association and develop standards, suggest educational programs, professional abilities in effective and efficient HIM in healthcare institutions. Conduct regular workshops, conferences and continued education to uplift the professional knowledge, skills and develop positive attitude towards loyalty, commitment and performing to the utmost level of standard criterion.

Chapter 4

Challenges of HIM Professionals with Emerging Technology and Reimbursement Methods

INTRODUCTION

The healthcare industry is undertaking a structural change by aligning Health Information Technology (HIT) with the delivery of care to improve quality, control costs, and enhance the efficiency of the system.

Healthcare organizations are promoting coordinated care to improve care and create savings. The health funders are moving away from fee for service reimbursement methodology to risk sharing and prospective payment models.

A majority of the Healthcare Organizations have realized the importance of Health Information Management (HIM) and their expectations are also growing day by day. The hospital management expects Health Information Managers to assume leadership roles and be part of the senior management team to support them in providing facts for business opportunities, clinical care improvement, efficient revenue cycle management, etc. This has lifted the status of the HIM professional to a new level, with different dimensions of roles and functionalities.

HIM role and challenges: In order to adhere with these changes, the present day role of HIM's role is expanded to managing medical records, studying health system to assist the health IT to implement EMR, playing a pivotal role for planning and executing data collection and performing big data analytics, educating physicians and care providers on documentation needs and providing extensive support in revenue cycle management.

The HI manager has lots of challenges in the day to day working of the organization and at the same time opportunities are also abundant in the present day Health Information Management market. HIM professionals have to face the challenges tactfully to progress. Challenges can be classified as ethical, health IT, information governance, coding and revenue cycle management, data analytics and healthcare finance.

Ethical challenges: Due to the continuous advancement and changes in the medical record documentation process, e.g. from paper based to electronic formats, etc., the HIM professionals have to be aligned with the changes and ensure that the fundamentals of documentation guidelines are followed. This can be achieved by having continuous audits and quality assurance programs involving all the healthcare providers. Although technology is taking over traditional methods, HI Managers have to be vigilant and ensure that medical record documentation principles such as quality, timeliness, etc. are managed properly.

Information technology (IT): With the digitizing of information systems in healthcare organizations, the role of HIM professionals have expanded into information technology (IT) and user support, which usually are the functions of IT support services. HIM professionals' training and experience in the intersection of clinical and management sciences as well as their knowledge about data quality equip them with the capability to maintain the integrity and accessibility of health information, although they may not necessarily have the particular skills to support technical operations of information technology systems.

Implementing electronic health records: A Health Information Manager will have to play a crucial role in software and vendor selection, as 80% of Health Information Systems are utilized by the HIM department. *Changes are pervasive, and many practices are ill prepared for the future, especially those lacking information management and technology support. HIM professionals could be great support to the institutions with their HIM skills in transforming the paper records into paperless or to electronic record systems. HIM professional has to involve in the complete system development life cycle starting from documenting the requirements, system designing to suit the needs of healthcare providers with user-friendly processes, till User Acceptance Testing. By this system, proper registration, scheduling, patient visit, pre-certification documentation, coding, and payment can be maintained.*

Coding and revenue cycle management (RCM): Healthcare is undergoing a fundamental shift from fee-for-service to value-based delivery and payment, creating a wrenching change in the markets. As you are all aware, accurate clinical documentation and coding reflects the actual care rendered which in turn represents the accurate reimbursement.

Getting it right at the first time is the biggest challenge in RCM. In order to achieve this, HIM professionals have to multi-task and monitor right from the beginning of the care until the claims are submitted. This whole cycle involves identity management, access management, documentation management, and revenue management. Health information management has to be very vigilant to ensure the coding processes are carried out accurately by conducting regular audits and be an active member in clinical documentation improvement teams.

Information governance: Though Electronic Medical Record is implemented widely, no hospital could achieve complete paperless medical records, instead it is less paperless record. Scanning and uploading of information, information through the medical equipment, etc. lead to a decentralized, isolated approach of information gathering which increases risk, duplication and cost though the information is stored in the electronic medium and reduces the storage and retrieval costs.

The generations old role to be the custodian of medical records have expanded now with emerging technologies as the HIM needs to develop the information governance policy meticulously taking into consideration the access rights, gathering patient information from various sources and collating it as part of the EMR and managing it safely and confidentially.

Data analytics: The reason for Health care Organizations to dependent on big data is to harness it, understand it and use it to cut costs, create more predictive healthcare and improve outcomes. The data analytics software available in the market gives more granular information with 360 degree view. The basic element of healthcare data originates from the

HIM department, right from the demographic, administrative, clinical, coding data and the results. Hence the HIM professionals have to spend a majority of time to ensure data collection, process, storage and analytical tools are properly managed and the required management information reports are generated regularly. Apart from regular reports generated by other departments, HIM being the bridge between administrative and clinical units of the healthcare organization, HIM professionals can help identify opportunities for the use of this data to improve business intelligence, clinical care, and decision-making throughout the organization.

Challenges of operating cost with decline income: Medical practices and health institutions are in transition in information management and technology as mentioned earlier; hence the HIM professionals have a big role to play during and beyond transition to electronic health records. The top challenges are increasing operating costs and waning reimbursement topped the list. This means spending more and getting less, if, this practice continues, the practitioner or the institution will be insolvent. The government institutions or hospitals are subsidized for the healthcare expenditure, while all the private practitioners and corporate hospitals, even though established with non-profit basis, have to survive and sustain the financial burden, otherwise will result into a low quality practice.

Cost justification: *HIM professionals working in small practices or big health institutions can research, help determine cost justifications, and support management in providing cost effective care. HIM professionals can help in ensuring compliance, analyze data and map clinical pathways and do utilization review. Firstly, an HIM professional can become well-versed on all aspects of electronic records; their cost, benefits, impact on workflow and efficiency, and revenue potential. It is the HIM's endeavor to show healthcare providers how they can save time, efforts, reduce operating cost, and sustain improved quality of care. Where there is a lack of good record system or inefficient management, there is a problem of declining reimbursement and increased operation cost. HIM professional plays an important role in bringing complete and relevant information coupled with efficiency of practice for prudent decision making are ways to successful implementation. Despite HIM not being IT educated, he is an expert in maintaining* proper content, documentation and workflow that can make a great difference and this knowledge serves as a valuable resource to help others to understand the importance of proper documentation, confidentiality, professionalism, and optimal care with the electronic record system.

Healthcare financing: The transition from traditional reimbursement models and toward pay-for-performance and prospective payment system will constitute a major paradigm shift for physician practices or health institutions.

The concept of the prospective payment system (PPS) is to have a cost fixed for homogeneous patient groups which are based on the documentation and coding. The Health Information Management team lead by the Manager, supported by the Clinical Documentation Improvement Specialist, Coders, Case Manager play a crucial role in case management, discharge planning which are the integral parts of the PPS. The intricacies of the clinical documentation and the coding will enable physician or hospital to receive accurate reimbursement.

HIM professional undertaking research: HIM professionals can help by researching and undertaking some case studies related to the subject. The abundant of information that technology supports, has revolutionized the image of many organizations and healthcare is one of them. With this facility, the HI Manager can play a good leadership role in improvements for financial benefits. Whenever, we suggest improvements, financial benefits, etc. it needs to be provided with meaningful data in terms of workflow and financial benefits to demonstrate the value of HIM field to the healthcare providers with all the justifications.

Leading the team: Leadership skills are vital for health information managers to excel in their profession. It is one of the important skills in educating personnel and advocating for products and procedures that enable the organization to provide quality care is possible. In a time of great transition for medical practices and health institutions, HIM professionals must be ready to change also. HIM professionals adopt a leadership framework that understands the emotional and mutual interdependence of workplace systems, the importance of effective relationships, and the effect of anxiety on an individual and organizational performance. To be successful, one has to be creative and adaptive to a constantly changing environment that requires the ability to assume leadership in multifaceted roles such as HIM practitioner, manager, educator, researcher and consultant.

HIM Preparedness: HIM professionals have to be abreast with current knowledge in clinical coding, data analytics, information governance, quality assurance and health costing to meet the needs.

AHIMA and other related Health Information Management associations, universities around the globe offer online courses to get the required qualification. Apart from the basic HIM qualification, one should dive deep and learn to the core of superspecialized HIM skills such as privacy, auditing, revenue cycle, clinical documentation, health data analysis, etc. to competently face the present day HIM challenges.

Conclusion: HIM professionals have to work with passion, dedication, and be a Good Samaritan. HIM professionals have to widen their focus and broaden their horizons. Everyone has to work dedicatedly and wait to seize the opportunity to prove their skills and climb the professional ladder. There are no shortcuts, the greater the efforts, better the future will be.

The role of a HIM profession is like the hub of the healthcare delivery wheel that has a central repository of rich information, and uses intellectual skills to explore the information and provide vision to the organization. Every challenge we meet on field is an important learning curve in our professional life. The more challenges we face, better we are equipped.

Chapter

5

Electronic Health Records (EHR) Functional Requirements and Specifications

The requirements for the functionality of the Electronic Health Record will vary and must function under ethical and legal principles specific to the time and place. Different countries may have diverging functional requirements for the content or usage of electronic health records, which can require radical changes of the technical makeup of the EHR implementation.

Health Level Seven, Inc. (HL7) defined the first EHR functional requirement standard in February 2007. The standard outlines important features and functions that should be contained in an EHR system. The standard functional model contains approximately 1,000 conformance criteria across 130 functions, including medication history, problem lists, orders, clinical decision support, and those supporting privacy and security. The function list is described from a user perspective and enables consistent expression of EHR system functionality, while the conformance criteria serves as a reference for purchasers of EHR systems and vendors developing EHR software.

The EHR standard functional model has proven to be a powerful tool for the Certification Commission for Health Information Technology (CCHIT). The HL7 standard for EHR systems has been extremely valuable for CCHIT's development of certification criteria.

EHR FUNCTIONAL REQUIREMENTS

Many of the requirements of an EHR are identified based on a fundamental functional understanding of what an EHR is intended to achieve, whether implemented as a middleware service or as a sub-component of a healthcare information system. The EHR must enable the communication of healthcare information to support shared patient care, improved quality of care, and effective resource utilization. This includes the support of evidence-based care and the rich ability to navigate and analyze EMRs for a wide range of purposes. Users must be able to access health record information from whichever system and in whatever format it is originally stored.

The functional requirements are classified as shown:

- Administration requirements
- Clinical documentation requirements
- Data export requirements

- Data import requirements
- Clinical decision support systems requirements
- E prescribing requirements
- Orders management requirements
- Reporting requirements
- Results management requirements
- Privacy protection and security requirements

A. **Administration requirements:** The clinical basis for this requirement is to provide comprehensive benefit eligibility (health plan, Medicaid, Medicare, etc.) information, to include managed care information. EHR will have the ability to conduct eligibility checking for all commercial health plans and Medicaid from within the application.

The functional requirement is that the EHR system can verify and document patient eligibility (e.g. insurance information) and patient demographic information. The system shall allow appropriate clinical staff to document and/or update patient identifying and financial information, and verify insurance eligibility. The system can print out medical summary including medication and diagnosis list.

B. **Clinical documentation requirements:** The clinical basis for this requirement is the clinical staff can document patient medication history electronically from patient. Clinician shall confirm previous medications and prescribe any potential new medications or make dose changes. Clinician shall come up with treatment plan and creates any new orders. Clinician shall have the ability to create treatment plans and create and electronically submit orders such as labs, radiology, physical therapy, and other supportive services. Specialist can document consult note, recommendations, and clearance. New medications or changes are ordered.

The functional requirement is that the EHR will have the ability to perform basic clinical documentation, including medication history. Current, active medications are viewable on demand. The system shall have the ability to display a complete medication history from information available within the EHR. The system can document a consultant note with appropriate clinical information from the medical record, recommendation, and clearance.

C. **Data export requirements:** The clinical basis for this requirement is that the provider will receive through their IT system, a complete and accurate medication history from multiple data sources in a single view. The medical history shall include the following in a clinically usable format: Differences between acute/chronic medication, sample history, different drug programs, medication reconciliation, and medication renewal history/compliance. Medication compliance includes drug name, dose, route, duration, prescribers name, area of prescription, prescription order date, prescription filled date, other chronic medications and so on.

The functional requirement is that the EHR will capture and export data elements required for defined medication reconciliation. Ambulatory EHR can export required medication reconciliation data elements, according to local standards and sharing rules. The system shall have the ability to capture patient medication and dispense history electronically from available electronic sources and render information to clinical user in a single view. This data should also be available for data export. It is strongly encouraged that EHR's immediately develop capability to export and import structured medical summary data, including medication histories.

D. **Data import requirements:** The clinical basis for this requirement is that the physician shall receive email alerts/messages directing her/him to a care consideration regarding one of her/his patients. A patient health record (PHR) system uses clinical decision support systems (CDSS) to create a set of Care Considerations for a patient. An alert can be sent either to the health insurance exception (HIE) or directly to the EHR that contains a link to the PHR for the provider to view the CC document.

The functional requirement is that the EHR shall import alerts from the HIE as per standards determined by the regional health information organization (RHIO). The EHR is able to retrieve (manual or automatic) aggregate clinical data to review. The system shall have the ability to incorporate data from another remote system's assessment tool data. It is strongly encouraged that EHR's immediately have capability to export and import structured medical summary data.

E. **Decision support system requirements:** The clinical basis for this requirement is the quality measurement. The system shall allow for frequent updates to the list of required data elements and numerator/denominator/exclusion statements for each measure. The system shall populate the EHR so that when a patient history of applicable life habit (nutrition, obesity, alcohol consumption, smoking, etc.) is documented, the indicator to advise the patient to stop behavior is automatic and there is a standard field with structured nomenclature for the documentation of advice.

The functional requirement is that the EHR system will allow additional required data elements to be added to the system based on enhancements to measures. The system shall populate the EHR so that when a patient history of applicable life habit is documented, the indicator to advise the patient to stop behavior is automatic and there is a standard field with structured nomenclature for the documentation of advice.

F. **ePrescribing requirements:** The clinical basis for this requirement is that the system shall have decision support capabilities. Technology allows cardiologist to determine if prescription drug is on formulary of patient's insurance plan. Formulary information provided through EMR or passed through the HIE by the RHIO. The system shall have decision support capabilities around medication alerts. The system shall be capable of allowing Emergency Department (ED) physician to verify known patient allergies prior to completion of ED prescription.

The functional requirement is that the EHR has Rx decision support for drug–drug interactions and allergy checking and has mandatory alerting for drug–drug interactions, allergies in the eRX process. The system shall have the ability to alert the provider to medication contraindications. The system shall support eRX capability according to standard protocols, and drug–allergy and drug–drug interaction checking, with real-time feedback to ordering clinician. The system shall be capable of allowing a physician to verify known patient allergies prior to completion of a prescription.

G. **Order management requirements:** The clinical basis for this clinician shall confirm previous medications and prescribe any potential new medications or make dose changes. Clinician shall come up with treatment plan and creates any new orders. Clinician shall have the ability to electronically submit orders such as labs, radiology, physical therapy, and other supportive services.

If electronic ordering is not live, system can create customized order forms for e-fax to relevant facility.

H. **Reporting requirements:** The clinical basis for this requirement is that the system shall have the capability to automatically identify patients who meet denominator requirements of each quality measure. Quality measures are still to be determined by projects. The system shall have the capability for the provider to manually select/deselect a patient as part of a panel of patients who are relevant/not relevant and qualified/not qualified for specific quality measures.

The functional requirement is that the system shall have the capability to automatically identify patients who meet denominator requirements of each quality measure. The system shall have the capability for the provider to manually select/deselect a patient as part of a panel of patients who are relevant/not relevant and qualified/not qualified for specific quality measures. Panel can be selected using ad hoc or embedded reporting functionality.

I. **Result management requirements:** The clinical basis for this requirement is that the system shall send the lab request electronically. Lab results are populated electronically into the EHR with flags for abnormal results; reminder is set in EHR for recommended time frame for the next lab test. All lab vendors must provide compendium with mapping to logical observation identifiers, names, and codes (LOINC), and must send LOINC mappings as determined by the RHIO.

The functional requirement is that the lab results are populated (imported) electronically into the EHR with flags for abnormal results. The EHR must accept electronically delivered lab results. The EHR must accept LOINC-mapped electronic lab results if available from the source lab.

J. **Privacy and security requirements:** The policy basis for this requirement is: In the event that a RHIO becomes aware of any actual or suspected privacy and/or security breach, either through notification by a participant or otherwise, the RHIO shall immediately investigate (or cause the applicable participant to investigate) the scope and magnitude of such actual or suspected breach, and promptly identify the root cause of the breach. Physician practices have a parallel requirement to investigate the scope, magnitude, and root causes of suspected breaches. In the event of a privacy and/or security breach, the RHIO shall mitigate (or cause the applicable participant to mitigate) to the extent practicable, any harmful effect of such privacy and/or security breach that is known to the RHIO or the participant.

The functional requirement is that the system must permit a person with administrative access to log into the system to investigate a potential breach. The system must have ad hoc query capability to assist in investigating potential breaches. The system must allow an administrator to terminate all users' access to a specific patient's data, or discontinue a user's access to the system in the event of a breach. The system must be able to determine when an "access" has occurred and log that event, in order to take corrective action, comply with state notification requirements and potentially inform patients of breach of their information.

FUNCTIONAL REQUIREMENTS VERSUS TECHNOLOGY

The technologies often included within requirements are difficult to generalize to any potential EHR implementation as they are often expressed in terms of the technology envisaged by the authoring project or team. However, there are a small number of themes that are probably generalizable to any kind of implementation, and are mentioned for completeness. A specification for the information model of an EHR would probably not explicitly demonstrate conformance in the areas listed below:

- Information models for messages
- Conformance to international standards
- Record server and persistence, interfaces and services
- Performance and concurrent use
- Version control
- Exceptions and errors.

Chapter 6

Tips for Evaluating the Pre-Implementation of Electronic Health Records Software

INTRODUCTION

The health industry around the world and particularly, developing countries are evolving quickly and many modern health institutions are working to advance the implementation and effective management of electronic health records (EHRs) by initiating and advocating consisted standards. Needs are evolving from simply translating data, to having access to intelligence that can drive clinical and administrative decision-making in real time. To have a right product is not that easy and most complex issue, hence one has to make efforts to ensure the product purchased or installed should not only fulfill the purpose for which it was procured but to meet the worth of the efforts and finance spent on the product.

SELECTION OF SOFTWARE

Selecting appropriate product is a herculean task and when it comes to electronic health record (EHR) systems; there are literally hundreds of products and quite good number of vendors in the market to choose one among them unless one established a well-defined comprehensive process for comparing products. The foremost, one should clear what type of product they need that would meet their requirements not only to meet for a shorter duration but also for long term. The following few tips would help in evaluation of pre-implementation EHR software that would meet and satisfy the organizational requirements.

1. First evaluate your set up, organization, size of practice, the specialty of the physicians, their typing skills and computer literacy, their attitude towards implementing EHR, infrastructure, budget and clear objective of implementing the EHR. In hospital set up, evaluate the OP, ED, and IP departments including OTs, ICU, CCU, NICU, etc.

2. Determine, whether tailor made in-house software required or vendor ready-made product.

3. Clearly create the institutional or individual physicians needs. Make a clear policy to review the required products. Most important to understand all aspects of products that required including software, hardware, network, PCs, and other equipment, storage capacity, servers, back-up mechanism, disaster plan, maintenance, vendor support, finance involved, interoperability, security, privacy and confidentiality, etc.

4. Discuss the institutional policies and plans with the concerned staff of the institution and obtain their views on entire plan and improve the policy document to meet the organizational set up.
5. Examine thoroughly the product that should contain the features that you are contemplating. Another exercise with the concerned staff is to get their concurrence. Once, this is done, look for an appropriate way of acquiring that is by 'in-house tailor made' or 'ready-made vendor product'.
6. If decided to have a vendor product, list in as much detail as possible every single feature you want in an ideal EHR. This should be a comprehensive and specific checklist.
7. Identify some appropriate vendors who can meet your requirements; and analyze on various aspects of issues such as economic vitality of the vendor, cost involvement, maintenance, etc. through web or communications.
8. Shortlist the vendor number and select a few with whom you can negotiate, get a demonstration copy of the software. A demonstration copy should perform like the real product. Fully relying on a demonstration copy would be disaster, one has to have many clarification cleared before agree to enter to contract of purchase or lease whatever.
9. Make a comparative statement of your required features and the different shortlisted vendors. Thoroughly examine and make problem-based selection properly. Compare the products side by side to see which works best for you. By this, you should be able to decide which one is close to your needs and select those vendors and be ready to site visit, where the product is being used. Have the views of using customers in all aspects; strengths and weaknesses, etc. In your visit team, there should be a well knowledgeable person who can evaluate and able to interpret the right way.
10. Finally, your experience with many vendors and lots of information should allow you to critically analyze with your team to prepare a very relevant list of questions you should ask about how well vendors respond to requests, training time, implementation difficulties, customization, upgrade frequency and specific features. How each system covers your general and specific required features? Of course, this is a sample; you will find many more issues to be tackled; it depends, on the size, type, specialty, vision and mission of the institution, etc.

EXPECTED OUTCOME OF ELECTRONIC HEALTH RECORD SOFTWARE (FEATURES OF SOFTWARE)

Increased productivity: Any software developed electronic health records (EHR) should meet the following so as able to get maximum benefit of enormously expensive element represents patient care. While practicing management systems should be capable of increasing overall productivity to meet the expected results. The integration of EHR software should be capable to customize for enhancing office workflow, maximizing paper-based redundancies and automating the selection of diagnosis and CPT codes based on chief complaints. Any software that deals with EHR should help provider more time spent with patients and enhance the automated data for future visits, patient care plans, etc.

Minimize paper records: Minimize the amount of paper records that physician's would keep on hand to maintain patient detailed histories and care provided. Minimize the manual work related to physician's daily practice, automatic International Classification and Current Procedure Terminology Coding. Need laboratory reports for reviewing timely for efficient decision making. Some physicians prefer customizable EHR software besides standard one for rendering efficient patient care. The system should able to significantly eliminate transcriptions costs. Interface with other practice management, suggestive for appropriate data entry and to prevent redundant data entry.

Easy navigation: Most important functionality should be easy navigation of the menu to increase usage speed streamlining the data input process. All the software installed should be easily interface, e.g. imaging systems, lab information system, and transcription, etc. Identify missing information, incomplete or unsigned progress notes and other orders for correction. Obviously, the security part should permit only the authorized users, password protection and automated signature for less sensitive areas.

Single screen: Another important aspect of consolidation of information from different sources, on a single screen, should facilitate care provider to observe his practical process much easier to complete his clinical work. The software should have internal massaging capabilities to assign tasks other staff for efficient communication.

Automated coder: Voice recognition and handwriting recognition software would be added advantage to enhance efficient and comprehensive documentation. Automated coder should capable of accurate coding and calculation of justifiable billing for service rendered. This includes ICD-10 CM and CPT codes, as well as the ability to add modifier codes and custom alternate descriptions or abbreviated descriptions. The system should capable of checking relevant information automatically and generate a bill and send to the insurance or other organization for payment.

Automatically update: As regards to encounter and admitted patient records, based on their medical histories, physical exam, the progress, additional edits and notes are automatically updated into the relevant sections of patient record. The software should have audit trails of patient data access by time, date and user name. The system should generate referral consultation notes, preview notes prior to completion, ability to import any other authorized information into patient record. Customize the software to automatically designate certain procedure and CPT codes for a specific diagnosis with identifying investigated lab tests and prescriptions for ordered for particular diagnosis. As well differential and complicated diagnoses are to be documented.

Side-side comparison: Precisely, the software related to patient administration should help the care provider to view side by side comparison of patient historical vital signs, investigation reports, scanned images, voice files and transcriptions. Recall notices, scheduling, tracking of different information including patient education, consulting physicians, and any information including order tests, physician consultations and surgical procedures from the patient record; track outstanding lab and other orders, flag abnormal lab results. That has been input to be easily analyzed and produced.

Multiple prescription templates: While prescription of drugs, the system should be able to show alert drug interactions and potential drug-drug, drug-allergy and drug-pregnancy or contraindications or conflicts. Electronically send prescriptions to specific pharmacies via a secured connection and multiple prescription templates include description of medication, dosage recommendations, patient education forms, drug ingredients, possible medication alternatives and more to assist patient care providers.

Integration of information: As regards to document management including storage and retrieval, the system should facilitate to search and retrieve easily the different images, and files could be easily indexed by patient unique number and date for faster retrieval. The system should integrate all related information for easy document management and image scanning. Image scanned documents can be automatically indexed based on templates using optical character recognition (OCR).

Data collection support: The EHR should support the collection of data for users other than clinical care, such as billing, quality management, outcomes reporting, and public health disease surveillance and reporting. As regards to attributes, essential requirements, and evidence; provide secured, reliable, real-time access to patient health record information, when and where it is needed to support care. For example: Essential requirements encompass guarantee the confidentiality and security of patient health information. Information should be reliable and available at all times that care is provided; capable of integrating the care provider's workflow, easily accessible all information related to patient's outpatient episodes or inpatient admissions. The system should meet complete HIPAA requirements.

Permit efficient data entry: Should be able to capture and manage episodic and longitudinal electronic health record information that should include time stamps, information source and audit trail for amendments. Permit efficient data entry of all orders and documentation by authorized clinicians including prescription writing and refill management and support electronic signature where permitted by law. Implemented EHR possess the evidence of message content standards for interoperable; such as DICOM, HL7, LOINC, Rx Norn, etc.

Integration of collected data: Essential functional requirements during the patient care should include patient problem list, patent history and physical exam, progress, nursing notes, consultation notes, and patient functional status, allergies, immunizations, medications dispensed and administered, diagnostic results and images in ER, ICU, OR, etc. most recent vital signs and input/output. All information collected previously for different episodic encounters, admissions, events etc. to be integrated and updated for easy reference of care providers prior to subsequent care for efficient decision making.

Assist in work planning: Assist with the work planning and delivering evidence-based care to patients: Provides tools for planning and organizing the clinician's work over a variety of time segments, such as on particular day and shift, and clinic session, etc. For hospital-based care, gather data and performs checking to support regulatory and accreditation requirement such as JCAHO safe care standards, Leapfrog standards for medication error prevention. Further, it should include decision support tools to guide and critique medication administration—right patient, right drug, right dose, right time, right route.

Support continuous quality improvement: Should be able to support continuous quality improvement, utilization review, risk management and performance management and provide flexible reporting tools for evaluating processes and outcomes of care by providing concurrent care, management level and on-line displays that enable easy access to summary views of pertinent information for groups (cohorts) of patients to support managers' detection and resolution of potential quality, staffing, and risk management issues.

Capture information without error: Should be able to capture the patient health-related information needed for reimbursement and billing, etc. without errors on claims, and should support clinical research, public health reporting, and population initiatives. This should provide disease management support for education, outreach and care to enrolled patients, support mandatory reporting, state health product liability reporting and social welfare reporting.

Summary

- Implementing an EMR system in the hospital is a daunting task. It requires good planning, strong leadership and supportive staff.
- Organizational issues need to drive for successful EHR implementation; poor choice of technology is the first step toward an unsuccessful project. System selection should be driven by the desired outcomes, technology adoption process.
- Technology evaluation can be centered around many different components, including reliability, performance measures, standards and interoperability, customized tradeoffs, usability, and usefulness.
- An environmental analysis of the organization that includes current process and workflow assessment, readiness to adopt new technologies, belief systems, and other human factor's concepts will identify the potential issues that could derail any EHR implementation.
- The pre-implementation evaluation accomplishes two things. First, it engages users in the implementation process, soliciting feedback and acting upon suggestions. Second, it can be used to identify any organizational constructs that could serve as roadblocks to successful implementation.
- Many EMRs are not designed to completely replace the paper record, so if "going paperless" is your goal must be to ensure that the software has all the tools required to accomplish it. The most important requirement for going paperless is to have a method of scanning outside documents as text or images and filing them in the EMR.
- Decide what to scan and what not; to scan selected important documents, such as Pap smears and radiology reports, and file the rest. Once the documents are scanned, keep them for at least a week to ensure reliable computer backup, and then they can be destroyed. Some documents that do not add useful information to the record, such as the fourth chest X-ray report for a hospitalized critically ill patient, are to be destroyed.
- Training should be in three phases—initial basic skills assessment, basic skills training and application-specific training—which has to be done in three months, two months and one week, respectively, before going live. Training session to be conducted by a vendor representative and hospital trainer. A summary document outlining key workflow changes to be distributed during the practice of training so that anyone who was unsure how to do a task with the new system had a quick reference.

Essentials for a successful EMR implementation but not limited to the following:

- Clear definition of goals
- Strong project leadership team to run the implementation
- Project manager with sufficient, dedicated time
- Strong physician leader to champion the project
- Detailed analysis of workflow
- High level of staff flexibility
- Commitment to "plan for the worst; hope for the best".

Chapter 7

Challenges of Hospital IT and Networking Design for Electronic Health Records

INTRODUCTION

Despite, the IT has been built-in into hospital system worldwide for nearly three decades; the full exploitation of IT has not been accomplished to the optimum. The author wishes to enlighten certain root causes that could be adding to the problem for delayed implementation. The hospital is a complex organization with diverse background with mixture of professionals, interact and co-ordinate their services to deliver best possible care ranging low to high risk patients. The implementation of IT in the hospital, as predicted, is not happening due to many hurdles that need to be tackled prudently.

Material and Methods

The patient is the nucleus, around which efforts of hospital policy-makers, administrators, departments, personnel of varied professional skills, knowledge revolve to provide best possible care. To be precise; the material is classified as: (i) Patient needs and demands, (ii) hospital functions, (iii) management, (iv) cost and finance, (v) information, and (vi) technology (3 Ts: Team, Tactics, and Technology). The methods include: The author's past experience of serving for 4 decades in GCC countries as Senior Consultant/ Adviser and WHO Consultant to the Ministries of Health of Kuwait, Saudi Arabia, Oman, Bahrain, Qatar and UAE, besides India, Afghanistan and Iran.

Discussion

There are many hospitals that have ideal standards, policies and procedures to ensure the system works effectively, while some hospitals, believe in running the system and tackling the issues as and when the situation demand, solutions are found and "show goes on". Many hospital policy makers, administrators, and care providers of later category, have felt that if IT is implemented in the hospital, all the problems would be resolved, instantly, everything will budge extremely well. The following are some of the challenges of hospitals to be reviewed thoroughly while developing and implementing the software for gaining optimum results.

Vision and Mission of the Hospital

Developing and implementing IT and network designing in the hospital

- Establishment of a new hospital or managing the existing hospital
- Meet the needs of modern highly demanding society
- Budgetary provision
- Running the hospital unhindered within legal and ethical limits
- Future hospital expansion scope vertically and horizontally
- Disaster plan and management control.

Hospital

- Need to study hospital functioning in-depth
- Running existing hospital within budget
- Ensure that the hospital meeting the set objectives with manual system (MS)

Hospital Organizational Needs

- Hospital resources including HR, other infrastructure
- Organization chart
- Standards, policies and procedures
- Quality of patient care proposed (standard operating procedures)
- Practice of professional ethics
- Developing and managing efficient information system
- Net work provision and needs for eHealth system
- Disaster plan.

Hospital Organization Structure

It is important to realize that each and every department and unit and individual in the system is contributing for effective management of hospital including providing swift, safe, quality improved and cost contained care to sick and injured. Hence, the IT and network design should incorporate and integrate every single aspect that adds the value in accomplishing the objectives of the hospital.

POTENTIAL CAUSES RELATED TO PATIENT

- Hospital-acquired infection
- Patient leaving against medical advice
- Mortality rate
- Patient repeated admissions
- Patient postoperative complications
- Incident cases
- Increased LOS (length of stay)
- Absconded patients
- Medication errors
- Transfusion reactions, wrong blood type
- Wrong site surgery (change of site procedure and organ)
- Obstetric and birth trauma
- Anesthesia and postoperative complications
- Hospital-acquired burns

- Change of investigations
- Wrong diagnosis, wrong medications
- Change of mother and child
- Safety, security of patient
- Protection of privacy of patient information
- Patient not improved.

Management

To streamline the administration:

- Ensure reduction of errors
- Improve care and save life
- Save time and dipping duplication
- Cost reduction
- Better resource utilization
- Billing and insurance settlements
- Provide medical education and research
- Medical legal issues and
- Timely submission of reports to various authorities

Cost and Finance Challenges

- 2/3rd expenditure on HR
- Indiscriminant ordering for costly and routine investigations
- Excessive prescription of drugs
- Costly equipment procuring with out optimum utilization
- Poor maintenance of equipment
- Wastage of hospital utilities
- Duplication of services and efforts
- Improper allocation of space, building
- Under utilization of services
- Increased hospital maintenance cost
- Ineffective utilization of beds and other resources
- *Not reviewing*: Blood usage, drug usage, pharmacy and therapeutic
- Not conducting peer review, surgical and invasive case review and medical records

Information Required

This being an era of information and knowledge, every stage of management whether clinical or non-clinical, needs accurate, complete and timely valid information. The expectations from electronic health records implementation are as follows:

- *Health information and data*: Having immediate access to key information—such as patients' diagnoses, allergies, lab test results, and medications—would improve caregivers' ability to make sound clinical decisions in a timely manner.
- *Result management*: The ability for all providers participating in the care of a patient in multiple settings to quickly access new and past test results would increase patient safety and the effectiveness of care.

- *Order management*: The ability to enter and store orders for prescriptions, tests, and other services in a computer-based system should enhance legibility, reduce duplication, and improve the speed with which orders are executed.
- *Decision support*: Using reminders prompts, and alerts, computerized decision-support systems would help improve compliance with best evidence based clinical practices, ensure regular screenings and other preventive practices, identify possible drug interactions, and facilitate diagnoses and treatments.
- *Electronic communication and connectivity*: Efficient, secure, and readily accessible communication among providers and patients would improve the continuity of care, increase the timeliness of diagnoses and treatments, and reduce the frequency of adverse events.
- *Patient support*: Tools that give patients access to their health records, provide interactive patient education, and help them carry out home-monitoring and self-testing can improve control of chronic conditions, such as diabetes.
- *Administrative processes*: Computerized administrative tools, such as scheduling systems, would greatly improve hospitals' and clinics' efficiency and provide more timely service to patients.
- *Reporting*: Electronic data storage that employs uniform data standards will enable health care organizations to respond more quickly to federal, state, and private reporting requirements, including those that support patient safety and disease surveillance."
- *Alignment of templates*: Methodical arrangement of templates and buttons should facilitate the users with much ease and as a normal flow that make user favorite.
- *Significant templates in one screen (area)*: Facilitate busy physician to scan quickly to have comprehensive picture of past and present; investigation results, medications and care status in one screen will help in making convincing decision.

THE IT DEPARTMENT

The IT department while making the software, should review the functions of the hospitals meticulously to address the problems and alert the management at every level of the hospital to provide best possible care to patient and to provide patient related reports, medicolegal, manpower staffing analysis, and allocation, quality assurance data; cost accounting information, insurance related information, management information besides clinical information for effective patient and improved quality care to patient.

The IT Department (development of HIS/EHR)

- IT is use >3 decades worldwide
- Not exploited IT to the optimum
- High hopes with IT implementation
- Review meticulously hospital functions
- It develops HIS, EHR, without understanding functional domains
- Assist in efficient management
- Aid in best possible care
- Clinical management, medical eduction and research
- Provide reports, insurance, MLC, HR, QA, CA

- EHR patient centric
- Easy accessibility, accuracy, completeness
- Evidence based decision making
- Real time point of care
- Streamline physician's workflow
- Provides clinical reminders
- Incorporating EHRR standards, e.g. HL 7, ASTM, PACS, DICOM, NCPDP, SNOMED, ICD, CPT, HIPAA and JACHO
- Alert reminding system

Development of Electronic Health Records

The EHR includes the process and functionality to allow collection of information and its integration with knowledge base to create decision support mechanisms, alerts, reminders, and other aids to clinical decision-making. The major value of EHR is the availability of electronically stored information online for access to the network to authorize at any station, at real-time, point of care and provide data for users other than direct clinical care, such as billing, quality management, disease surveillance and reporting. Further it should be capable of reduction of errors, duplication, time saving, easy accessibility, convenience, accuracy and completeness, cost reduction and research and education.

While developing software, most important aspect is meticulous preparation of domain of all functions related to physician's office, outpatient, ER., inpatient, OT, ICU, CCU, Lab, Radiology, other imaging sections, medication; e-prescription nursing, clinical reminders, medical specialties, documentation, flowchart and screen by database administrators and web designers prior to technical involvement, such as research and development, coding by programmers, incorporating EHR-related standards, for example; HL7, ASTM, PACS, DICOM, NCPDP, SNOMED, ICD, CPT, HIPAA and JCAHO recommended accreditation standards, testing and re-testing, mock and live operation by varied users before the software finally released for live.

Integration of Network Infrastructure

Those hospitals that have network infrastructure, but there are several physically separate networks, supporting clinical data, non-clinical data, voice, research, educational equipment, and departmental staff, for manageability, efficiency, costs, there is a need to converge these separate networks into one physical infrastructure, while still providing the isolation, security, and responsiveness needed by the organization. And those hospitals are newly implementing IT and networking design should integrate all networks to have optimum benefits.

Need to Exchange Clinical Knowledge

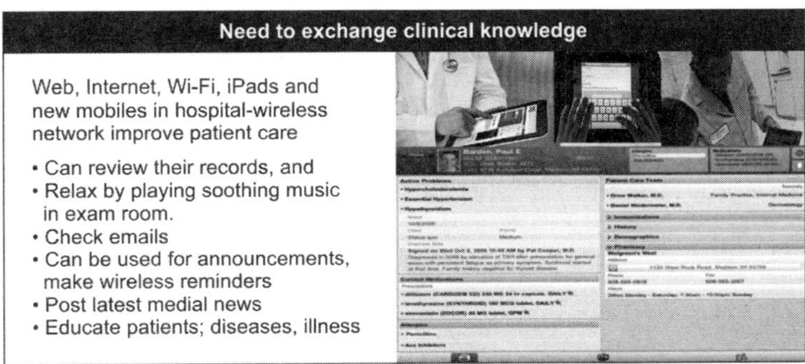

Electronic Health Records

- **Advantages of electronic medical records**
- **There are numerous advantages of EMR**

Patient's perfective

- Improved diagnosis and treatment
- Significantly fewer errors found within personal health records
- Faster care and decision-making responses from assigned medical professionals.

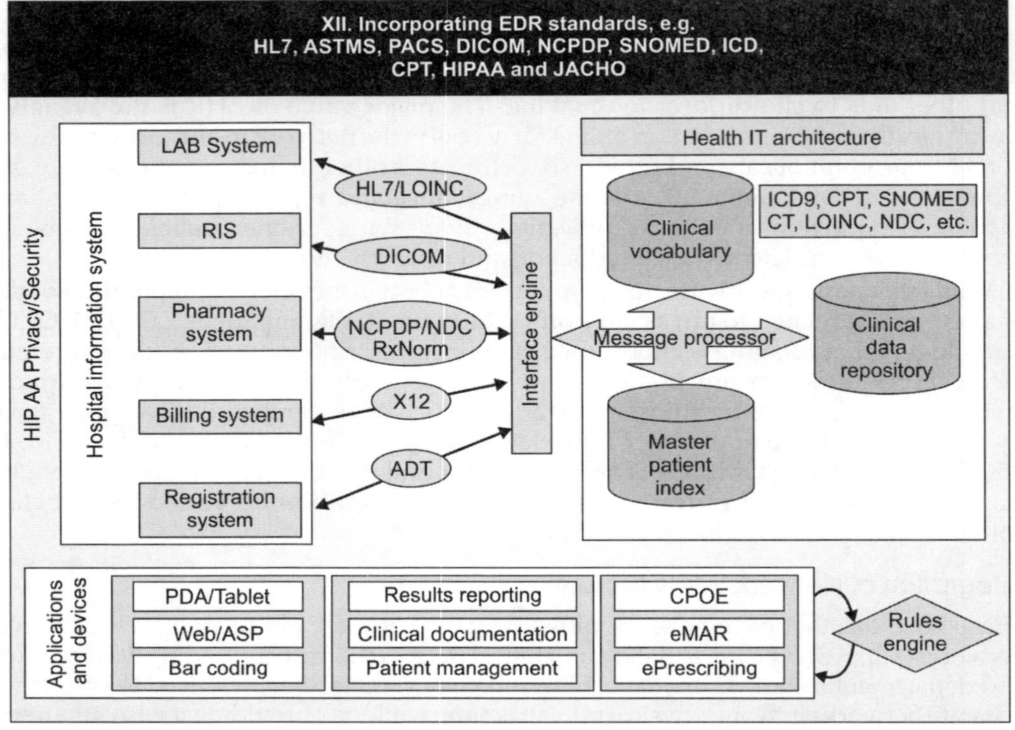
XII. Incorporating EDR standards, e.g.
HL7, ASTMS, PACS, DICOM, NCPDP, SNOMED, ICD,
CPT, HIPAA and JACHO
HIP AA Privacy/Security
Hospital information system
LAB System
RIS
Pharmacy system
Billing system
Registration system
HL7/LOINC
DICOM
NCPDP/NDC
RxNorm
X12
ADT
Interface engine
Health IT architecture
Clinical vocabulary
ICD9, CPT, SNOMED CT, LOINC, NDC, etc.
Message processor
Clinical data repository
Master patient index
Applications and devices
PDA/Tablet
Web/ASP
Bar coding
Results reporting
Clinical documentation
Patient management
CPOE
eMAR
ePrescribing
Rules engine

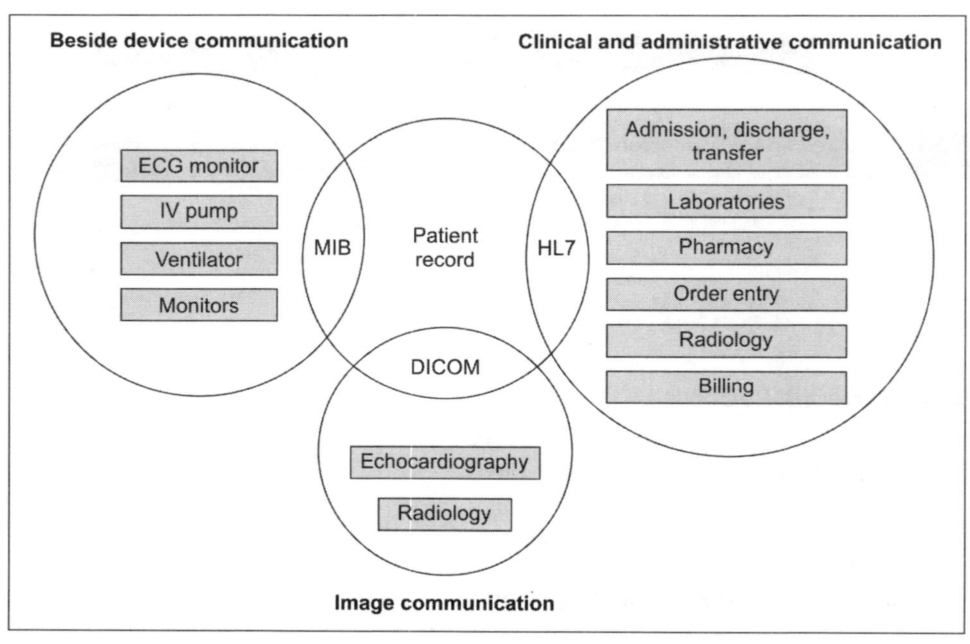
Beside device communication
Clinical and administrative communication
ECG monitor
IV pump
Ventilator
Monitors
MIB
Patient record
HL7
Admission, discharge, transfer
Laboratories
Pharmacy
Order entry
Radiology
Billing
DICOM
Echocardiography
Radiology
Image communication

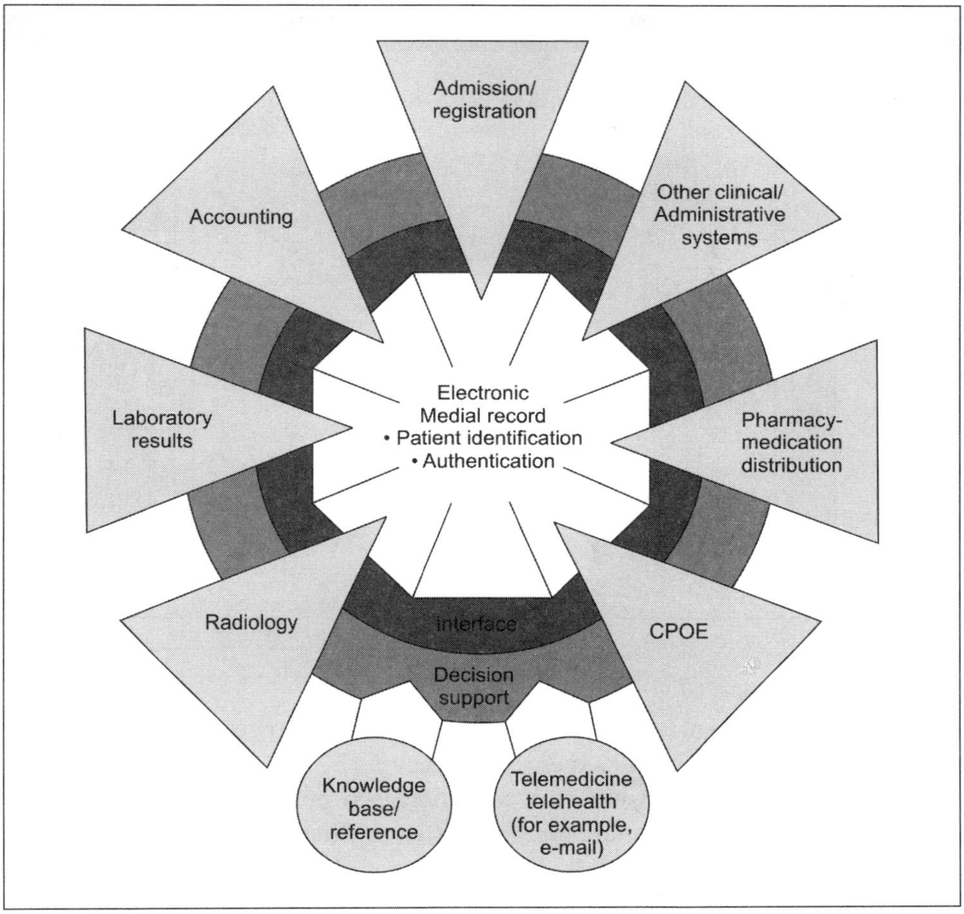

Admission/
registration
Accounting
Other clinical/
Administrative
systems
Laboratory
results
Electronic
Medial record
• Patient identification
• Authentication
Pharmacy-
medication
distribution
Radiology
interface
CPOE
Decision
support
Knowledge
base/
reference
Telemedicine
telehealth
(for example,
e-mail)

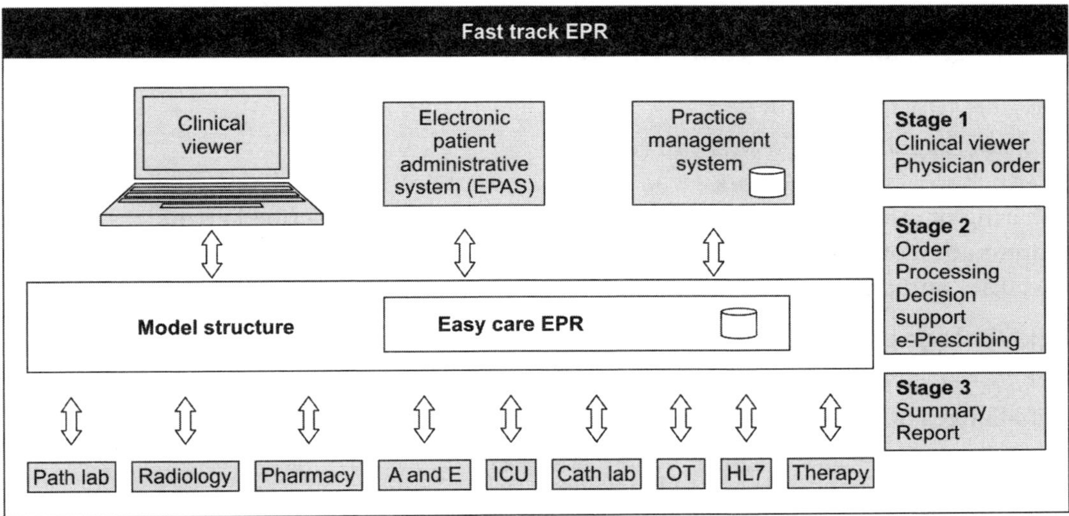
Fast track EPR
Clinical
viewer
Electronic
patient
administrative
system (EPAS)
Practice
management
system
Stage 1
Clinical viewer
Physician order
Stage 2
Order
Processing
Decision
support
e-Prescribing
Model structure
Easy care EPR
Stage 3
Summary
Report
Path lab
Radiology
Pharmacy
A and E
ICU
Cath lab
OT
HL7
Therapy

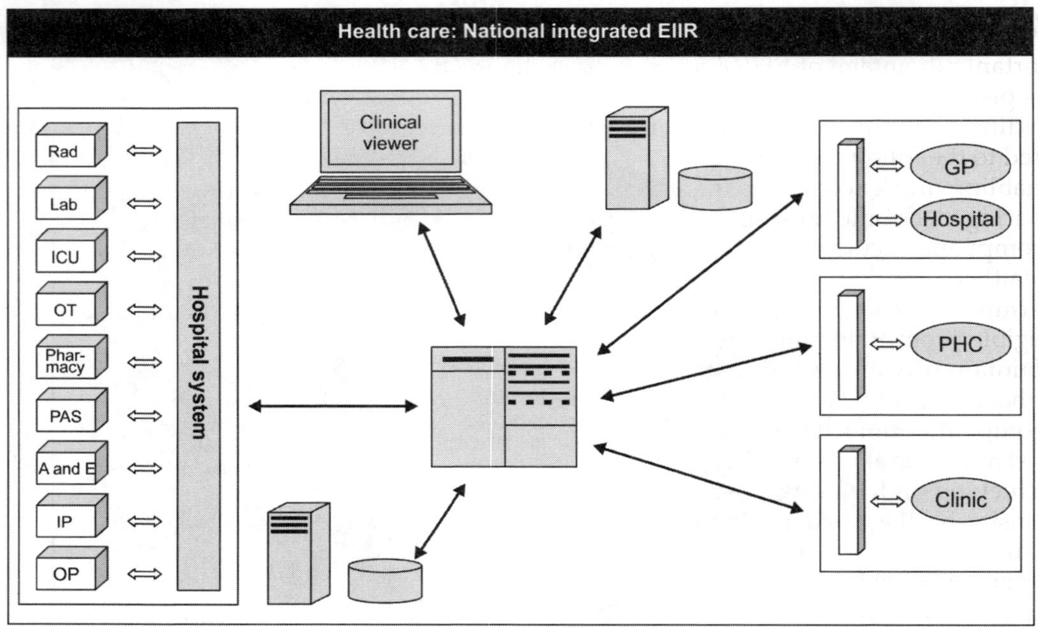

Medical practice perspective

- The ability to quickly transfer patient data from one department to another.
- The digital records environment saves the space
- The ability to enhance patient workflow and increased productivity
- Improved results patient care management with a decline in errors in medical practice
- Reduced operational costs such as transcription services and overtime labor expenses
- Customizable and scalable electronic medical records that can grow with your practice
- Efficient e-prescribing and clinical documentation capabilities
- More accurately and efficiently processed patient billing
- Exchange of information easily and promtly.

Patient safety perspective

- Patient diagnosis and security of records
- Reduction of medical errors
- Sharing of information within medical practice reduces transcribed errors
- Elimination of lost or misplaced patient records
- Security and privacy of record is maintained.

Disadvantages of Electronic Medical Records

There are numerous disadvantages of EMR:

- Challenges of investment, preparation and training
- Transition of old paper record to electronic records
- Big obstacle for medical staff to have computer skills
- Physician spend more time with computer than patient.

ADVANTAGES OF ELECTRONIC HEALTH RECORDS

Important advantage of EHRs is ability to exchange health information electronically that helps provide better managed care resulting higher quality and safer care to patient. And providing accurate and complete information at the point of patient care enhances and not limited to the following:

- Enabling quick access to patient records for more coordinated resulting efficient care
- Sharing electronic information with patients and other clinicians securely
- Prompt and accurate diagnosis of patients, reduce medical errors, and provide safer care
- Healthcare provider interaction and communication help quick treatment
- Permit safer and reliable prescribing prevent adverse of effects of medicine
- Legible prompt documentation enable coding and billing
- Maintain privacy and security of patient data
- Enhances healthcare providers productivity of quality patient care
- Prompt attentions help provider's efficiency in improving quality reduce errors
- Cost reduction affects by minimizing the duplication of testing, documenting and paper work.
- Achieving high quality, cost efficient
- Consistent diagnosis is a must
- Standard care for all
- Organized care is possible
- Medical errors or minimized
- Integrated delivery system
- Converting data into meaningful information for standing trends of healthcare operations and patient safety issues and output will help in decision-making
  - HIM professionals can have strong partnership with healthcare providers due to their unique knowledge
  - Accurate, complete and timely data can help the healthcare provider to render better care.
  - To eliminate, e.g. adverse events, injuries caused by medical management, etc. need greater diligence.
  - Data must be transparent and honest documentation practice, standardization of content and definitions
  - HIM should collaborate with IT to develop and use appropriate system for care providers
  - Unit record concept of all information related to single patient should be in one central database

Conclusion

The benefits of IT can be fully realized; only when the existing deficiencies of hospital manual system are meticulously tackled by management. The IT developers with the help of concerned to ensure that integrated IT and networking design developed should meet all the functions and challenges of hospitals with special reference to patient care. Ironically, most of IT experts devote their efforts towards Hospital Information System (HIS) and especially on EHR either without understanding or ignoring the intricacies of functional domain.

The main objective of this presentation is to explain the role of IT in managing the Hospital Information System (HIS). The author has brought out several challenges that are part of hospital functioning and without addressing them appropriately, the eHealth system in the hospital will not be effective. The purpose of an HIS is to achieve the best possible support of patient care and administration by electronic data processing. The information that is readily accessible, timely, complete, accurate, legible, and relevant is critical to health care providers for efficient patient care. In order to ensure adequate access, the need for comprehensive information is much greater today.

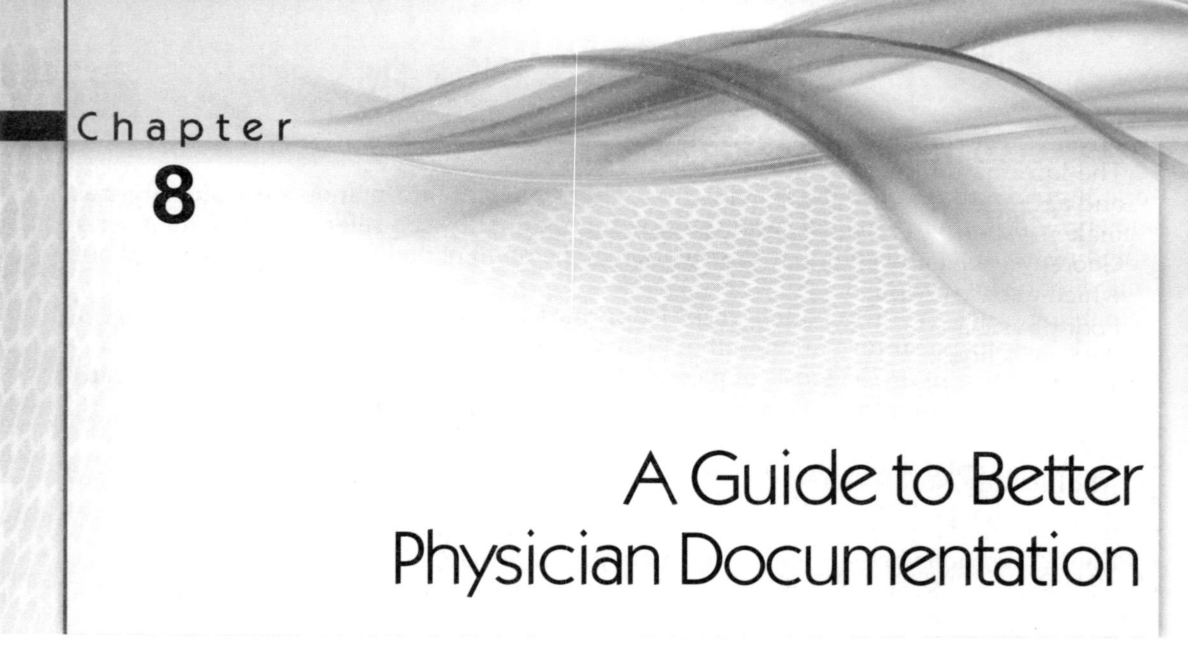

Chapter 8

A Guide to Better Physician Documentation

The Recommendation on Physician Documentation was presented by Expert Panel Chair: Kern MD, MHSc, FRCP ©, Asst. Professor, Neurology Program Director, University of Toronto, Canada.

As chair of the Physician Documentation Expert Panel and on behalf of my fellow panel members, I am pleased to present you with this guide to better physician documentation. It reflects the collective input and recommendations of a panel of your peers, representing a range of disciplines, and the profession's regulator and association as well as stakeholders, who came together in the fall of 2005 because of concerns about the deficiencies in patient health records due to incomplete, inaccurate and lengthy delays in physician documentation.

- As physicians, the health and care of our patients are our greatest concerns, and it is clear to us that inadequate documentation impacts on both patient care and outcomes. A family doctor treating a patient without the benefit of a discharge summary from an acute care physician is working at a disadvantage in a potentially life-threatening situation.
- Quality physician documentation shared in a timely manner can help avoid negative consequences, such as adverse medication events.
- These are some of the concerns that brought us together to devise strategies and tools to improve physician documentation primarily in acute and ambulatory care episodes. This is an issue that impacts on the quality of patient care and the overall health care needs of Ontarians.
- The patient health record is a physician's most powerful communication tool. It is the key to exchanging critical information with all members of the clinical team. It is an essential communication vehicle, not only in a hospital setting, but also in other health care settings.
- The health record links acute care physicians with primary care physicians and allows for the transfer of potentially life-saving information. The health record is paramount to the continuity of care. When there is a breakdown in this communication, due to delays in the transfer of information or incomplete and inaccurate information, the consequences can be negative.

- Physician documentation also drives the quality of data within the health care system. The information written and maintained in patient health records, once it is collected and aggregated, is used by clinicians, health system planners, researchers, and decision-makers as the basis for important decisions related to the health care needs of Ontarians. Good physician documentation ensures that a better quality of data will be available on which to base critical health care sector decisions.
- Poor physician documentation can, in part, be linked to the lack of focus on this issue in medical schools.
- This inattention to good documentation procedures continues through the internship and residency phase of medical training, which means that physicians are not being adequately equipped to document effectively in the course of their medical training.
- Additionally, studies have raised concerns about deficiencies in the documentation of patient charts at Ontario's hospitals, including issues of accuracy and lack of completeness.
- To support the goal of improving the quality of physician documentation, a group of my esteemed colleagues and I were asked by the Ministry of Health and Long-Term Care's Health Results Team Lead for Information.
- Information Management Strategy. In conjunction with the Health Results Team, the panel spent several months creating an information package for physicians, which includes:
  - This comprehensive guide, detailing the impact of good physician documentation on patient care and outcomes, as well as the consequences of poor communication
  - Chart completion policy templates to serve as a standard guide to physicians and hospitals, that will help facilitate the accurate and timely completion of patient chart.

A slide presentation on physician documentation emphasizing the key points from the guide:

- It is the hope of the panel that these documents will be useful to you and your colleagues in providing a foundation for improving the quality of physician documentation. Complete, accurate and timely physician documentation will enhance patient care and greatly benefit Ontario's health care system.
- We would encourage you to share these materials with your medical colleagues. Through better physician documentation we can enhance our most powerful communication tool, the health record, to optimize patient care and ensure that a better quality of data is available for critical health care decisions.

Chapter

9

Personnel Requirements and Job Description

This section deals with the following:

I. Personnel requirements according to the bed strength of the hospital.

II. Job descriptions for three important categories of medical record department personnel, e.g. medical record officer, medical record technician and assistant medical record technician.

PERSONNEL MANAGEMENT IN MEDICAL RECORD (HEALTH INFORMATION) DEPARTMENT

The staff of medical record department gives their best service to the department only when their morale is high. The points furnished below are important and should be observed meticulously to build up high morale among departmental employees.

- Selection of suitable persons is vital.
- Salaries must be commensurate with their qualifications and training.
- Periodic orientation of staff to policies and procedures is necessary.
- Written policy and procedure manuals with organization charts, department functions and staff job descriptions are necessary.
- Good interdepartmental and intradepartmental relationships and effective communication systems are essential.
- Medical record officers (Health Information Manager) should be dynamic, unbiased, judicious, firm and flexible.
- The medical record officer should be source of encouragement to his staff.
- The medical record officer should spend substantial time on plans relating to the improvement of existing services as well as on future developments. Objectives of the department should be clearly specified.
- The entire department should function as a team to maintain confidentiality, to protect the facility from legal action and to provide the best service to the hospital in general and the patient in particular.
- Accommodations for employees to improve their educational and professional status should be provided.

- Active participation by the staff in all the activities of the department coupled with good incentives enhances the interests of the staff and consequently provides excellent output.
- Practice of good ethics and discipline makes a model department for the hospital.

Norms for Developing the Number of Personnel

Formula for deploying the number of personnel to furnish around the clock service:

Working days × number of shifts = number of persons required to be posted man days

Man days are actual working days available, i.e. after subtracting the number of holidays to which the staff is entitled. For example, out of 365 days, each member of the staff is entitled to 148 days, so 365–148 = 217 man days for one person. For instance, the admissions office must function during shifts with one clerk/technician posted on each shift. Then the number of persons to be deployed would be 5 persons.

$$\frac{365 \times 3}{217} = 5 \text{ approx.}$$

Formula for calculation of personnel required for MRD (given below)

A minimum of two persons for any size of the hospital + 1 person for every 100 beds (50–100) + 1 person for every 10 beds, e.g. number of staff required for medical record department:

i. *Of 100 bedded hospital*: 2 + 1 +10 = 13 personnel

ii. *Of 500 bedded hospital*: 2 + 5 + 50 = 57 personnel

Categories of staff for MRD according to bed strength

Category	*Bed*					
	30	*50*	*100*	*250*	*500*	*750*
Medical record officer	–	–	1	1	1	1
Medical record technician	1	1	2	6	12	14
Asst. Med. rec. technician	4	7	10	23	44	70
Total	**5**	**8**	**13**	**30**	**57**	**85**
Med. sec./transcription	–	1	2	4	7	8
Quality assurance specialist	–	–	1	1	1	1
Grand total	5	9	16	35	65	94
OP. average (daily)	120	280	400	1000	2000	3000
Inpatient admissions (yearly)	1080	1800	3600	9000	18000	27000

JOB DESCRIPTIONS MEDICAL RECORD OFFICER (HEALTH INFORMATION MANAGER): QUALIFICATION

Bachelor Degree in Health Information Management from any recognized university or Indian context:

- One year diploma in medical records after university graduation with 3 years experience in medical records. Organization and management of the medical record department .

University degree in medical records with at least 4 years experience in medical records.

or

Four-year Health Information Management (HIM) Bachelor's degree program from authorized university.

Line of Promotion

- Responsible to the director of central information department or hospital director (medical).
- Supervise Assistant MRO or medical record technicians.
- Appointed or promoted to this job by fulfilling the required qualifications.
- Eligible to for promotion to senior medical record officer or medical record specialist.

Duties and Responsibilities

- To establish, organize and manage a medical record department with appropriate systems to provide an effective service in the hospital.
- To develop policies and procedures relating to the medical record department in accordance with the Health directorate/Ministry of Health.
- To assist the medical record committee in the design and development of different forms required for hospital use.
- To review the medical records of outpatients admitted patients and emergency patients to ensure that they include all important documents and pertinent information.
- To cooperate with the medical, nursing and other staff persons in completing patient medical records.
- To participate and assist in quality assurance, utilization review, infection control and other committees and programs.
- To prepare and maintain medical reports, medical certificates and birth and death registers and to notify concerned authorities in duly completing the required procedures.
- To prepare monthly statistical reports concerning the hospital activities carried out, and to submit to concerned authorities any suggestions for improvements.
- To observe professional ethics and to protect the confidentiality of information from unauthorized persons; to keep medical legal records under safe custody and to attend court whenever required.
- To participate and assist in research programs to develop new methods and procedures for improving administrative activities and financial control.
- To select appropriate personnel for the medical record department and train them for performing their jobs efficiently.
- To prepare and carryout educational and training programs such as certificates, diplomas and degrees for medical record personnel.
- To accept the responsibility for the safe preservation of patient property during hospitalization.
- To effectively carryout registration systems and to control the movement of patient files in order to achieve a unit record.
- To introduce computer services for the effective function of the outpatient, inpatient and emergency registration systems to collect clinical and administrative statistics. Medical Records Organization and Management.
- To supply patient files in accordance with the established procedures for medical care, medical education, medical training, and medical care evaluation management and legal purposes.
- To maintain and protect medical records in accordance with the policies relating to preservation and destruction.

- To cooperate with the medical nursing, heads of departments, patients, health agencies, other hospitals and legal authorities for smooth and efficient functioning of the hospital in general and of the medical record department in particular.
- To supervise the work of the medical record department staff, medical secretaries, and medical transcriptionists.
- To participate in educational programs such as seminars, workshops and conferences related to the medical record profession.
- To carryout any other duties and functions related to medical record services as instructed by the immediate chief.

MEDICAL RECORD TECHNICIAN (HEALTH INFORMATION TECHNICIAN): QUALIFICATION

Two-year Diploma in Health Information Management (HIM) from any recognized institute or university. Or from Indian context:

- High school diploma or certificate with practical training in the medical records field for at least 6 months with 8 years experience as assistant medical record technician, or
- Certificate or diploma in medical records after an intermediate education, or
- Two-year Diploma in Medical Records after high school graduation or technical school graduation.

Line of Promotion

- Responsible to medical record officer (Health Information Manager) or his representative.
- Appointed or promoted to this position by fulfilling the required qualifications.
- Eligible for promotion to a higher grade in the same position.
- Supervise assistant medical record technicians.

Duties and Responsibilities

- To carryout technical analysis and evaluation of medical records in accordance with hospital standards.
- To collect medical, administrative and other statistics required by the hospital and to provide health information for planning and evaluation of healthcare.
- To code and index diseases, surgical operations and therapeutic procedures according to international classification of diseases and operations or according to criteria set forth by the health directorate/Ministry of Health.
- To provide medical record services including reception, registration, appointments and inpatient, outpatient and emergency department filing and retrieving systems. Organization and management of the medical record department
- To implement the transcription of medical and other reports in the medical record department or clinical units or wards.
- To evaluate documentation for deficiencies in the outpatient and inpatient medical files and to arranging for completion of records with the cooperation of medical and nursing staff.
- To feed patient care information into the computer for processing, storage and retrieval when required.
- To assist medical education and medical research programs by providing required information.
- To cooperate with all departments related to medical record services in order obtain acceptable records for providing efficient services.

- To protect medical records specially medical legal cases from unauthorized disclosure so as to maintain confidentiality.
- To assist the medical staff and their committees in the hospital in executing the quality assurance program.
- To supervise one or more medical record units and to assist in departmental educational and administrative systems.
- To observe medical ethics as recommended for medical record professionals.
- To participate in educational programs such as seminars, workshops and conferences related to medical record field.
- To work any one of the three shifts as required.
- To perform any other work related to medical records as instructed by his or her direct or immediate chief.

Assistant Medical Record Technician: Qualification

High school qualifications with at least 6 months training in medical records.

Line of Promotion

- Responsible to medical record technician.
- Appointed to this post by fulfilling the required qualifications.
- Eligible for promotion to a higher grade within the same position.
- Eligible for promotion to medical record technician.

Duties and Responsibilities

- To prepare prenumbered folders with color coding.
- To collect basic identification data from the patient and record it on the patient medical file.
- To register new and old (follow-up) patients and arrange appointments for both outpatients and inpatients.
- To help and direct patients in the outpatient clinic.
- To prepare patient master index cards, to arrange them according to alphabetical order, to file them in the index cabinets, and to retrieve them when required. Medical Records Organization and Management
- To collect investigation reports from the laboratory, X-ray and other investigation departments and to arrange and mount them in the appropriate records.
- To receive patient records and X-rays and to arrange and file them in the appropriate location.
- To retrieve records and X-rays and send them to the required department.
- To be capable to work in all units of the medical record department as well as the outpatient clinic, the admissions office and any ward or unit and to carryout the work of that unit as per recommended procedures.
- To assemble and process records as per the established procedures.
- To be familiar with microfilm or computers and other mechanical devices for maintaining records.
- To collect and prepare statistics of outpatients, emergency patients and inpatients.
- To strictly observe instructions given in the procedure manual to carryout assigned duties and responsibilities.
- To work on any of the three shifts as required.

- To index previously coded disease and operation cases on the disease and operation index cards.
- To maintain confidentiality of patient information and prevent disclosure to unauthorized persons.
- To register birth, death and infectious disease cases in the appropriate manner.
- To participate in educational programs, e.g. seminars, workshops and conferences related to the medical record field.
- To observe professional ethics as recommended for the medical record profession.
- To perform any work given by immediate or direct chief.

The following information is relevant to the **American Health Information Management Association** (AHIMA) of USA.

Medical Records (or Health Information) Technician: Registered Health Information Management Technician (Technologist).

Technicians assemble patients' health information including medical history, symptoms, examination results, tests, and treatments.

Medical records and health information technicians, commonly referred to as health information technicians, organize and manage health information data by ensuring its quality, accuracy, accessibility, and security in both paper and electronic systems. They use various classification systems to code and categorize patient information for insurance reimbursement purposes, for databases and registries, and to maintain patients' medical and treatment histories.

Duties: *Health information technicians typically do the following:*

- Review patient records for timeliness, completeness, accuracy, and appropriateness of data
- Organize and maintain data for clinical databases and registries
- Track patient outcomes for quality assessment
- Use classification software to assign clinical codes for reimbursement and data analysis
- Electronically record data for collection, storage, analysis, retrieval, and reporting
- Protect patients' health information for confidentiality, authorized access for treatment, and data security.

All health information technicians document patients' health information, including their medical history, symptoms, examination and test results, treatments, and other information about healthcare services that are provided to patients. Their duties vary with the size of the facility in which they work.

Although health information technicians do not provide direct patient care, they work regularly with registered nurses and other healthcare professionals. They meet with these workers to clarify diagnoses or to get additional information to make sure that records are complete and accurate.

The increasing use of electronic health records (EHRs) will continue to change the job responsibilities of health information technicians. Federal legislation provides incentives for physicians' offices and hospitals to implement EHR systems into their practice. This will lead to continued adoption of this software in these facilities. Technicians will need to be familiar with, or be able to learn, EHR computer software, follow EHR security and privacy practices, and analyze electronic data to improve healthcare information as more healthcare providers and hospitals adopt EHR systems.

Health information technicians can specialize in many aspects of health information, e.g. some work as medical coders, sometimes called coding specialists, or as cancer registrars.

Medical coders typically do the following:

- Review patient information for pre-existing conditions such as diabetes
- Retrieve patient records for medical personnel
- Work as a liaison between the health clinician and billing offices

Cancer registrars typically do the following:

- Review patient records and pathology reports for completeness and accuracy
- Assign classification codes to represent the diagnosis and treatment of cancers and benign tumors
- Conduct annual follow-ups to track treatment, survival, and recovery
- Analyze and compile cancer patient information for research purposes
- Maintain facility, regional, and national databases of cancer patients

Ten Health Information Technology Skills employers are looking for in their Health Information Technology candidates:

The qualified HITs must acquire the skills that are not limited to the following to gain a job easily.

- Training
- Communication skills
- Organizing skills
- Writing skills
- Computer skills
- Microsoft excel
- Research skills
- Quality assurance and control
- Oriented well in the profession
- Problem solving skills

The HM professionals must possess all the required skills to be a proficient professional and to carryout his given responsibilities effectively and efficiently. As HIT has varieties of tasks perform, such as collection, analyzing the reports, medical diagnostic and procedure coding, dealing with medical, nursing and other allied healthcare providers to ensure that patient document is complete and accurate in all aspects. Need to coordinate with many in accomplishing the day-to-day work for which he should be well equipped with required skills to carryout his job efficiently.

Job Responsibilities

- Utilizes all applicable electronic systems.
- Assists medical staff with chart completion. Appropriately tracks records to and from incomplete record area. Checks all applicable systems for reports. Inserts reports into medical records and updates accordingly. Sends weekly notifications to physicians. Updates chart tracking system with new physician profiles.
- Ensures receipt of all records and documents in accordance with departmental policies. Accurately tracks charts and communicates with other departments to ensure all records and documents are received. Follows up in a timely manner for missing charts or parts. Organizes discharge paperwork prior to analysis. Creates new file folders if applicable and ensures proper chart size. Assembles medical records in standardized format in accordance with departmental procedures. Analyzes medical records in accordance with departmental procedures. Checks all appropriate systems for documentation.

- Transports medical records and assists walk-in requestors in a courteous manner. Answers the telephone in a polite manner, identifying themselves and the department. Takes messages thoroughly and accurately. Answers calls promptly and gives out accurate information to routine questions while following hospital confidentiality policies. Transfers calls to the correct individual based on content of inquiry.
- Retrieves medical records. Delivers medical records to appropriate location. Transports medical records in a timely fashion. Safeguards medical records during transport to ensure confidentiality and integrity.
- Maintains permanent file area and storage area. Locates and retrieves and files medical records as required. Files information according to departmental filing systems in designated areas. Maintains files in a well-organized manner. Retrieves charts and other records from files as requested in a timely manner. Obtains medical records from electronic system, when applicable. Follows established procedures for completing productivity form.
- Performs other duties as assigned.

ESSENTIAL FUNCTIONS AND RESPONSIBILITIES

1. Reviews the electronic health record to determine principal diagnoses, secondary diagnoses and significant procedures to assign appropriate ICD and CPT codes for data retrieval, research and reimbursement purposes.
2. Uses 3M electronic encoder and hardcopy coding book to determine appropriate coding guidelines.
3. Abstracts inpatient and outpatient date into 3M Health Data Management abstract for research projects, quality improvement studies, and statistical reporting.
4. Utilizes 3M Audit Expert, NCCI and OCE edits, LCD's and NCD's to determine appropriateness and completeness of coding and health record documentation.
5. Codes accounts on a timely basis by payor's cut-off dates under the "Just-in-Time" philosophy.
6. Investigates and tracks unbilled accounts to determine reason for incomplete status and works with appropriate resources for completion.
7. Enters observation, infusion, injection charges in powerchart charge set as appropriate, using compliant physician orders.
8. Utilizes software systems for identification of patients/workload to include Vista, 3M HDM, and health quest.
9. Collaborates with medical staff and clinical documentation specialists to ensure that documentation in health record support services provided to accurately and compliantly assign codes.
10. Facilitates communication and processes/resolves patient billing and service issues.
11. Collaborates with members of various ancillary departments to complete special projects, also may serve on both intradepartmental and interdepartmental committees and task forces.
12. Utilizes written communication skills to respond to recommended coding changes made by external auditors.
13. Serves as a resource for coding issues to other members of the organization/healthcare team.
14. Maintains continuing education credits for certification.
15. Maintains good rapport and cooperative relationships. Approaches conflict in a constructive manner. Helps to identify problems, offer solutions, and participates in their resolution.
16. Maintains the confidentiality of information acquired pertaining to patient, physicians, employees, and visitors to Saint Joseph Mercy Health System. Discusses patient and

hospital information only among appropriate personnel in appropriately private places.

17. Assumes responsibility for performance of job duties in the safest possible manner, to assure personal safety and that of coworkers, and to report all preventable hazards and unsafe practices immediately to management.
18. Behaves in accordance with the Mission, Vision and Values of Saint Joseph Mercy Health System.
19. Provides quality patient care by considering the age specific, development and cultural needs through competent clinical practice. Demonstrates unit/area competencies.
20. Maintains competency by attending and participating in webinars, seminars and training sessions as assigned.

Methods to Ensure Data Quality

The accuracy of data depends on the manual or computer information system design for collecting, recording, storing, processing, accessing and displaying data as well as the ability and follow-through of the people involved in each phase of these activities. Everyone involved with documenting or using health information is responsible for its quality. According to AHIMA's Data Quality Management Model, there are four key processes for data:

Application: The purpose for which the data are collected.

1. **Collection:** The processes by which data elements are accumulated.
2. **Warehousing:** The processes and systems used to store and maintain data and data journals.
3. **Analysis:** The process of translating data into information utilized for an application.

Each aspect is analyzed with 10 different data characteristics:

- **Accuracy:** Data are the correct values and are valid.
- **Accessibility:** Data items should be easily obtainable and legal to collect.
- **Comprehensiveness:** All required data items are included. Ensure that the entire scope of the data is collected and document intentional limitations.
- **Consistency:** The value of the data should be reliable and the same across applications.
- **Currency:** The data should be uptodate. A datum value is uptodate if it is current for a specific point in time. It is outdate if it was current at some preceding time yet incorrect at a later time.
- **Definition:** Clear definitions should be provided so that current and future data users will know what the data mean. Each data element should have clear meaning and acceptable values.
- **Granularity:** The attributes and values of data should be defined at the correct level of detail.
- **Precision:** Data values should be just large enough to support the application or process.
- **Relevancy:** The data are meaningful to the performance of the process or application for which they are collected.
- **Timeliness:** Timeliness is determined by how the data are being used and their context.

Employment Opportunities for Qualified HIM Professionals. The Following are some of the Titles and not Limited to

- Domain manager
- Medical language and classification manager

- Information security manager
- Reimbursement manager
- Clinical application coordinator
- Clinical project manager
- Clinical research associate
- Optical imaging coordinator
- Risk management specialist
- Senior document coordinator
- Systems analyst
- Insurance specialist
- Medical records manager
- Network analyst
- Program analyst
- HIM director or manager
- Clinical data analyst
- Health data/information resource manager
- Health information system application designer
- Compliance officer
- Chief or Director, clinical information officer
- Quality improvement analyst
- Program director
- Data integrity analyst
- Data quality manger
- Medical office administrator
- Revenue cycle manager
- Coder or coding specialist
- Assistant HIM director
- Business process engineer
- Health information specialist or administrator
- Patient information coordinator
- HIM project manager
- Clinical data analyst
- HIM systems manager
- Information security officer
- Privacy officer
- Regional HIM director
- Assistant HIM director
- Information privacy coordinator.

Places for Employment Opportunities for Qualified HIM Professionals

- Hospitals
- Nursing homes
- Physician practices
- Research institutes
- Medical legal dealing with healthcare issues
- Software companies

- Consulting companies
- Insurance companies
- Healthcare educational institutes
- Pharmaceutical companies
- Government ministries
- Corporate hospitals
- Finance dealing with healthcare system
- Accreditation organizations
- Rehabilitation centers
- Project manager
- Systems analyst
- Web developer
- Insurance specialist
- Medical records supervisor
- Healthcare consultant
- Network analyst, and
- Program analyst
- Compliance officer
- Quality improvement analyst
- Program director
- Professor
- Data integrity analyst
- Director of clinical informatics
- Data quality manger
- HIM manger
- Medical office administrator
- Revenue cycle manager
- Coder

HIM Professionals Need to Possess the Following Skills but not Limit to for Better Employment Opportunities

- Leadership skills
- Communication skills
- Analytical skills
- Organizing skills
- Managerial skills
- Writing sills
- Computer skills
- Collaborating skills
- Research work solution finding skills
- Quality assurance and control skills
- Well orientated
- Problems identifying skills
- Problem solving skills
- Health cost contained skills
- Project management skills

- Team building skills
- Planning skills
- Risk management skills
- Disaster management skills
- Internal communication management
- Develop interviewing processes
- Direct and conduct recruitment, hiring and training of personnel
- Develop coaching strategies
- Limit conflict and encouraging workplace unity
- Overcome barriers in communication with staff and outside healthcare administrators

Some other operational skills necessary to healthcare leaders' job include:

A large part of a healthcare administration is financially and managerially focused, as most of healthcare manager's work in an office environment. They are in-charge of managing hospitals, community health centers, clinics, private medical group practices, managed care organizations, nursing homes, and other healthcare facilities. Analytical skills necessary to responsibly manage the business side of a clinic, hospital, or other healthcare-based companies include:

- Information systems management and troubleshooting
- Maintain awareness of advances in data processing technology, medicine, computerized diagnostic and treatment equipment, financing options, and health insurance changes
- Logistics and research
- Patient administration
- Maintain quality of service offered to patients
- Team performance measurement and motivation
- Facilities development and enhancement
- Project and operations management
- Fiscal operations, which can span from accounting, planning budgets, planning and authorizing to expenditures, establishing rates for services, and coordinating financial reporting
- Economic knowledge and insight
- Consultation
- Supply ordering and inventory management
- Human resources management
- Direction, supervision and evaluation of medical, technical, nursing, service, clerical, maintenance and other personnel
- Education and training management
- Public relations and marketing
- Knowledge of current government regulations, legal and ethical practices, policies and standards
- Strategic planning
- Development and execution of organizational procedures
- Efficient and accurate administration of finance, diet of patient, engineering, and distribution of medical aid. It helps to view a broad picture of hospital growth
- Improved monitoring of drug usage, and study of effectiveness. This leads to the reduction of adverse drug interactions while promoting more appropriate pharmaceutical utilization.
- Enhances information integrity, reduces transcription errors, and reduces duplication of information entries.

- Hospital software is easy to use and eliminates error caused by handwriting. New technology computer systems give perfect performance to pull up information from server or cloud servers.

EFFECTIVE HEALTHCARE LEADERSHIP NEEDS AND STAYING FOREFRONT OF THE COMPETITION

Today's healthcare landscape is a dynamic, unpredictable sea of legislative and economic transformation needs for highly educated and motivated administrators who maintain cutting-edge information system skills and managerial expertise as they oversee huge healthcare operations. A strong business orientation coupled with sharp leadership and communication skills are vital for today's healthcare administrators. Healthcare leaders, especially those in administrative and management roles, need a wide range of operational, relational, and analytical skills to effectively carryout their responsibilities. Healthcare administrators' abilities to do their jobs well, directly affect the quality and availability of affordable healthcare. The following traits of highly successful general and specialized healthcare industry leaders, not limited to the following include:

- Having a strong business orientation—private healthcare is more than a calling, it is also a business that needs to accomplish financial goals and stay out of the red.
- Maintaining a positive attitude—this keeps workplace morale up. Leaders have dreams and goals for their staff, and spreading positivity helps create an environment where these visions can come to pass.
- Varying work hour's acceptance—nurses and doctors work the floor 24 × 7; emergency situations that call on the insurance and medical financing expertise of healthcare administrators do not may occur at any point in the day.
- Willingness to out-market the competition—other healthcare facilities and vying for patients' business. Administrators with a proactive approach to marketing will ensure success of the organization.
- Approaching work proactively—managers lead by example, and a proactive attitude is contagious in the workplace. Staying motivated and encouraging others to perform at their best is crucial for reaching goals and maintaining quality patient care.
- Having strong leadership skills—leaders have to focus on how well employees are performing and evaluate healthcare processes. Possessing the confidence to independently direct the organization and make important decisions to benefit overall patient care.
- Making strong employment decisions— in the name of good time management, managers task employees with the jobs they are most capable of handling efficiently.
- Understanding priorities and staying organized—overseeing use of information data systems, computer programs and healthcare machines requires extensive organizational habits and ruthless prioritization.
- Improving them and their staff consistently—leaders should continuously push for improved hospital procedures and strive for higher quality patient care. Implementing and working to accomplish set goals can increase team collaboration and build relationships.
- Being available to professional and honest with their staff—being an accessible and efficient leader who fulfills his or her duties while assisting others will create bonds of trust between administrators and staff.
- Continuing an education—professionals never stop learning, and a voracious appetite for up-to-the-minute information and research about modern healthcare issues in technology, economics, finance, management, or legal and ethical issues will keep an administrator relevant to the industry.

Chapter

10

Diploma in Medical Record Technology (Health Information Management) Training Program

INTRODUCTION

The Diploma in Medical Record Technology Training Program functions within the philosophy and policies of the Ministry of Health of the nation or state that reflect the nation's/state's view and beliefs of self-development of indigenously trained people in the context of their sociocultural background. The program generally supports the National Health Policy; to have adequate professional manpower to contribute in the program upholds the right of every individual to receive safe and quality healthcare.

In addition, the faculty subscribes to the following belief statements which are fundamental principles upon which the Diploma Medical Record Technology Training Program was developed.

The faculty believes in the worth of the human being and respects the uniqueness of the individual who are active partners in their own healthcare.

The faculty accepts the World Health Organization definition of health, which states, in part, that: Health is state of complete physical, mental and social well-being and not merely the absence of disease or infirmity. The faculty believes that spirituality is also component of health.

The faculty believes that medical record management (health information management) is dynamic profession whose goal is the promotion, maintenance of an optimum level of health and the prevention of illness in individuals, families, groups and communities throughout the life span by maintaining good medical records at par with international standards. Medical record department accomplishes its goal by creating and maintaining individual patient medical record to perform those activities, which meet their basic patient, doctors, nursing and other allied health professional need and which they would do unaided if they had the necessary knowledge, skill and motivation. Medical record profession is carried out through the use of the medical record process. Medical record function in cooperation and collaboration with members of the healthcare team and other related professions at primary, secondary and tertiary levels and in a variety of settings: Primary health center, extended primary health center, secondary and tertiary care hospitals outpatient, inpatient and accident and emergency services.

The faculty believes that personal growth and professional development of the student is achieved through multidisciplinary education. This approach encourages students to synthesize knowledge from the humanities and the natural, behavioral and medical record science in the practice of adequate, safe and high quality medical record maintenance for those in need. Students learn problem solving methodologies and decision-making skill in an environment that fosters responsibility, creativity, critical thinking, leadership potential and a positive attitude toward persons, health, society and the profession.

The faculty believes that evaluation is continuous process of appraisal of the faculty, students, curriculum, administration, and resources and is necessary to determine the effectiveness of the program in meeting its objectives.

The faculty believes it is accountable for the quality of the educational program in the role of a teacher, faculty guide learners through activities in order to achieve the objectives of the program. As teachers, faculty members are resource persons, planners' facilitators, and evaluators of the learning process. In the role of researcher, faculty members serve as resource persons to those in medical record education and medical record service. Faculty members indirectly contribute to the health of the community as trainers.

PURPOSE

The goal of the Diploma in Medical Record Technology Training Program is to prepare a Medical Record Technologist who is able to function efficiently and effectively, as a member of the health care team and who is qualified to meet the medical record profession needs of the people of a nation. The medical record technologist is competent to practice in the primary, secondary and tertiary healthcare institutions. The program provides a basis for further development and continued learning of the graduate.

CONCEPTUAL FRAMEWORK OF THE CURRICULUM

The primary concept guiding the curriculum is that of the individual patient needs. The individual patient is understood to be a biological, psychological, social and spiritual human being in continuous interaction with the environment. The individual is composed of systems and each system is a subsystem of the larger system of which it is a part.

Individuals must meet their human needs in order to maintain life. They do so through voluntary actions and involuntary process. A voluntary action is a behavior of an individual that is deliberate and is intended to affect something to which it is directed, moving it to a condition that differs from its condition prior to being acted upon. It is regulated by will and by choice. An involuntary process is a continuous and regular action or succession of action occurring in a definite manner and is independent of will or choice.

These voluntary actions and involuntary processes result, in the individual, in either homeostasis or adaptation or actual or potential alterations in health. When the voluntary actions and involuntary processes are positive for the individual, they result in homeostasis and adaptation, when they are negative for the individual; they result in actual or potential alterations in health.

Actual alterations in health are changes in the existing health state or condition of the individual. Potential alterations are possible changes that may occur in the existing health state or condition of the individual. Actual alterations in health are defined as illness—an abnormal process in which aspects of the biological, psychological, social and spiritual components of the individual are diminished or impaired compared with that individual's previous condition.

Homeostasis refers to "the necessary adjustments that the body can make rapidly" to maintain internal composition "within limits precisely defined for each organism." Adaptation refers to the responses the individual makes to function adequately under "changed conditions of the environment."

Medical record technologist is required when individuals experience actual or potential alterations in health, which prevent them from performing those activities, which meet their basic human needs. Medical Record Technologist assists individuals to meet their needs which they would do unaided if they had the necessary knowledge, skill or motivation.

TERMINAL PROGRAM OBJECTIVES

Upon completion of the diploma in medical record technology program, the graduate will be able to:

Utilize cognitive, psychomotor and affective abilities derived from the humanities and the natural, behavioral and medical record sciences to provide medical record services to individual, families, groups and communities.

Utilize the medical record process to deliver safe and effective medical record service at primary, secondary and tertiary levels.

Assess the ability of individual, family, group and community—at primary secondary and tertiary levels—to meet basic patient needs and healthcare team to accomplish the activities of daily patient care.

Formulate a medical record policies and procedures to basic patient need for individuals, families, groups, and communities at primary, secondary and tertiary levels.

Develop an individualized medical record service plan for individuals, families, groups and communities at primary, secondary and tertiary levels.

Implement the plan of medical record service for individuals, families, groups, and communities at primary, secondary and tertiary levels.

Evaluate the response of an individual's, family, group, and community to proper medical record documentation.

Evaluate the effectiveness of the techniques and principles of communication and counseling strategies in working with individuals, families, groups, communities, and significant others as well as members of the healthcare team.

Assume responsibility for implementation of ethical, legal, sociocultural and professional standards in the provision of medical record service.

Evaluate the effectiveness of health teaching to promote health, maintain well-being and prevent illness in individuals, families, groups and communities.

Demonstrate an awareness of the role of research in medical record practice and support the research activities of others.

Manage the medical records service of small group in a structural environment.

Apply policies and procedures related to the economical use of supplies and equipment in the health care delivery system.

Evaluate own personal and professional growth and development.

COURSE OUTLINE

Course Title: English Language I (EL101)
English Language II (EL102)

Course Credits:

English Language I (EL101)

Theory	6 Cr. hours	270 hours
Laboratory	———	———
Practical	———	———
Total	6 Cr. hours	270 hours

English Language II (EL102)

Theory	5 Cr. hours	225 hours
Laboratory	———	———
Practical	———	———
Total	5 Cr. hours	225 hours

Course Placement: Year - 1, semester - 1 = 6 credit hours (270 hours)
Year - 1, semester - 1 = 5 credit hours (225 hours)

COURSE DESCRIPTION

This course refers to the English language course taught in various semesters throughout the year of study in both basic and post basic programs. The course is designed to address linguistic skills necessary to support the student with his studies in the Diploma Medical Record Technology Program. The course emphasizes on English as a second language and aims to strengthen the linguistic skills necessary to grasp the essentials of the professional studies. The course is designed to move from simple too much more complex skills through the study of basic grammar to pronunciation, conversation, reading, comprehension, writing and so on.

COURSE OBJECTIVE

At the end of the course students will be able to:

Basic english language grammar such as parts of speech
Phrases and clauses
Improve and strengthen the listening skills
Improve and strengthen the reading skills
Sentence types and structure and formation of simple sentences formation
Sentence analysis and formation of compound and complex sentences
Improve and strengthen the written and spoken English language skills
Improve and strengthen the communication skills
Develop spoken language skills
Develop written language skills such as paragraph and story writing

Hints development to help in taking notes in the classes
Develop letter and essays writing
Advance communication skills in health field
Understand the meaning of basic sciences, medical sciences, and allied health sciences terminology
Increase the vocabulary skills.

TEACHING STRATEGIES

Teaching strategies will include lectures, handouts and multiple-choice question to reinforce theoretical knowledge.

Unit	*Course contents*	*Number of hours*
1	Basic English language grammar such as parts of speech, phrases and clauses	50
2	Listening practice and skills	50
3	Reading skills	50
4	Sentence types and structure and formation of simple sentences formation	25
5	Sentence analysis and formation of compound and complex sentences	50
6	Spoken english language such as short and long conversation	50
7	Written language skills such as paragraph and story writing	50
8	Communication skills such as formal and informal	30
9	Hints development to help in taking notes in the classes	20
10	Letter and essays writing	50
11	Advance communication skills in health field	30
12	Basic sciences, medical sciences, and allied health sciences terminology and meaning	30
13	Vocabulary skills	10

EVALUATION SCHEME

Continuous assessment	20%
Mid term and pre-final examination (written)	30%
Final examination (written and oral)	50%

RECOMMENDED TEXTS

Communicative Grammar 1, 2, and 3 (3 books) by Ann Brumfit/Scott Wendeatt

A course in Intermediate Scientific English Frank Chaplen - 1983,
Denmark House, 37–39 Queen Elizabeth Street London SEI 2QB
ISBN 07135 14167

Mystery Tour Activity Book, Peter Viney & Karen Viney 1988
Oxford University Press, Walton Street, Oxford OX2 6DP, UK

Essential grammar in use—A self-study reference and practice book for *elementary students of english with answers* by Raymond Murphy, 2nd Edition 1998, Cambridge University Press,

The Edinburgh Building, Cambridge CB2 2RY, UK,
Cambridge University Press, 40 West 20th Street, New York, NY 10011 - 4211, USA
Cambridge University Press, 10 Stamford Road, Oak Leigh, Melbourne 3166, Australia

ISBN 0521 55928 6 (with answers) ISBN 0521 55927 8 (without answers)

New English grammar in use, *Supplementary Exercises with Answers* by Louise Hashemi with Raymond Murphy – 11th Edition, 1998
ISBN 0521 44954 5 (with answers) ISBN 0521 44955 3 (without answers)
ISBN 0521 43684 X (with answers) ISBN 0521 43681 8 (without answers)
Focus on Preliminary English Test by Daniel L Fried Booth, Nelson 1991
Trans Nelson and Sons Ltd, Nelson House, Mayfield Road, Walton-on-Thames Surrey, KT12 5PL, UK ISBN 0 17 556500 7

Headway, Work Book Elementary, 1998, LTZ & John Soars, Oxford University Press, Great Clarendon Street, Oxford OX2 6DP, UK
ISBN 0 19 433993 9 (with key) ISBN 0 19 433999 8 (without key)

Study Skills in English–1997 by Michael J Wallace, student book,
Cambridge University Press, the Edinburgh Building, Cambridge CB2 2RY, UK,
Cambridge University Press, 40 West 20th Street, New York, NY 10011 - 4211, USA
Cambridge University Press, 10 Stamford Road, Oak Leigh, Melbourne 3166, Australia
ISBN 0 521 22110 2 (Student's book) ISBN 0 521 22109 9 (Tutor's book)
ISBN 0 521 22108 0 (Cassette)

Study Reading: A Course in reading skill for academic purposes by Erik H. Glendining Beverly Holm Strom
Cambridge University Press, 40 West 20th Street, New York, NY 10011 - 4211, USA
Cambridge University Press, 10 Stamford Road, Oak Leigh, Melbourne 3166, Australia
ISBN 0 521 39974 2

Study Speaking—A course in spoken English for Academic Purposes by Tony Lynch and Kenneth Anderson – 5th Editions, 1998
Cambridge University Press, 40 West 20th Street, New York, NY 10011 - 4211, USA
Cambridge University Press, 10 Stamford Road, Oak Leigh, Melbourne 3166, Australia
ISBN 0 521 39551 8 (Book) ISBN 0 521 42259 9 (Cassette)

Study Listening—Understanding Lectures and Talks in English by Tony Lynch 1998 - Guide for teachers and self-study
Cambridge University Press, 40 West 20th Street, New York, NY 10011 - 4211, USA
Cambridge University Press, 10 Stamford Road, Oak Leigh, Melbourne 3166, Australia
ISBN 0 521 27314 3 (Guide for Teacher and Self-Study) ISBN 0 521 27314 5 (student book)
ISBN 0 521 25331 4 (Cassette)

Teacher's Manual—Academic Listening Encounters Listening Note Taking, and Discussion, Content Focus: Human Behavior by Miriam Espeseth
Cambridge University Press, 40 West 20th Street, New York, NY 10011 - 4211 USA
Cambridge University Press, 10 Stamford Road, Oak Leigh, Melbourne 3166, Australia
ISBN 0 521 57821 5 (Guide for Teacher and Self-Study) ISBN 0 521 57821 3 (student book)
ISBN 0 521 57819 1 (Cassette)

Teacher's Manual—Academic Listening Encounters Reading, Study, Skills and Writing, Content Focus: Human Behavior by Bernard Seal

Cambridge University Press, 40 West 20th Street, New York, NY 10011 - 4211, USA
Cambridge University Press, 10 Stamford Road, Oak Leigh, Melbourne 3166, Australia
ISBN 0 521 47660 7 (guide for teacher and self-study) ISBN 0 521 47658 5 (student book)

Longman Photo Dictionary by Marilyn S. Rosenthal and Daniel B. Freeman 1990
Cambridge University Press, 40 West 20th Street, New York, NY 10011 - 4211, USA
Cambridge University Press, 10 Stamford Road, Oak Leigh, Melbourne 3166, Australia
ISBN 0 582 89371 2

The Lost Secret by Robert O' Neill & Marrin Shovel, BBC English Class Room Edition BBC English, PO Box No. 76, Bush House, London WC2B 4PH, UK, 1990

Learning Medical Terminology, 8th Edition, by Miriam G. Austrin, Harvey R Ausstrin, Mosby Lifeline, Mosby - year book in 1991, 11830 West Line Industrial Drive, St Louis, Missouri 63146 (9430060 CIP)

An Introduction to Medical Terminology—A Self-Teaching Package, 1999, by Andrew R. Hutton, Churchill Livingston, Robert Stevenson House, 1-3 Boxter's Place, Leith Walk, Edinburgh EH1 3AF UK

Nucleus, English for Science and Technology, General science by Martin Bates/Tony Dudley - Evans - Teachers Manual, Longman, Longman House, Burnt Mill, Harlow Essex CM20, 2JE, England, ISBN 0 582 55247 8

Nucleus—English for Science and Technology, Nursing science by Martin Bates/Tony Dudley - Evans - Teachers Manual, Longman, Longman House, Burnt Mill, Harlow Essex CM20, 2JE, England, ISBN 0 582 51309 X

English for Nurses by David Austin and Tim Crisfield 1976, ISBN 0 582 55019 X, Longman House, Burnt Mill, Harlow Essex CM20, 2JE, England

Introduction to Biology by DG Mackean, 1998, Published by John Murray (Publishers) Ltd, 50, Albemarle Street, London WIX 4BD, UK, ISBN 0 719 2831 3

English for Nurses by D Thomas and J. Thomas, Edward Arnold (Publishers) Ltd, 1977, 25, Hill Street, London WIX 8LL, UK

Special English Book 1 Nursing by Donald Dallas, Collier Macmillan International Inc., 866, Third Avenue, New York, NY 10022 ISBN 0 02 972800 2

English to English Dictionary Webster's, USA, and Oxford, UK, and *Dorland's Medical Dictionary* - big size (for reference), Medical Dictionary English

Course Title:	Mathematics and Hospital Information I (HI 101)		
Course Credits:	Theory	3	45 hours
	Laboratory	———	———
	Practical	———	———
	Total	3	45 hours
Course Placement:	Year - 1, Semester - 1		
Course Title:	Mathematics		
Course Credits:	Theory	1 cr. hr	15 hours
	Laboratory	———	———
	Practical	———	———
	Total	1 cr. hr	15 hours

COURSE DESCRIPTION

This course will comprise basic calculation, which is essential for medical record technologist. It is designed to develop mathematical skills, concepts and the ability to apply them with confidence in medical record service. By the end of the course, students should be able to plan and present a realistic sequence of operation to solve given problems, which they encounter during their career.

Skills

At the end of the course, trainees should be able to achieve the following

Develop their knowledge and understanding of innumeracy to the full extent of their capabilities, solving mental arithmetic and practical problems in arithmetic in a manner, which encourages confidence.

Solve problems, present solutions clearly, check and interpret the results.

Develop an ability to apply numeracy in other subjects, particularly statistical calculations.

Acquire a foundation appropriate to their further study of other disciplines

COURSE OBJECTIVES

On successfully completion of the course, the medical record technologist trainee will be able to use non-calculator methods to solve mental arithmetic

Add, subtract, multiply, divide—whole numbers, decimals and fractions

Reduce fractions to its lowest terms and solve problems based on fractions

Convert fractions to decimals, percentages and *vice versa*.

Calculate percentages of quantities through problem solving

Approximate using significant figures or decimal places.

Understand and operate in the metric unit/standard international unit of measurement and apply the conversion of one unit of measurement to another

Use electronic calculator.

Algebra, calculus, trigonometry calculation

TEACHING STRATEGIES

Teaching strategies will include lectures, handouts and multiple-choice question to reinforce theoretical knowledge.

Unit	*Course contents*	*Number of hours*
1	Solve problems, present solutions clearly, check and interpret the results	2
2	Add, subtract, multiply, divide—whole numbers, decimals and fractions	2
3	Reduce fractions to its lowest terms and solve problems based on fractions	2
4	Convert fractions to decimals, percentages and *vice versa*	2
5	Calculate percentages of quantities through problem solving	1
6	Approximate, using significant figures or decimal places	1
7	Understand and operate in the metric unit/standard International unit of measurement and apply the conversion of one unit of measurement to another	1
8	Use electronic calculator	1
9	Algebra, calculus, trigonometry calculation	3

EVALUATION SCHEME

Continuous assessment	20%
Mid term and pre-final examination (written)	30%
Final examination (written and oral)	50%

RECOMMENDED TEXTS

A. Greer. A Complete GCSE Mathematic for General Course (2000), Stanley Thornes (Publishers) Ltd, Cheltenham, England

Robert Powel GCSE Mathematics—National Curriculum Key Stage 4(2000), Letts Educational Ltd, London England.

Course Title:	Hospital Information I (HI 101) (Statistics)		
Course Credits:	Theory	2 cr. hr	30 hours
	Laboratory	———	———
	Practical	———	———
	Total	2 cr. hr	30 hours

COURSE DESCRIPTION

This course consists of general statistics, definitions, methods of collection of data, types of data, rates, ratios, measures of central tendency, mean, median, mode, measures of dispersion, standard deviation and reporting, presentation and analysis of statistical data.

COURSE OBJECTIVES

At the end of the course, the student should be able to:
Define statistics
Know different methods of collection of data
Understand different types of data, rates and ratios
Calculate simple averages, mean, median and mode
Calculation mean deviation, standard deviation
Provide graphic presentation

TEACHING STRATEGIES

Teaching strategies will include lectures, handouts, continuous practice, multiple-choice, one line, and brief, essay types of question and answers to reinforce theoretical knowledge.

Unit	*Course contents*	*Number of hours*
1	Introduction to general statistical history and definition	3
2	Purposes of collection of statistics and their values	3
3	Methods of collection of data	3
4	Types of data	2
5	Calculation of rates and ratio	3
6	Measures of central tendency—simple average, geometric Mean, harmonic mean, median, and mode	10
7	Measures of dispersion—mean deviation, standard deviation, range	10
8	Graphic presentation of statistics—bar, pie, histogram	5
9	Use of calculator and computers	3
10	Uses of statistics	3

LABORATORY

The above course content is covered simultaneously through laboratory practice. The theory classes are followed by practical laboratory work.

Evaluation Scheme

Continuous written assessment and mid term examination	50%
Written assessment and final examination	50%

Course book, charts, worksheets and library resources

Students are required to pass (50%) in these components.

Course Title:	Information technology I (IT 102)		
Course Credits:	Theory	2 Cr hrs	30 hours
	Laboratory	2 Cr hrs	60 hours
	Practical	———	———
	Total	4 Cr hrs	90 hours
Course Placement:	Year - 1, Semester - 1		

COURSE DESCRIPTION

This course is designed to provide students with a basic understanding of computer terminology, programming concepts, use of ready-made package of software with option to extend their learning once basic requirements are met. The course will equip them with the skill essential for operating a personal computer, LAN and WAN including keyboard, mouse and printer. They will learn to simple tasks using word processing and spreadsheet applications and how to communicate with other computers using the internet/e-mail/ World Wide Web. The course will be almost totally laboratory based with students being guided through a series of computer-based lessons and additional learning task sheets. Theoretical concepts will be integrated where appropriate. Whenever possible material used will integrate and reinforce learning in other courses.

COURSE OBJECTIVES

At the end of the course students will be able to:

- Demonstrate keyboarding and mouse skills to a minimum of 45 words per minute with 99% accuracy.
- Explain the basic functions of a computer.
- Identify the types and key components of personal computers.
- Utilize the operating (Widow 98/2000) to perform all the level 1 tasks listed in the unit 3 objectives especially accessing application software and managing files.
- Create, save and print simple documents using the level 1 features listed in the unit 4 objective (Word 2000).
- Create, save and print a spreadsheet using the level 1 features listed in the unit 5 objectives (Excel 2000).
- Create, save and print a power point using level 1 features listed in the unit 6 objectives. Produce short on-screen slide shows using the facilities of power point 2000 listed the optional unit.

- Work with internet, email and www and access Internet and www. Send and receive email communications as per unit 7. Use the www to find and retrieve data.

Level 2 (Mandatory)

Understand the concepts of basic ready-made hospital information packages as per MOH or individual hospital policies. Trainees able to work with read-ymade hospital information database packages. Update, patient sociological, history, clinical information in the computer data base, save and print the patient registration with label, other reports as and when required.

It is recognized that students undertaking the course will enter with varying levels of prior computing experience. There will also be significant differences in laboratory/ computer access between institutes initially. To accommodate for these discrepancies the course has been developed on two levels. A set of competencies identified as essential for beginning computer literacy are presented as required learning and these will be assessed. Additional, optional material is provided in most units for students ready to extend their skills further. A learning unit on using ready-made hospital information package as per MOH or hospital policies to create, save and print patient registration prints the labels, and other reports as and when required also included as a Level 2 option (*see* mandatory unit learning objectives)

It is anticipated that as computer access increases for all students the time given to teaching keyboarding skills will be reduced. Gaining keyboard proficiency should be increasing undertaken as a self-learning activity out of class time using the typing tutor package supplied. This will allow for the completion of more second level options in class time.

TITLE OF UNITS

Level 1 (Basic)

Unit 1	Introduction to microcomputers
Unit 2	Using the keyboard and mouse
Unit 3	Data versus information
Unit 4	Working with windows (Widows 98/2000)
Unit 5	Working with Microsoft words or word processing (Word 98/2000)
Unit 6	Working with spreadsheets numbers (Excel 2000)
Unit 7	Presentation of graph
Unit 8	Working power point (2000)
Unit 9	Data base concepts
Unit 10	Working on-line (MS explorer) internet, email and www
Unit 11	Basic concepts of development of computer application (software)—special reference to health information

Level 2 (Mandatory Leaning Unit)

Unit 12	Understand the concepts of basic ready-made hospital information data base packages as per MOH or hospital policies and access and work with ready-made hospital information packages. Create, save and print the patient registration with label, other reports as and when required.

TEACHING STRATEGIES

Unit	*Course contents*	*Number of hours*
1	Level 1 (basic) Introduction to microcomputers	3
2	Using the keyboard and mouse	12
3	Data versus information	5
4	Working with windows (Widows 98/2000)	5
5	Working with Microsoft words or word processing (Word 98/2000)	10
6	Working with spreadsheets numbers (Excel 2000)	10
7	Presentation of graph	5
8	Working power point (2000)	5
9	Data base concepts	5
10	Working on-line (MS explorer) internet, email and www	5
11	Basic concepts of development of computer application (software)—special reference to health information	5
12	Level 2 (mandatory leaning unit) Understand the concepts of basic ready-made hospital information data base packages as per MOH or hosital policies and access and work with ready-made hospital information packages. Create, save and print the patient registration with label, other reports as and when required	20

Students will almost entirely in the computer laboratory. They will use:

Interactive software packages and off-line internet lessons to

- Develop keyboarding skills
- Learn about the use of computers and their component
- Identify and learn to use main functions of the MS Window 98/2000 operating system
- Understand and perform key features of MS Excel 2000
- Learn about the power point and presentation
- Learn about and use the internet
- Teacher guided tutorials, which will support the computer-based lessons by facilitating the performance of assigned learning tasks and monitoring student progress
- Student paced learning exercises to practice and master the required competencies in word, excel and power point 2000.

A project designed to utilize ready-made hospital information data base package, access all the hospital information medical record modules, and prepare hospital statistical reports and other reports, internet skills and to integrate and consolidate other skills learned.

EVALUATION METHODS

Continuous Assessment

15% keyboard skill (to be completed by week 12 or before)

Minimum required achievement 30 words per minutes and will be awarded 10%

Desirable achievement 40 words per minutes and will be awarded 15%

(Word per minute will adjusted to include accuracy, i.e. 99% or better is required 15% computing concepts and working with widows.

FINAL ASSESSMENT

25% on word-processing, excel, power point 2000, and internet access

25% on hospital information package access and create the hospital

Statistical reports

Final assessment based on 2 hours computer-based exam.

PROJECT

35% a project designed to demonstrating use of the hospital information medical record module package from Level 2 mandatory unit will be completed on time. It is anticipated that work from units 4, 5, and 6 may be used in the project.

- The assessment of keyboard skills can be taken at any time agreed to by the teacher
- Students are required to pass (50%) in these components.

RESOURCES REQUIRED

Multi-media Laboratory Providing

Individual student access to a personal computer for all class periods, additional access for practice is highly desirable.

Individual network login providing secure student access to workspace on the server

Internet access—for class time and for project work

Software uniformly installed as below

Required System and Application Software

Windows 98/2000

MS office professional

MS internet explorer (as supplied with windows)

MOH Hospital Information Data Base software

Interactive Teaching Packages

Typing tutor

Type master typing test (to be used for standardizing keyboard testing)

Leaning windows

Leaning Office 2000

Learning hospital Information Data Base Package

Course Title:	Medical Record Sciences - MR 102		
	(Theory Part and Laboratory Part)		
Course Credits:	Theory	2 Cr hr	30 hours
	Laboratory	1 Cr hr	30 hours
	Practical	————	————
	Total	3 Cr hr	60 hours

Theory Part:

Course Credits:	Theory	2 Cr hr	30 hours
	Laboratory	———	———
	Practical	———	———
	Total	2 Cr hr	30 hours
Course Placement:	Year - 1, Semester - 2		

COURSE DESCRIPTION

The course is designed to provide students with a basic understanding of history of medical records, concepts of medical records, role of medical records in health care delivery system, and development of medical records forms. An introduction to the history of medicine and the historical development of the healthcare field with emphasis on the organizational structures of health institutions in USA, UK, India, etc. an introduction to the medical records department and an overview of the medical record contents, from and profession.

COURSE OBJECTIVES

At the conclusion of this unit the student should be able to:

Identify the important personnel in medicine and their major contributions.

Trace the historical development of the health care facilities of different countries.

Trace the historical development of the medical records in different countries.

Define medical record, hospital, doctors, nurses, allied health, paramedical staff and their profession.

Organizational chart diagram showing the relationship of hospital, administrator, medical record staff, professional and administrative services, corporate/private hospital chart/structure.

Identify major allied health professions and their functions.

Discuss the new trends in health care delivery and role of medical records.

State the educational requirement and responsibilities for different levels of medical record professionals.

Top level:	Director/Manager/Head of Medical Records Department (MRD) or Medical Records Officer (MRO).
Middle level	Supervisor level
Operational level	Assistant Medical Record Technician (AMRT), and Medical Record Technician (MRT)—day-to-day functions

Apply principles of medical ethics as practitioner, both in professional relationship and in the professional organization.

Define "Medical Record" and state the criterion for a good medical record.

Define the value of medical records from the standpoint of the

- Patient
- Physician
- Hospital

- Medical legal
- Research
- Medical education
- Public health (national)
- International

Name the major functions of Medical Record Department

Name the four (4) sections of the MRD and whose responsibility—they are

- Medical Record Officer (MRO)
- Assistant Medical Record Officer (AMRO)
- Medical Record Technician/Medical Record Supervisor
- Assistant Medical Record Technician/Clerk Administrator

Name the contents of medical record

- Sociological information
- Clinical information

Cite the criterion for the adequacy of sociological data obtained for the medical record and apply this criterion to sample records for evaluation purposes.

Form a list of items to be taken from the sociologic section various medical records, identify listing, which are poorly recorded and rewrite the item in better form.

Define the term "Clinical Information"

- Provisional diagnosis
- Principal diagnosis
- Secondary diagnosis
- Final diagnosis
- Deferential diagnosis
- Procedures—diagnostic/operative
- Anaesthesia—local, general, epidural, and spinal
- Result—alive, or dead less than (<)48 hours and more than (>)48
- Hours/cured, improved, same, worst, referred to other hospital.

Delivery information

Type of delivery:	Spontaneous or LSCS or vacuum or forceps
Outcome of delivery:	Male or female/single or twin or more/alive or dead

Name the different types of medical record format

- Integrated Medical Record System
- Source Oriented Medical Record System
- Problem Oriented Medical Record (POMR) System

Medical record committee formation and its functions

Designing form

- Paper quality
- Paper size
- Paper colour
- Paper standardisation

Basic, common and important medical record forms used in the hospitals in different services

- Medical forms/computerized modules
- Nursing forms/computerized modules
- Diagnostic request and report forms/computerized modules
- Paramedical service forms/computerized modules
- Administrative forms/computerized modules
- Medical record department forms/computerized modules
- Register/computerized module

TITLE OF UNITS

Unit 1. History of Medicine

Historical development of medicine and medical records—ancient history, stone-age, Indian history, ancient Greek and Roman history, medieval history, etc.

Important historical general development in different countries

Unit 1a. Historical Development of Healthcare Field

Development and organizational structure of health institutions in different countries such as hospitals health clinics and others.

Unit 2. Concepts of Medical Records and Introduction to MRD

Definition of medical record, uses of medical record, property—medical record

Agencies and organizations that set standards for medical records

Formation and purposes of health agencies and organization

Computerization of medical records

Unit 2a. Medical Record Administration and the Professional Organization

Medical record administrator, medical record technologist, assistant medical record technician

- Functions
- Educational qualifications
- Employment opportunities

Ancillary medical record personnel—medical secretaries, medical transcriptions and others

Ethics—definition, and medical ethics, pledges and codes of ethics

Hippocratic oath, code of ethics relating to medical record profession

Professional conduct—relationship with professional staff and public

International federation and development of medical record organization

Unit 2b. Functions of MRD

Accident and Emergency Service Registration

Outpatient service

- Central registration
- Appointment

Inpatient (ward) service

- Admission office
- Waiting list

Medical records department

- Medical record review
- Assembling and deficiency check
- Doctor's conference room
- Completion and accuracy

Coding of diseases as per ICD-10 (WHO) and diagnostic and operative procedures as per ICP (WHO).

Indexing of coded diseases, diagnostic and operative procedures

Compiling of statistics

Filing storage methods and retrieval of records

Outpatient and late inpatient laboratory report mounting

Research (assisting medical staff) study

- Special studies
- Data for research
- Committees

Medical transcription service

Release of information

Maintenance of forms/registers or computerized on line system

Retention of records as per retention policy

Preparation of official report and correspondence

Maintenance of department library

Unit 3. Role of Medical Records in Healthcare Delivery System

Medical services, allied health services, diagnostic services—laboratory, radiology (X-ray/CT scan/ultrasound/ECG, echocardiogram, EEG, EMG, endoscopies, nursing service, paramedical services, administrative services, and support services.

Unit 3a. Medical Record Department and Inter Departmental Relationship

Hospital administrator

Heads of the department of different services

Medical services staff

Nursing services staff

Ancillary services staff

Allied health services staff

Support services staff

Unit 3b. Quality of Assurance Plan

Medical record screening indicators

Quality assurance worksheet

Concurrent chart review

Monthly mortality and morbidity

Problem identification and corrective plan

MRD function analysis

Cost analysis worksheet

Unit 3c. Nursing Service

Introduction maintenance of medical record in the ward

Record relating to the care and treatment of patient

Maintenance of stock books

Hospital administrative records

Ward maintenance register

Attendance register of working staff in the ward

Nurse treatment registers (day and night reports of the condition of patient)

Nurses records

Nurses observation chart

Graphic (TPR) chart

Intake and output charts

Chart for special cases

Unit 3d. Medical Records in Infection Control

Infection control prevents or stops the spread of infection in healthcare settings. Medical Records information helps in identifying the infection and measures to control—whether it was developed in the hospital as nosocomial infection.

Unit 3e. Medical Records in Long-Term Care

Rehabilitation records

Medical health records

Content of mental health records

Assessing the patient

- Physical assessment
- Emotional assessment and behavioral
- Assessment item to be included
- Social assessment
- Recreational assessment
- Legal assessment
- Vocational assessment
- Nutritional assessment
- Other assessments

Unit 4. Development of Medical Record Forms

Contents and format of different types of medical record format

- Source oriented medical record system
- Integrated medical record system
- Problem oriented medical record system (POMR)

Basic sections of a conventional records/computerized records

Sociological or identification

- Contents
- Items common to all forms/modules

Medical section—clinical information

- Types of reports
- Responsibility for each

Nurses section—clinical information

- Nurse's notes
- Graphic charts
- Other special reports

Component parts of a conventional record (each part discussed as to content, responsibility for writing departments involved, standards governing)

Unit 4a. Basic Inpatient Medical Record Forms and Computerized Modules

Summary or face sheet or admission and discharge record

History and physical examination

Consultation record

Progress notes

Physician order record

Diagnostic record

- Clinical laboratory
- Radiology
- Tissue report
- Other special examination reports
  - ECG, echocardiogram, EEG, EMG, endoscopies, haemodialysis, radioactive isotopes, etc.

Operative record

Anaesthesia record

Obstetrical record

Prenatal record

Labour record

Delivery record

Newborn record/birth notification form

Newborn identification record

Physical therapy record

Occupational therapy record

Nursing record
- Nurse's record
- Graphic chart
- Intake and output record

Discharge summary or death summary (clinical resume)
Other correspondence record
Short stay record for day care patient
Accident and emergency record
Medicolegal record
Autopsy report

Unit 4b. Basic Outpatient Records and Computerized Modules

History and physical examination
Clinical progress record
Laboratory mount sheet

Unit 4c. Administrative Records in the Medical Record

Clothes and/or valuable record
Social service record
Unusual occurrence or incident report record
Administrative—often not a part of the record
Transport record

Unit 4d. Medical Record Format Types. Standard Assembling Order—merits and demerits

Integrated
Source oriented
Problem oriented

Unit 4e. Forms Control and Design

Control programs
- Methods
- Objectives
- Functions

Standardization programs
- Purpose
- Examples of some current level of standardization
  - Order of assembly
  - Forms
  - Others

Design
- Colour
- Paper
- Printing
- Brand
- Block

Data
- Arrangement and grouping
- Sequence
- Captions and wording
- Input

Spacing
- Horizontal and vertical
- Marginal

Lines
Instructions, guides and routing
Physical consideration
- Size
- Weight
- Printing
- Punching and binding
- Lamination
- Enforcement
- Speciality form
- Photocoping and microfilming
- Review and comparison of sample forms

TITLE OF UNITS—THERORY PART

Unit 1 History of medical records
Unit 2 Concept of medical records
Unit 3 Role of medical records in healthcare delivery system
Unit 4 Development of medical records forms

TEACHING STRATEGIES—THEORY AND LABORATORY PART

TITLE OF UNITS—THEORY PART

Unit	*Course contents*	*Number of hours*
1	**History of medicine:** Historical development of medicine and medical records—ancient history, stone-age, Indian history, ancient Greek and roman history, medieval history, etc. Important historical general development in different countries	2
1a.	**Historical development of healthcare field:** Development and organizational structure of health institutions in different countries such as hospitals health clinics and others	1
2	**Concepts of medical records:** And introduction to MRD historical developments and concepts of early medical record, and development of medical record department, definition of medical record, uses of medical record, property—medical record, agencies and organizations that set standards for medical records—formation and purposes of health agencies and organization, computerization of medical records	2

Contd...

Unit	Course contents	Number of hours
2a.	**Medical record administration and the professional organization:** Medical record administrator, medical record technologist, assistant medical record technician functions, educational qualifications, and employment opportunities. Ancillary medical record personnel—medical secretaries, medical transcriptions and others, ethics—definition, and medical ethics, pledges and codes of ethics, Hippocratic oath, code of ethics relating to medical record profession, professional conduct—relationship with professional staff and public international federation and development of medical record organization	4
2b.	**Functions of MRD:** Accident and emergency service registration, outpatient service, inpatient (ward) service medical records department—medical record review, coding, indexing, discharge analysis, statistics, filing and retrieving, research, lab mounting, release of information, medical transcription, retention policy, and preparation of reports and correspondences	2
3	**Introduction to healthcare delivery system:** Medical services, allied health services, diagnostic services—laboratory, radiology (X-ray/CT scan/ ultrasound/ECG, echocardiogram, EEG, EMG, endoscopies, nursing service, paramedical services, administrative services, and support services	2
3a.	**Medical record department inter departmental relationship:** To hospital administrator, heads of the department of different services, medical services staff, nursing services staff, ancillary services staff, allied health services staff, support services staff	2
3b.	**Quality of assurance plan:** Medical record screening indicators, quality assurance work sheet, concurrent chart review, monthly mortality and morbidity, problem identification and corrective plan, MRD function analysis, cost analysis worksheet	2
3c.	**Nursing service:** Introduction maintenance of medical record in the ward record relating to the care and treatment of patient, maintenance of stock books, hospital administrative records, ward maintenance register, attendance register of working staff in the ward, nurse treatment register (day and night report of the condition of patient, nurses records, nurses observation chart, graphic (TPR) chart, intake and output chart, chart for special cases	2
3.d.	Medical records in infection control	1
3e.	Medical records in long-term care hospital—rehabilitation records, psychiatry records, infectious diseases records	2
4	**Development of medical record forms:** Contents and format of different types of medical record format, types of records and reports of medical, allied health, diagnostic, nursing, paramedical, administrative and other support services. Component parts of a conventional record (each part discussed as to content, responsibility for writing departments involved, standards governing	2
4a.	Basic inpatient medical record forms and computerized modules	1
4b.	Basic outpatient records and computerized modules	1
4c.	Administrative records in the medical record	1
4d.	Medical record format types (standard assembling order) merits and demerits	2
4e.	Forms control and design	1

Contd...

Course Title:	Medical record sciences - MR 102 (Laboratory Part)		
Course Credits:	Theory	———	———
	Laboratory	1 Cr hr	30 hours
	Practical	———	———
	Total	1 Cr hr	30 hours
Course Placement:	Year - 1, Semester - 2		

COURSE DESCRIPTION

This laboratory experience is designed to offer experience in a medical department that develop the student's cognitive, affective and psychomotor skills to produce a medical record technologist.

COURSE OBJECTIVES

At the conclusion of this semester laboratory experience the students should be able to carry out the following specific tasks with 90% competency.

Demonstrate through their laboratory experience, an understanding the importance of medical records and the standards.

Demonstrate through their laboratory experience, uses and values of medical records

Develop ethics for a model medical record department

State the educational requirement and responsibilities for different levels of medical record professionals.

Produce organizational charts of: (a) MOH or hospital, (b) hospital, (c) medical records department.

To recognize all forms and their importance of each in relation to the medical record

Demonstrate their laboratory experience, types of format of medical records, standard medical record assembling order and the merits and demerits.

Demonstrate to assemble and analyze the medical records

Design forms for medical records and develop forms control methods.

TEACHING STRATEGIES

TITLE OF UNITS: LABORATORY PART

Unit	*Course contents*	*Number of hours*
1	Demonstrate through their laboratory experience, an understanding the importance of medical records and the standards	2
2	Demonstrate through their laboratory experience, uses and values of medical records	2
3	Develop ethics for a model medical record department	2
4	State the educational requirement and responsibilities for different levels of medical record professionals	3
5	Produce organizational charts of: (a) Ministry of health, (b) hospital, (c) medical records department	2
6	To recognize all forms and their importance of each in relation to the medical record	3
7	Demonstrate their laboratory experience, types of format of medical records, standard medical record assembling order and the merits and demerits	4
8	Demonstrate to assemble and analyze the medical records	10
9	Design forms for medical records and develop forms control methods	4

Lectures, laboratory practice, directed practice (hospital visit) OIMRIT charts, reference books, textbook, audio-visual presentation, video tapes, group discussion, seminars, role-play exercise.

Evaluation Methods

Continuous assessment	20%
Laboratory practice assessment	20%
Directed practice assessment	10%
Final examination	
• Written examination	30%
• Practical examination	10%
• Oral and viva examination	10%

Required and Recommended Textbooks

"Managing Medical Records" by Dr. GD Mogli, Channel Publication, Nevada, USA.

"Medical Record Organization and Management—2nd Edition" by Dr. GD Mogli, Jaypee Brothers, Medical Publishers (P) Ltd., New Delhi India.

"Certification on Cause of Death" by Dr. GD Mogli, Channel Publication, Nevada, USA.

Medical Records Management by Edna K. Huffman, Publication: Physician Record Company, Berwyn, Illinois, USA.

"Patient Care Research" by GD Mogli, Jaypee Brothers, Medical Publishers (P) Ltd., New Delhi, India.

"Health Records Paper to Paperless" by GD Mogli, Jaypee Brothers, Medical Publishers (P) Ltd., New Delhi, India.

Course Title:	Hospital Information II (HI 102)		
Course Credits:	Theory	2	30 hours
	Laboratory	———	———
	Practical	———	———
	Total	2	30 hours
Course Placement:	Year - 1, Semester - 2		

COURSE DESCRIPTION

This course consists of public health and vital statistics as well as in-depth study of hospital statistics including source of data, definition, and collection of information, reporting presentation and analysis of statistical data.

COURSE OBJECTIVES

At the end of the course, the student should be able to:

State the legal requirements for reporting vital statistics and the procedures for completion of birth and death certificates and the notification of infection diseases.

State principles of discharge analysis and service assignments

Understand the purpose of collections and depth of collection for different levels of users.

Define all terms and formulae related to hospital statistics

Compute hospital statistics derived from the daily bed returns and census figures.

Collect statistical data and present it in acceptable format

Prepare and present statistical data for monthly and annual reports

Describe the source of health statistics in Ministry of Health and types of information available for collection.

TEACHING STRATEGIES

Teaching strategies will include lectures, handouts, continuous practice, multiple-choice, one line, and brief, essay types of question and answers to reinforce theoretical knowledge.

Unit	*Course contents*	*Number of hours*
1	Introduction to health statistics, history of definition	2
2	Types and purposes of health statistics—vital statistics—birth certificate and notification, death certificate and notification, perinatal death certificate and notification, morbidity statistical collection, cancer notification and statistical collection	3
3	Hospital statistics, definition of statistics	3
4	Source of statistics, units of measurement	3
5	Inpatient statistics—service wide discharges, nationality wide discharges (local and non-local), age and sex classification, geographical classification, discharges alive and dead, inpatient diseases and operations—minor, intermediate, and major, bed utilization (general and private if any)	5
6	Commonly computed rates and percentage—average daily census, percentage of occupancy, average length of inpatient, fetal death rate, gross death rate, net death rate, fetal death rate, neonatal death rate, perinatal death rate, anesthesia death rate, postoperative death rate, maternal death rate, autopsy rate, consultation rate, caesarean section rate, infection rate, hospital infection rate, and postoperation rate	5
7	Turn over or discharges per bed, and turn over interval between discharges to admission	2
8	Collection of outpatient statistics—new cases, follow-cases, daily averages, age and sex classification, nationality classification, service classification, geographical wide distribution	3
9	Collection of accident and emergency (AE) statistics—daily cases, sex and age classification, medico-legal cases, emergency admission, AE referrals, service classification, classification of AE cases such as RTA, burns, poisonings, and other cases	3
10	Collection of other department statistics—laboratory, radiology, dietary, blood bank, physiotherapy, occupational therapy	3
11	Administrative statistics—collect the following information from various administrative units: number of medical staff—senior, junior by specialty, number of dentist, seniors and juniors, number of nursing personnel (cadre wide and student nurses, if any), number of paramedical workers, administrative staff, expenditure, income	3
12	Reporting hospital statistics—preparation reports, presentation reports, analysis of data, uses of hospital and health data, administration health services—hospital, planning, evaluating, reporting, utilization review	10

LABORATORY

The above course content is covered simultaneously through laboratory practice. The theory classes are followed by practical laboratory work.

Evaluation Scheme

Continuous assessment	20%
Mid term examination and pre-final examination	30%
Final examination (written, and practical)	50%

Course book, OIMRT's, charts, worksheets and library resources

Students are required to pass (50%) in these components.

Course Title:	Anatomy and physiology I (AP-102)		
Course Credits:	Theory	3 Cr. hr	45 hours
	Laboratory	———	———
	Practical	———	———
	Total	3 Cr. hr	45 hours
Course Placement:	Year - 1, Semester - 2		

COURSE DESCRIPTION

The anatomy and physiology I course is 15 weeks long and is an introduction to the study of the structure and function of the human body. This part I of the anatomy and physiology course introduces the student to the concepts of anatomy and physiology as subjects in the medical record curriculum and begins with an explanation of how the body is structurally organized from the chemical/cellular level through the tissue, organ and system level and finally to the organism level.

A description of the various cells and tissue types follow and then the student is introduced to the individual body systems. The part 1 of the curse covers the muscular, skeletal, respiratory, digestive and cardiovascular systems. The other body system will be covered on part II of the course. Practical and simulated exercises are an integral part of this course.

COURSE OBJECTIVES

At the end of this course the student should be able to:

Define the terms 'anatomy' and 'physiology'

Describe the organization of the body from cells to the whole organism

Describe and explain the structure and functions of the skeletal system

Describe and explain the structure and functions of the muscular system

Describe and explain the structure and functions of the respiratory system

Describe and explain the structure and functions of the digestive system

Describe and explain the structure and functions of the cardiovascular system

TITLE OF UNITS

Unit 1 The basic structure and chemistry of cells and tissues
Unit 2 Surface anatomy
Unit 3 The skeletal system
Unit 3 The muscular system
Unit 4 The respiratory system
Unit 5 The digestive system
Unit 6 The cardiovascular system

TEACHING STRATEGIES

Unit	*Course contents*	*Number of hours*
1	Introduction The cell and biological organization, body fluids and electrolytes. The elementary tissues of the body blood constituents and functions, red blood cells, white blood cells, platelets, blood clotting, blood groups	10
2	Surface anatomy	5
3	Skeletal system Major bones of the body Structures and functions of major joints	10
4	Muscular system Muscle tissues, muscle physiology, major muscles of head, neck, arm, and leg	5
5	Respiratory system Anatomy—respiratory passage, lungs Physiology of respiration Pulmonary ventilation Tissue respiration Gaseous exchange and transport Regulation of respiration	10
6	Digestive system Anatomy—food passage, structure and function of mouth, larynx, pharynx, epiglottis, esophagus, stomach, small and large intestine, anus rectum mechanical and chemical breakdown of food and absorption digestive system Accessory organs structure and functions liver, gall bladder, and pancreases	10
7	Cardiovascular system Heart structure and functions, circulation of blood, cardiac cycle, cardiac output, blood pressure, principles blood vessels	10

Course book, OIMRT's, anatomical charts, student handouts, worksheets, anatomical software system wide and library resources

EVALUATION METHODS

Continuous assessment	20%
Mid term examination and pre-final examination	30%
Final examination (written, and practical)	50%

Recommended Texts

Dr. Tony Smith (1995) The Human Body	Dorling Kindersley
Clancy J & McVicar A (1995) Physiology & Anatomy	Edward Arnold
Govan A. et al (1992) Pathology Illustrated	Churchill Livingston
C. Scanlon & T. Sander (1995) Essentials of Anatomy and Physiology	F.A. Davis Company - Philadelphia, USA
Anatomy and physiology for Paramedical students Jaypee Brothers (P) Ltd..www.jaypeebrothers.com	Prof. Dr. G D Mogli
Paramedics 6-in-1 Handbook; Jaypee Brothers (P) Lrd., www. Jaypeebrothers.com	Prof. Dr G D Mogli

Course Title:	Medical Terminology I (MT- 102)		
Course Credits:	Theory	1 Cr. hrs	15 hours
	Laboratory	1 Cr. hrs	30 hours
	Practical	———	———
	Total	2 Cr. hrs	45 hours
Course Placement:	Year - 1, Semester - 2		

COURSE DESCRIPTION

The course is designed to provide the student with the medical terminology necessary to understand and interpret the information contained in the medical record and medical literatures and assist the student in writing term correctly abstracted medical material or taking dictation, medical record analysis especially deficiency check.

COURSE OBJECTIVES

At the end of the course student will be able to:

Know the source of medical words
Know the element of medical words such as prefixes, roots, suffixes and combining forms
Use a medical dictionary, and pronounce medical terms
Gain an understanding of standard medical terms and its usage including abbreviations
Understand the relationship between medical terms and their synonyms in common language
Acquire the ability to spell medical words
Develop the ability to give an intelligent reading from medical literature
Acquire the ability to analyze the meaning of unfamiliar words
Analyze and define medical and surgical terms
Convert lay terms to their equivalent medical terms
Use medical terms in their appropriate context
Define term relating to the musculoskeletal system
Define term relating to the cardiovascular system
Define term relating to the respiratory system
Define term relating to the digestive system
Define term relating to the urinary system
Define term relating to the reproductive system
Define term relating to the central nervous system

TITLE OF UNITS

Unit 1	Objectives and values of medical terminology
Unit 2	Basic concepts—sources of medical words, deviation of words
Unit 3	Element of medical terms—suffixes and compounding elements, diagnostic suffixes, operative suffixes, symptomatic suffixes
Unit 4	Element of medical terms—roots
Unit 5	Element of medical terms—prefixes
Unit 6	Colors, numerals, symbols and phobias
Unit 7	General terms, body as a whole study of the body—anatomy, physiology, pathology, biology, histology, embryology, anatomical planes, and position of a body, regions, cavity, body fluids and chemicals
Unit 8	Study of the structure of body—cell, tissues, organs, system
Unit 9	Study of the term relating to the musculoskeletal system and its disorder
Unit 10	Study of the term relating to the cardiovascular system and its disorder
Unit 11	Study of the term relating to the respiratory system and its disorder
Unit 12	Study of the term relating to the digestive system and its disorder
Unit 13	Study of the term relating to the urinary system and its disorder
Unit 14	Study of the term relating to the reproductive system and its disorder
Unit 15	Study of the term relating to the central nervous system and its disorder

TEACHING STRATEGIES

Unit	*Course contents*	*Number of hours*
1	Objectives and values of medical terminology	1
2	Basic concepts—sources of medical words, deviation of words	2
3	Element of medical terms suffixes and compounding elements, diagnostic suffixes, operative suffixes, symptomatic suffixes	5
4	Element of medical terms—roots	4
5	Element of medical terms—prefixes	4
6	Colors, numerals, symbols and phobias	3
7	General terms, body as a whole study of the body—anatomy, physiology, pathology, biology, histology, embryology, anatomical planes, and position of a body, regions, cavity, body fluids and chemicals	3
8	Study of the structure of body—cell, tissues, organs, system	2
9	Study of the term relating to the musculoskeletal system	2
10	Study of the term relating to the central nervous system	2
11	Study of the terms relating to the sense organs	2
12	Study of the term relating to the respiratory system	2
13	Study of the term relating to the cardiovascular system	2
14	Study of the term relating to the digestive system	3
15	Study of the term relating to the urinary system	1
16	Study of the term relating to the reproductive system	3
17	Study of the term relating to the endocrine system	2
18	Study of the term relating to the lymphatic system	2

Teaching strategies will include course book, OIMRT's, anatomical charts, student handouts, worksheets, anatomical software system wide and library resources lectures, continuous practice, multiple-choice, one line, brief, essay types of question and answers to reinforce theoretical knowledge.

LABORATORY

The above course content is covered simultaneously through laboratory practice. The theory classes are followed by practical laboratory work.

Evaluation Scheme

Continuous assessment	20%
Mid term examination and pre-final examination	30%
Final examination (written, and practical)	50%

Students are required to pass (50%) in these components.

RECOMMENDED BOOKS

Learning Medical Terminology, 8th Edition, by Miriam G. Austrin, Harvey R Ausstrin, Mosby Lifeline, Mosby—Year Book in 1991, 11830 West Line Industrial Drive, St Louis, Missouri 63146 (9430060 CIP)

An Introduction to Medical Terminology—A Self-Teaching Package, 1999, by Andrew R. Hutton, Churchill Livingston, Robert Stevenson House, 1–3 Boxter's Place, Leith Walk, Edinburgh EH1 3AF UK

Anatomy and physiology for Paramedical students Jaypee Brothers (P) Ltd.www.jaypeebrothers.com	Prof. Dr. G D Mogli
Paramedics 6-in-1 Handbook; Jaypee Brothers (P) Lrd., www. Jaypeebrothers.com	Prof. Dr. G D Mogli

Course Title:	Anatomy and Physiology II (AP 201)		
Course Credits:	Theory	2 Cr. hr	30 hours
	Laboratory	———	———
	Practical	———	———
	Practical	2 Cr. hr	30 hours
Course Placement:	Year - 2, Semester - 1		

COURSE DESCRIPTION

The anatomy and physiology I course is 15 weeks long and is an introduction to the study of the structure and function of the human body. This part I of the anatomy and physiology course introduces the student to the concepts of anatomy and physiology as subjects in the medical record curriculum and begins with an explanation of how the body is structurally organized from the chemical/cellular level through the tissue, organ and system level and finally to the organismic level.

A description of the various cells and tissue types follow and then the student is introduced to the individual body systems. The part 1 of the curse covers the nervous, sensory, genitourinary, reproductive, endocrine and lymphatic systems. The other body system will be covered on part II of the course. Practical and simulated exercises are an integral part of this course.

COURSE OBJECTIVES

At the end of this course the student should be able to

Describe and explain the structure and functions of the nervous system
Describe and explain the structure and functions of the sensory system
Describe and explain the structure and functions of the genito-urinary system
Describe and explain the structure and functions of the reproductive system
Describe and explain the structure and functions of the lymphatic system

TITLE OF UNITS

Unit 1 The nervous system
Unit 2 The sensory system
Unit 3 The genitourinary system
Unit 4 The reproductive system
Unit 5 The lymphatic system

TEACHING STRATEGIES

Unit	*Course contents*	*Number of hours*
1	The nervous system Neurons—structure and functional unit, structure and functional and functions of parts of the brain and spinal cord, autonomic nervous system, parasympathetic and sympathetic nervous system	15
2	The sensory system Structure and functions of eye, ear, nose, tongue and skin	10
3	The genitourinary system Structural and functional unit of nephron, structure and blood supply of urinary system, structure and function of kidney, ureter, urinary bladder, and urethra. Formation of urine and maturation function	5
4	The reproductive system Male reproductive system—structure and functions Female reproductive—system structure and functions	10
5	The lymphatic system Structure and function of lymph, lymph nodes, lymphatic vessels and spleen.	5

Course book, OHT's, charts, worksheets and library resources

EVALUATION METHODS

Continuous assessment	20%
Mid term examination and pre-final examination	30%
Final examination (written, and practical)	50%

Students are required to pass (50%) in these components.

RECOMMENDED TEXTS

Dr. Tony Smith (1995). The Human Body	Dorling Kindersley
Clancy J & McVicar A (1995). Physiology and Anatomy	Edward Arnold

Govan A. et al (1992). Pathology Illustrated — Churchill Livingston

C. Scanlon & T. Sander (1995). Essentials of Anatomy and Physiology — FA Davis Company - Philadelphia, USA

Anatomy and Physiology for Paramedical Students Jaypee Brothers (P) Ltd..www.jaypeebrothers.com — Prof. Dr. G D Mogli

Paramedics 6-in-1 Handbook; Jaypee Brothers (P) Lrd., www. Jaypeebrothers.com — Prof Dr GD Mogli

Course Title:	Medical Terminology II (MT- 201)		
Course Credits:	Theory	2 Cr. hr	30 hours
	Laboratory	1 Cr. hr	30 hours
	Practical	———	———
	Total	3 Cr. hr	60 hours
Course Placement:	Year - 2, Semester - 1		

COURSE DESCRIPTION

The course is designed to provide the student with the medical terminology necessary to understand and interpret the information contained in the medical record and medical literatures and assist the student in writing term correctly abstracted medical material or taking dictation, medical record analysis especially deficiency check.

COURSE OBJECTIVES

At the end of the course student will be able to:

Know the element of medical words such as prefixes, roots, suffixes and combining forms of various system of human body

Use a medical dictionary, and pronounce medical terms

Gain an understanding of standard medical terms and its usage including abbreviations of various specialty services

Understand the relationship between medical terms and their synonyms in common language of various systems of human body

Acquire the ability to spell medical words of various systems of human body

Develop the ability to give an intelligent reading from medical literature, medical records.

Acquire the ability to analyze the meaning of unfamiliar words

Analyze and define medical and surgical terms

Convert lay terms to their equivalent medical terms

Use medical terms in their appropriate context

Define anatomical, symptomatic, pathological/diagnostic, and operative terms relating to the musculoskeletal system

Define anatomical, symptomatic, diagnostic, and operative terms term relating to the central nervous system and psychiatric disorders.

Define anatomical, symptomatic, pathological/diagnostic, and operative terms/term relating to the sense organs

Define anatomical, symptomatic, pathological/diagnostic, and operative terms/term relating to the respiratory system

Define anatomical, symptomatic, pathological/diagnostic, and operative terms/term relating to the cardiovascular system

Define anatomical, symptomatic, pathological/diagnostic, and operative terms/term relating to the digestive system

Define anatomical, symptomatic, pathological/diagnostic, and operative terms/term relating to the urinary system

Define anatomical, symptomatic, pathological/diagnostic, and operative terms/term relating to the reproductive system

Define anatomical, symptomatic, pathological/diagnostic, and operative terms/term relating to the endocrine system

Define anatomical, symptomatic, pathological/diagnostic, and operative terms/term relating to the lymphatic system

Define anatomical, symptomatic, pathological/diagnostic, and operative terms/term relating to the immunology, integumentary and blood and blood forming organs.

TEACHING STRATEGIES

Unit	*Course contents*	*Number of hours*
1	Define anatomical, symptomatic, pathological/diagnostic, and operative terms relating to the musculoskeletal system	5
2	Define anatomical, symptomatic, diagnostic, and operative terms term relating to the central nervous system and psychiatric disorders	7
3	Define anatomical, symptomatic, pathological/diagnostic, and operative terms/term relating to the sense organs	3
4	Define anatomical, symptomatic, pathological/diagnostic, and operative terms/term relating to the respiratory system	5
5	Define anatomical, symptomatic, pathological/diagnostic, and operative terms/term relating to the cardiovascular system	7
6	Define anatomical, symptomatic, pathological/diagnostic, and operative terms/term relating to the digestive system	7
7	Define anatomical, symptomatic, pathological/diagnostic, and operative terms/term relating to the urinary system	5
8	Define anatomical, symptomatic, pathological/diagnostic, and operative terms/term relating to the reproductive system	5
9	Define anatomical, symptomatic, pathological/diagnostic, and operative terms/term relating to the endocrine system	5
10	Define anatomical, symptomatic, pathological/diagnostic, and operative terms/term relating to the lymphatic system	5
11	Define anatomical, symptomatic, pathological/diagnostic, and operative terms/term relating to the immunology, integumentary and blood and blood forming organs	6

Teaching strategies will include course book, OIMRT's, anatomical charts, student handouts, worksheets, anatomical software system wide and library resources lectures, continuous practice, multiple-choice, one line, brief, essay types of question and answers to reinforce theoretical knowledge.

LABORATORY

The above course content is covered simultaneously through laboratory practice. The theory classes are followed by practical laboratory work.

Evaluation Scheme

Continuous assessment	20%
Mid term examination and pre-final examination	30%
Final examination (written, and practical)	50%

Students are required to pass (50%) in these components.

RECOMMENDED TEXTS

Learning Medical Terminology, 8th Edition, by Miriam G. Austrin, Harvey R Ausstrin, Mosby Lifeline, Mosby—Year Book in 1991, 11830 West Line Industrial Drive, St Louis, Missouri 63146 (9430060 CIP)

An Introduction to Medical Terminology—A Self-Teaching Package, 1999, by Andrew R. Hutton, Churchill Livingston, Robert Stevenson House, 1–3 Boxter's Place, Leith Walk, Edinburgh EH1 3AF UK

Anatomy and Physiology for Paramedical Students
Jaypee Brothers (P) Ltd..www.jaypeebrothers.com Prof Dr G D Mogli

Paramedics 6-in-1 Handbook; Jaypee Brothers
(P) Lrd., www. Jaypeebrothers.com Prof Dr G D Mogli

Course Title:	Medical record sciences directed practice (MR 201)		
Course Credits:	Theory	———	———
	Laboratory	———	———
	Practical	4 Cr. hrs	180 hours
	Total	4 Cr. hrs	180 hours
Course Placement:	Year - 2, Semester - 1		

COURSE DESCRIPTION

Supervise learning experience in well-organized and staffed medical record departments of hospitals, under the supervision of experience medical record administrators. Students are assigned to Ministry of Health Hospitals or corporate, or any hospitals selected for specified period of training practice.

Through the experience the student develops insight, understanding and skills in medical record procedures, accepts responsibilities and recognizes the need for preserving for confidential nature of the medical record recognizes contributors of and learns to work with professional and non-professional personnel.

Student assignments are planned so that experience is gained in all procedures previously studied through classroom presentation and laboratory.

COURSE OBJECTIVES

At the conclusion of the practical experience the student should be able to perform the functions of a medical record technologist with 90% of competency.

CLINICAL EXPERIENCE

Unit 1 Outpatient registration—hospital number control, registration of new cases, master patient index, filing, retrieving, typing and up dating, other related procedures (30 hours)

Unit 2 Outpatient registration—appointment—new, old, answering phone calls, preparation of new records or modules (21 hours)

Unit 3 Outpatient clinics—appointment system, collection of new and old records, collection of X-rays and diagnostic reports, collection of pharmacy prescription sheets, referrals, and admissions (30 hours)

Unit 4 Accident and emergency registration—accident and emergency number control, registration, diagnostic reports, referrals, registration of medico-legal "cases, other related procedures (15 hours)

Unit 5 Admission and discharge procedures—admission procedures waiting list maintenance, bed occupancy, in-house, discharge procedures, discharge patient information, special cases and other related procedures.

Unit 6 Ward management—maintenance of records/X-ray, admission and discharge register/module, investigation reports/module, census reports/module, other related function.

Unit 7 Medical record filing area—filing of records, filing of X-rays, collection and mounting reports, processing of outpatient reports, retrieval of records, retrieval of X-rays, coding and indexing of diagnostic and operative procedures (I)

COURSE DESCRIPTION

The course is designed to provide students with a basic understanding of medical record standards, general policies, legal aspects, legislative process, court system, patient rights, advance directives, primary versus secondary records, security and confidentiality, release of information, monitor change in regulation and accreditation standards on release/ retentions of patient records.

COURSE OBJECTIVES

At the conclusion of this unit the student should be able to:

Understand and define medical record standards

Ethics—definition, and medical ethics, pledges and codes of ethics, Hippocratic oath, code of ethics relating to medical record profession, professional conduct—relationship with professional staff and public

Responsibility of medical record specialist, and technologist

Identify the rules and regulations of the MOH/private relating hospitals

Understand and explain general policies of medical records at par with national and international standards

Understand the different legal systems on which the laws of Oman are based

Define medical legal aspects of medical records and strictly follow the medico-legal procedures.

Register the medico-legal cases

Discuss the importance of having laws to protect the patient, doctors, hospital, and Ministry of Health.

Recognize the legislative process and court system procedures and follow the same strictly.

Discuss the patient rights/advocacy and advance directives

The patient has the right to the health record information.

Understand and differentiate primary versus secondary records and its protection including other statistics protection.

Discus the retention policy and procedures of medical records

Discuss the importance of confidentiality and how it is related to medical records in all of its aspects.

Discuss the importance of authorization and informed consent.

Discuss all aspects relating to the release of information to the patient, doctor, other health facilities and Ministry of Health.

Forms for release of information

Release of drug and alcohol abuse patient information

Cite the medico-legal laws that exist at present in Oman (requirement, release) responsible, confidentiality actual laws for treatment and how they affect the Ministry of Health, healthcare facilities, doctors, patient and medical records department.

Describe the role of Ministry of Health, hospitals, doctors, and medical records departments can play in the creation enforcement and defence of medico-legal laws.

Discuss the importance of security, confidentiality and reliability of data in automated medical record system.

Explain area for mishandling medical records, which may result in potential liability for the health care facility.

Discuss the responsibility of MRD in regard to maintenance retention, ownership and protection.

Monitor change in regulations and accreditation standards on releases/retention of patient records

TITLE OF UNITS—THEORY PART

Unit 1	Medical record standards
Unit 2	Ethics—definition, and medical ethics, pledges and codes of ethics, hippocratic oath, code of ethics relating to medical record profession, professional conduct—relationship with professional staff and public
Unit 3	Responsibility of medical record specialist, and technologist
Unit 4	Identify the rules and regulations of the MOH/private relating hospitals
Unit 5	General rule and regulation—the different legal systems, on which the laws of Oman are based, define medico-legal aspects of medical records and strictly follow the medico-legal procedures. Medico-legal cases registration procedures, Discuss the importance of having laws to protect the patient, doctors, hospital, and ministry of health. Medico-legal case registration, temporary permission to leave the hospital, consent—general, special, emergency operation, patient leaving the hospital against medical advice.

Unit 6 Recognize the legislative process and court system procedures and follow the same strictly. Documentary evidence, insurance cases, workmen's compensation, personal injury suits, malpractice suits, will cases. Authorization for operation, completion of records, specific consents for amputation of a part, patient against medical advice, proper birth and death registration and notification, criminal cases.

Unit 7 Impact of the Consumer Protection Act in medical field—who is a consumer? Why the Consumer Protections Act? What is service? What is deficiency?

Unit 8 Medical Malpractice/Negligence—standard of care, maltreatment, mismanagement, how the medical record the patient, doctor, hospital, malpractice law suit, liability of omission, execution of the consumer protection act, powers of consumer agencies, place and time limit for filing a complaint, duty under court of law.

Unit 9 Discuss the patient rights/advocacy and advance directives, the patient right to the health record information.

Unit 10 Understand and differentiate primary versus secondary records and its protection including other statistics protection.

Unit 11 Discus the retention policy and procedures of medical records, discuss the responsibility of MRD in regard to maintenance retention, ownership and protection.

Unit 12 Discuss the importance of security and confidentiality and how it is related to medical records in all of its aspects. Discuss the importance of security, confidentiality and reliability of data in automated medical record system

Unit 13 Discuss all aspects relating to the release of information to the patient, doctor, other health facilities and Ministry of Health. Form for release of information. Release of drug and alcohol abuse patient information

Unit 14 Cite the medico-legal laws that exists at present in your country (requirement, release) responsible, confidentiality actual laws for treatment and how they affect the Ministry of Health, healthcare facilities, doctors, patient and medical records department.

Unit 15 Describe the role of Ministry of Health, hospitals, doctors, and medical records departments can play in the creation enforcement and defence of medico-legal laws.

Unit 16 Explain area for mishandling medical records, which may result in potential liability for the health care facility.

Unit 17 Monitor change in regulations and accreditation standards on releases/retention of patient records.

TEACHING STRATEGIES

Lectures, laboratory practice, directed practice (hospital visit) charts, reference books, textbook, audio-visual presentation, video tapes, group discussion, seminars, role-play exercise.

TITLE OF UNITS—LABORATORY PART

Unit 1 Discuss medical record standards

Unit 2 Discuss ethics—definition, and medical ethics, pledges and codes of ethics, Hippocratic oath, code of ethics relating to medical record profession, professional conduct—relationship with professional staff and public

Unit 3 Explain the responsibility of medical record specialist, and technologist

Unit 4 Identify the rules and regulations of the MOH/private relating hospitals

Unit 5 General rule and regulation—the different legal systems, on which the laws of Oman are based, define medical legal aspects of medical records and strictly follow the medico-legal procedures. Medico-legal cases registration procedures, discuss the importance of having laws to protect the patient, doctors, hospital, and ministry of health. Medico-legal case registration, temporary permission to leave the hospital, consent—ceneral, special, emergency operation, patient leaving the hospital against medical advice.

Unit 6 Recognize the legislative process and court system procedures and follow the same strictly. Documentary evidence, insurance cases, workmen's compensation, personal injury suits, malpractice suits, will cases. Authorization for operation, completion of records, specific consents for amputation of a part, patient against medical advice, proper birth and death registration and notification, criminal cases

Unit 7 Impact of the consumer protection act in medical field— who is a consumer? Why the Consumer Protections Act? What is service? What is deficiency?

Unit 8 Medical malpractice/negligence—standard of care, maltreatment, mismanagement, how the medical record the patient, doctor, hospital, malpractice law suit, liability of omission, execution of the Consumer Protection Act, powers of consumer agencies, place and time limit for filing a complaint, duty under court of law

Unit 9 Discuss the patient rights/advocacy and advance directives, the patient right to the health record information.

Unit 10 Understand and differentiate primary versus secondary records and its protection including other statistics protection.

Unit 11 Discus the retention policy and procedures of medical records, discuss the responsibility of MRD in regard to maintenance retention, ownership and protection

Unit 12 Discuss the importance of security and confidentiality and how it is related to medical records in all of its aspects. Discuss the importance of security, confidentiality and reliability of data in automated medical record system

Unit 13 Discuss all aspects relating to the release of information to the patient, doctor, other health facilities and ministry of health. Form for release of information. Release of drug and alcohol abuse patient information

Unit 14 Cite the medico-legal laws that exists at present in Oman (requirement, release) responsible, confidentiality actual laws for treatment and how they affect the Ministry of Health, healthcare facilities, doctors, patient and medical records department.

Unit 15 Describe the role of Ministry of Health, hospitals, doctors, and medical records departments can play in the creation enforcement and defence of medico-legal laws.

Unit 16 Explain area for mishandling medical records, which may result in potential liability for the health care facility.

Unit 17 Monitor change in regulations and accreditation standards on releases/retention of patient records

Evaluation Methods

Continuous assessment	20%
Laboratory practice assessment	20%
Directed practice assessment	10%
Final examination	
• Written examination	30%
• Practical examination	10%
• Oral and viva examination	10%

Required and Recommended Textbooks

"Managing Medical Records" by Dr GD Mogli, Channel Publication, Nevada, USA.

"Medical Record Organization and Management 2nd Edition" by Dr GD Mogli, Jaypee Brothers, Medical Publishers (P) Ltd., New Delhi, India.

"Certification on Cause of Death" by Dr GD Mogli, Channel Publication, Nevada, USA.

Medical Records Management by Edna K. Huffman, Publication: Physician Record Company, Berwyn, Illinois, USA.

"Patient Care Research" by GD Mogli, Jaypee Brothers, Medical Publishers (P) Ltd., New Delhi, India.

"Health Records Paper to Paperless" by GD Mogli, Jaypee Brothers, Medical Publishers (P) Ltd., New Delhi, India.

Course Title:	Information Technology II (IT)		
Course Credits:	Theory	1 Cr. hr	15 hours
	Laboratory	2 Cr. hr	60 hours
	Practical	———	———
	Total	3 Cr. hr	75 hours
Course Placement:	Year - 2, Semester – 1		

PREREQUISITE

Introduction to information technology, key boarding skills a minimum of 30 words per minute.

COURSE DESCRIPTION

This course is designed to provide medical record technology students with a basic understanding of the MOH or hospital policy planning concerning using the electronic patient file. The students will learn the basic functions of the Hospital Information Management System (HIMS) and its application modules (subsystem). The student will be briefly introduced to the features of each subsystem mainly those modules which are linked with the medical record module. The major focus of this course will on medical record module.

The course will equip student with essential skills needed to use the medical record module. It will allow students to enter patient identification data and clinical information into the computer. The students will the process of creating indent template, creating a query based on a single or multiple criteria and preparing statistical report and other reports. The course will be totally laboratory based with students being guided through a series of computer based lessons and additional learning task sheet. All data sets used in this course, are simulated cases and are not specific to a real patient or location; they developed to help student interact with the system in an effective way. Theoretical concepts will be integrated where appropriate. Whenever possible material used will integrate and reinforce learning in other courses.

COURSE OBJECTIVES

At the end of the course student will be able to:

Demonstrate understanding of MOH/hospital policy and planning concerning the use of an electronic patient medical record module

Demonstrate understanding of HIMS and its main applications

Utilize the windows 2000 perform HIMS basic functions

Document medical record intervention/procedures other relevant care rendered to patient

Create a query based on a single or multiple criteria such patient name, age, sex, doctor name, clinic name, admission date, discharge date, etc.

Able to prepare, modify and print admissions, discharges list, other required reports and duty roster

Understand the structured problem solving methods in computer by developing algorithms and flowchart

Able to developing simple computer application (software) on hospital information system

Introduction to networking, data integrity, security and confidentiality

Able to coordinate other relevant functions with appropriate departments, creating and handling database inventory of all data components, maintain integrity of patient numbering system.

Able to document imaging, electronic record storage and backup

Understand the concept and development of electronic medical records

Understand the concept of automatic identification and voice recognition technology

TITLE OF UNITS

Unit 1 Understanding of MOH/hospital policy and planning concerning the use of an electronic patient file

Unit 2 Demonstrate understanding of HIMS and its main application

Unit 3 Utilize the windows 2000 perform HIMS basic functions

Unit 4 Document medical record interventions/procedures and other relevant care rendered to patient

Unit 5 Create a query based on a single or multiple criteria such as patient name, age, sex, doctor name, clinic name, admission date, discharge date, etc.

Unit 6 Prepare, modify and print admission, discharge, duty roaster and other required reports

Unit 7 Structured problem solving methods in computer by developing algorithms and flowchart

Unit 8 Developing simple computer application (software) on hospital information system

Unit 9 Introduction to networking, data integrity, security and confidentiality

Unit 10 Coordinate other relevant functions with appropriate departments, creating and handling database inventory of all data components, maintain integrity of patient numbering system.

Unit 11 Document imaging, electronic record storage and backup

Unit 12 Concept and development of electronic medical records

Unit 13 Automatic identification and voice recognition technology

TEACHING STRATEGIES

Unit	*Course contents*	*Number of hours*
1	Demonstrate understanding of MOH policy and planning concerning the use of an electronic patient medical record module	5
2	Demonstrate understanding of HIMS and its main applications	10
3	Utilize the windows 2000 perform HIMS basic functions	5
4	Document medical record intervention/procedures ot her relevant care rendered to patient	10
5	Create a query based on a single or multiple criteria such patient name, age, sex, doctor name, clinic name, admission date, discharge date, etc.	2
6	Able to prepare, modify and print admissions, discharges list, other required reports and duty roster	3
7	Understand the structured problem solving methods in computer by developing algorithms, and flowchart	2
8	Able to developing simple computer application (software) on hospital information system	5
9	Introduction to networking, data integrity, security and confidentiality	3
10	Able to coordinate other relevant functions with appropriate departments, creating and handling database inventory of all data components, maintain integrity of patient numbering system	10
11	Able to document imaging, electronic record storage and backup	5
12	Understand the concept and development of electronic medical records	10
13	Understand the concept of automatic identification and voice recognition technology	5

Students will almost entirely in the computer laboratory. They will use:

Interactive software packages and off-line Internet lessons to

Develop keyboarding skills

Learn about the use of computers and their component

Identify and learn to use main functions of the MS Window 98/2000 operating system

Understand and perform key features of MS Excel 2000

Demonstrate understanding of MOH policy and planning concerning the use of an electronic patient medical record module

Demonstrate understanding of HIMS and its main applications

Utilize the windows 2000 perform HIMS basic functions

Document medical record intervention/procedures other relevant care rendered to patient

Create a query based on a single or multiple criteria such patient name, age, sex, doctor name, clinic name, admission date, discharge date, etc.

Able to prepare, modify and print duty roaster

Understand the structured problem solving methods in computer by developing algorithms and flowchart

Able to developing simple computer application (software) on hospital information system

Introduction to networking, data integrity, security and confidentiality

Able to coordinate other relevant functions with appropriate departments, creating and handling database inventory of all data components, maintain integrity of patient numbering system.

Able to document imaging, electronic record storage and backup

Understand the concept and development of electronic medical records

Understand the concept of automatic identification and voice recognition technology

Teacher guided tutorials, which will support the computer-based lessons by facilitating the performance of assigned learning tasks and monitoring student progress

Student paced learning exercises to practice and master the required competencies in word, excel and power point 2000 and MOH Hospital Information Management System (HIMS)

A project designed to utilize ready-made hospital information data base package, access all the hospital information medical record modules, and prepare hospital statistical reports and other reports, internet skills and to integrate and consolidate other skills learned.

EVALUATION METHODS

Continuous Assessment

Continuous assessment	30%
Project work	20%

FINAL ASSESSMENT

10% on word-processing, excel, power point 2000, and internet access
40% on hospital information package access and create the hospital statistical reports

Final assessment based on 3 hours computer-based exam.

Project

20%, a project designed to demonstrating use of the Hospital Information Medical Record Module Package from level 2 mandatory unit will be completed on time. It is anticipated that work from Units 4, 5, and 6 may be used in the project.

The assessment of keyboard skills can be taken at any time agreed to by the teacher

Students are required to pass (50%) in these components.

RESOURCES REQUIRED

Multi-media Laboratory Providing

Individual student access to a personal computer for all class periods, additional access for practice is highly desirable.

Individual network login providing secure student access to workspace on the server

Internet access—for class time and for project work

Software uniformly installed as below

Required System and Application Software

Windows 98/2000
MS office professional
MS internet explorer (as supplied with windows)
MOH hospital information management system data base software

Interactive Teaching Packages

Typing tutor

Type master typing test (to be used for standardizing keyboard testing)

Leaning windows

Leaning office 2000

Learning hospital information data base package

Course Title: Medical Terminology-III (MT-202)

Pathology

Biochemistry

Microbiology

Radio-diagnosis

- Forensic medicine
- Pharmacology
- Sociology
- Psychology
- Health education

Course Credits:	Theory	3 Cr. hr	45 hours
	Laboratory	———	———
	Practical	———	———
	Total	3 Cr. hr	45 hours
Course Plaement:	Year - 2, Semester – 2		

COURSE DESCRIPTION

The course consists of basic fundamental of pathology, biochemistry, microbiology, radio-diagnosis, forensic medicine, pharmacology, sociology, psychology and health education

COURSE OBJECTIVES

At the end of course the learner should be able to:

Define and classify diseases

Classify various types of lesions/tumors (benign and malignant)

Classify broadly the various types of bacterial and its proportion

Different types of virus and types of diseases brought by them

Understand the chemistry in body, in health and diseases, clotting mechanisms of blood, enzymes, vitamins, hormones, protein, nitrogen's, carbohydrates, water metabolism, and acid balance urine, etc.

Knowledge about imaging science and technology such as X-rays, special radio-diagnostic procedures such as ultrasound sonogram, CT scan, magnetic resonance imaging, etc.

Know the legal procedures related to medico-legal aspects of cases and deaths.

Pharmacology includes systemic pharmacology, CNS drugs, autonomic cardiovascular, gastrointestinal tract, endocrine glands, anti-infective, urinary and respiratory system drugs. This subject is to provide medical record students with essential information about certain groups of drugs commonly used.

Sociology includes structure community, human dynamic group relationship, and interaction within the society. Identify the various areas of development, e.g. cognitive, moral and language. Identify individual differences; identify the factors that influences individual health factor.

Psychology includes types counseling, psychotherapies, and psychological disorders. Psychological factors in stress and relationship.

Health education includes concepts, scope, characteristics and principles of health education, effectiveness of the techniques and principles of communication and counseling strategies in working with individuals, families, groups as well as members of healthcare team. Demonstrate skill in health education to promote health, maintain well-being and prevent illness among individuals, families, and groups in the community.

COURSE DESCRIPTION

Pathology

Introduction to clinical pathology

Definition and classification of diseases

Broad outline and classification of various types of clinical lesions/tambours (benign and malignant)

Microbiology

What is a bacterium—broad classification of various types of bacterial and its properties?

Broad discussion about viruses and types of diseases brought about by them.

Name and purposes of some important tests conducted in laboratories.

Biochemistry

Chemistry in health

Chemistry in body, in health and in disease

Clotting mechanisms of blood

Enzymes

Gastrointestinal tract

Vitamins

Hormones
Protein and non-protein
Nitrogenous substances
Carbohydrates
Electrolytes
Water and metabolism
Acid–base balance
Urine

Forensic Medicine

Introduction
Legal procedures, medical law and ethics
Identification, medico-legal autopsy
Death and postmortem changes
External cause of injuries and medico-legal aspects (case studies)

Pharmacology

General information about drugs
Drugs used to control infections
Drugs acting on the central nervous system
Drugs acting on the autonomic nervous system
Drugs used for disorders of the respiratory system
Drugs used for disorders of gastro intestinal tract
Drugs used for disorders of cardiovascular system
Drugs used for disorders of the blood forming organs
Drugs used for disorders of the urinary system
Drugs used for disorders of endocrine glands

Sociology

Structure of community
Human dynamic group relationship and interaction within the society
Identify the various areas of development, e.g. cognitive, moral and language. Identify individual differences
Identify the factors that influence individual health.

Psychology

Identify the individual differences
Psychology includes types counseling
Types of psychotherapies
Psychological disorders
Psychological factors in stress and relationship

Health Education

Concepts, scope, characteristics and principles of health education, effectiveness of the techniques and principles of communication and counseling strategies in working with individuals, families, groups as well as members of healthcare team.

Demonstrate skill in health education to promote health, maintain well-being and prevent illness among individuals, families, and groups in the community.

TEACHING STRATEGIES

Unit	*Course contents*	*Number of hours*
1	Pathology define and classify diseases classify various types of lesions/ tumors (benign and malignant)	5
2	Biochemistry understand the chemistry in body, in health and diseases, clotting mechanisms of blood, enzymes, vitamins, hormones, protein, nitrogen's, carbohydrates, water metabolism, and acid balance urine, etc.	5
3	Microbiology classify broadly the various types of bacterial and its proportion different types of virus and types of diseases brought by them	5
4	Radio-diagnosis knowledge about imaging science and technology such as X-rays, special radio-diagnostic procedures such as ultra sound sonogram, CT scan, magnetic resonance imaging, etc.	5
5	Forensic medicine legal procedures related to medico legal aspects of cases and deaths	5
6	Pharmacology includes systemic pharmacology, CNS drugs, autonomic cardiovascular, gastrointestinal tract, endocrine glands, anti-infective, urinary and respiratory system drugs. This subject to provide medical record students with essential information about certain groups of drugs commonly used.	5
7	Sociology includes structure community, human dynamic group relationship, and interaction within the society. Identify the various areas of development, e.g. cognitive, moral and language. Identify individual differences; identify the factors that influences individual health.	5
8	Psychology includes types counseling, psychotherapies, and psychological disorders. Psychological factors in stress and relationship	5
9	Health education includes concepts, scope, characteristics and principles of health education, effectiveness of the techniques and principles of communication and counseling strategies in working with individuals, families, groups as well as members of health care team. Demonstrate skill in health education to promote health, maintain well-being and prevent illness among individuals, families, and groups in the community	5

Evaluation Methods

Continuous assessment	20% written assignments or group projects
Mid term assessment	30%
Final examination	50%

Required and Recommended Reference

Required curriculum task force, biochemistry, student course books

Essential anatomy and physiology

Biochemistry for Nurses, by Anthikad J

Fredric A Bettelheim, Jerry March (1999), Introduction to Organic and Biochemistry, Third Edition – Harcourt College Publishers.

MEDICAL RECORD TECHNOLOGIST PROGRAM EVALUATION (GUIDELINES FOR EVALUATING STUDENTS AND ALLOCATE THE INTERNAL MARKS)

The following points are to be carefully noted by the teaching faculty, e.g. demonstrator, hospital medical records officer, clinical practice supervisor.

QUALTITY OF WORK

Considering the student's degree of familiarity with the facility procedure and the assigned task, does the student produce a technically accurate product? Complete product?

APPLICATION TO WORK

Was student attentive?

Willing to do work?

Show enthusiasm in the learning task?

KNOWLEDGE OF MEDICAL RECORD PRINCIPLES

Does the student relate or display his/her knowledge of medical record principles and apply them in their proper context?

UDERSTANDING WHERE ASSIGNED AREA FITS WORK INTO FLOW OF DEPARTMENT

This is an integral of "Pulling it all together" and makes a clinical experience much more meaningfully. Your reinforcement in this area will identify the relationship of the assigned task to the overall facility health information system.

PROFESSIONALISM

Did the student exhibit tact and discretion interacting with other professionals, peers, and area personnel?

Was the student considered so as not to disrupt the workflow of the department?

Was the student neat in appearance?

INITIATIVE

Does the student ask for other work when assigned task has been completed?

Do not downgrade the student on this point, it will only be considered a plus if present, not a minus if absent.

MEDICAL RECORD TECHNOLOGIST OF CLINICAL EXPERIENCE LOG

PART A

Student Name: ______________________________ Roll No. ________

Hospital Name: ________________________ Section: ________________

Medical Record:

PART B

Date	Time		Activities
	From	*To*	

INSTRUCTION FOR COMPLETION OF CLINICAL EXPERIENCE LOG

This long is to be completed by the students on a daily basis giving detailed outlines of all the activities/procedures performed step by step. In order to, the clinical instructor can evaluate the level of knowledge and performance of the student. The log is an important document for evaluation of the student in clinical experience.

PART A

The student must complete the identification section giving full name, student roll number. Circle the correct course number and write the name of the hospital and name of the assigned section.

PART B

This form has to be filled to reflect the different activities on a daily basis.

Date: Write the date in the date column daily.

Time: State the starting and ending time of each function.

Times used for other activities, which are not related to, say functions, i.e. for coffee break, telephone call and in activity time.

Activities: The detailed step-by-step report on the clinical experience has to be written.

EXAMPLE

Date	*Time*		*Activities*
	From	*To*	
2.9.2015	09.00 am	09.45 am	Received a referral form, checked PMI for previous admission, and assigned a register number. Completed a master index… ..
	09.45 am	10.00 am	In active (no patients)
	10.00 am	10.15 am	Break for coffee
	10.15 am	11. 00 am	Audit: Checking lab report for wrongly filed reports ————

Return of log: This log has to be returned by the student to the clinical instructor on a weekly basis.

Clinical instructor: To write comments and signed and discuss with faculty members the student progress before returning to the student.

Faculty: The faculty members at the completion of each section shall also be responsible for any and all problems arising from the students, clinical instructors and hospital.

MEDICAL RECORDS TECHNICIAN PROGRAM

(CLINICAL INSTURCTOR STUDENT PROGRESS REPORT)

Student Name: ______________________________ Roll No.______

Hospital Name: ______________________ Section: ______________

Medical Record:

INSTRUCTIONS

For clinical instructor to be based on observation and activities log.

Part—I tasks performed	*Acceptable*	*Needs more practice*	*Not performed*

Comments: Signature

MEDICAL RECORD TECHNOLOGIST LAB AND CLINICAL PRACTICE EVALUATION

Student Name:

Student Roll No: Area of Clinical Instruction:

Quality of Work:

Comments: ____

____

____

Application to Work:

Comments: ____

____

____

Understanding of Assigned Tasks

Comments: ______________________________

____

____

KNOWLEDGE OF MEDICAL RECORD PRINCIPLES

Comments: ______________________________

____

____

UNDERSTANDING WHERE ASSIGNED AREA FITS INTO FLOW OF DEPARTMENT

Comments: ______________________________

____

PROFESSIONALISM (ATTITUDE)

Comments: ______________________________

____

____

Initiative: Yes ____________ No ____________

Comments: ______________________________

____

Excellent	(A)	(90% and Above)
Very good	(B)	(80 to 89%)
Good	(C)	(70 to 79%)
Average	(D)	(60 to 69%)
Failure	(F)	(Less than 60%)

BASE GRADE AND COMMENTS

Assessment sheet
Written reports by students
Student logs
Observation of a job duties explanation
Written test bases on above

Signature of:

I. Clinical instructor
II. Faculty member

TWO-YEAR DIPLOMA IN HEALTH INFORMATION MANAGEMENT TECHNOLOGY PROGRAM

Training Program

The two year Diploma Health Information Technology Program will be conducted by the Ministry of Health under the direct supervision of qualified professionals at the recognized universities or institutes. It should provide instructions and clinical experience to assist students in developing the technical skills necessary to maintain components of health information systems consistent with the medical, administrative, ethical, legal accreditation and regulator requirements of the health care delivery system of the Government of India Ministry of Health (MOH).

The teaching faculties of the health information management (HIM) institute and Hospitals should committed to provide the best possible learning environment for the students by providing an educational experience that meets the individual needs of all candidates. The students should be provided with the tools necessary to meet the requirements of the program, and are expected to accept responsibility for their education and to make full utilization of the learning opportunities offered to them.

Duration: The course is of two years. The course will consist of four semesters, the first from September to January and second from February to June.

Commencement of the course: First week of September, every year.

No. of admissions: 20–30 candidates per course will be admitted.

Medium of instruction: The medium of instruction offered should be in English language

Admission Requirements

Essential

1. Passed General Secondary Education Certificate with minimum 65% aggregate marks or equivalent.
2. Qualified candidates of six month assistant medical record technician (AMRT) program of any recognized institute or MOH with good academic and excellent working performance experience can also be considered OR equivalent as approved by the MOH educational programs.

Desirable

Experience in computer word processing knowledge. Already working in HIM department with minimum of one year experience and meeting the required qualifications.

Selection procedure: Applications to the course will be invited by the MOH or authorized regional authorities of Government of India or authorized organizations. An ad-hoc selection committee will select the candidates purely on merit basis as per the criteria laid down.

Evaluation: Continuous periodical written tests will be conducted in each subject monthly or in each chapter of study. Assignments and performance in seminars, viva voce will be awarded marks. At the end of each semester, final written tests as per the subjects taught will be conducted.

Credits: The credit ratios are set at:

15 hrs theory = 1 credit

30 hrs laboratory = 1 credit

45 hrs practical at the hospital = 1 credit

45 hrs English lecture = 1 credit

Grade points:			*Points*	
A	85% and above	....	Excellent	 4
B	75–84%	....	Very good	 3
C	65–74%	....	Good	 2
D	50–64%	....	Pass	 1
E	less than 50%	....	Fail	 0

Grade points are calculated as follows:

Grade points = Credit hours × Points

Grade point average is calculated as follows:

Total Grade Points Earned

Total Credits Attempted

Pass: A candidate will be deemed to have been passed in each subject, if he secures not less than 40% in internal and as well as external examinations with an aggregate of not less than 50%. The internal assessment marks are based on overall performance of the candidate's characteristics and traits such as punctuality, attitude, devotion, industrious, seriousness, etc. A candidate is deemed to be successful in completing the diploma in health information management program provided if he passes in all the subjects.

Award of diploma: Successful candidates will be awarded diploma in health information Management by the authorized institute of HIM or by collaborative university.

Location of the programme: All theoretical classes and Laboratory sessions will be conducted at the HIM institute and practical training will be imparted at recognize hospitals or health institutions.

Attendance: Each candidate should put in attendance of at least 85%.

Discipline: Each candidate shall observe discipline according to rules and regulations laid down by the HIM institute. Any violation of discipline the candidate may run the risk of removal from the HIM training program.

Analysis of semester and credit hours in each subject

S. No	*Subjects*	*Total hours in each semester*					*Total credits in each semester*				
		I	*II*	*III*	*IV*	*Total*	*I*	*II*	*III*	*IV*	*Total*
1	English language	135	45	–	–	180	3	1	–	–	4
2	Medical records science	45	180	210	75	510	2	6	6	3	17
3	Basic allied sciences	75	45	–	–	120	4	3	–	–	7
4	Hospital information	45	45	–	–	90	2	2	–	–	4
5	Anatomy and physiology	45	45	–	–	90	2	2	–	–	4
6	Healthcare delivery	30	–	–	30	60	2	–	–	2	4
7	Information technology	45	–	75	–	120	2	–	3	–	5
8	Medical terminology	–	45	90	–	135	–	2	4	–	6
9	Organization and management	–	–	30	30	60	–	–	2	2	4
10	Classification and indexing methods of diseases and procedures	–	–	15	90	105	–	–	1	4	5
11	Quality assurance and research methodology	–	–	–	30	30	–	–	–	2	2
12	Internship including seminars	–	–	–	165	165	–	–	–	4	4
	Total	**420**	**405**	**420**	**420**	**1665**	**17**	**16**	**16**	**17**	**66**

SEMESTER—WIDE SYLLABUS

FIRST SEMESTER							
Subject	*Code*	*Lectures*	*Lab*	*Practical*	*Total hr.*	*Credit hrs.*	*Prerequisite*
English language	EL-101	3		–	135	3	
Medical records science I	MR-101	1	1		45	2	
Basic allied sciences I (mathematics, biology, physics and chemistry)	AS-101	3	1		75	4	
Hospital information I (general statistics)	HI-101	1	1	–	45	2	
Anatomy and physiology I	AP-101	1	1		45	2	
Healthcare delivery I	HD-101	2	-	–	30	2	
Information technology (computer science) I	IT-101	1	1	–	45	2	
Total		**12**	**5**		**420**	**17**	

SECOND SEMESTER							
Subject	*Code*	*Lectures*	*Lab*	*Practical*	*Total hr.*	*Credit hrs.*	*Prerequisite*
English language II (pre-requisite)	EL-102	1		–	45	1	
Medical record science II	MR-102	2	2	2	180	6	MR-101
Basic allied sciences II (pathology, biochemistry, microbiology, radio-diagnosis, forensic medicine, pharmacology sociology, psychology, health education)	AS-102	3			45	3	
Hospital information II (hospital statistics)	HI-102	1	1		45	2	HI-I01
Anatomy and physiology II	AP-102	1	1		45	2	
Medical terminology I	MT-102	1	1		45	2	AP-I01
Total		**9**	**5**	**2**	**405**	**16**	

THIRD SEMESTER							
Subject	*Code*	*Lectures*	*Lab*	*Practical*	*Total hr.*	*Credit hrs.*	*Prerequisite*
Medical records science III	MR-201	1	2	3	210	6	MR-102
Organization and management-II business administration and principles of economics	OM-201	2			30	2	
Medical terminology II	MT-201	2	2		90	4	MT-102
Information technology (computer science II	IT-201	1	2		75	3	IT-101
Classification and indexing methods of diseases and procedures -I	CI-201	1			15	1	AP-101
Total		**7**	**6**	**3**	**420**	**16**	

FOURTH SEMESTER

Subject	*Code*	*Lectures*	*Lab*	*Practical*	*Total hr.*	*Credit hrs.*	*Prerequisite*
Medical records science IV	MR-202	1	2		75	3	MR-201
Classification and indexing methods of diseases and procedures II	CI-202	2	2		90	4	CI-201
Organization and management II (human resource management)	OM-202	2			30	2	
Quality assurance and research methodology	QA-202	2			30	2	
Healthcare delivery II	HD-202	2	–	–	30	2	HD-101
Internship including seminars	IN-202		1	3	165	4	
Total		**9**	**5**	**3**	**420**	**17**	

COURSE DESCRIPTION

S. No	*Subject*	*Code*	*Syllabus*
1.	English language	EL-101	Fundamentals of english language, including grammar.
2.	Health information management (HIM) I	MR-101	History of medical records, concept of medical records, role of medical records in health care delivery, development of medical record forms.
3.	Basic allied sciences I	AS-101	Basic mathematics including, algebra, geometry, trigonometry, calculus. Introduction to biology, physics and chemistry.
4.	General statistics and biostatistics I	GS-101	Introduction to general statistics, collection and presentation of data. Central tendency—mean, median, mode, standard deviation, ratios, range, rates.
5.	Anatomy and physiology I	AP-101	Fundamentals of anatomy and physiology—to develop understanding of the clinical knowledge through study of the structure and function of the healthy human body. cell, skeletal system, muscular system, respiratory system and digestive system, cardiovascular system.
6.	Healthcare delivery I	HD-101	Structure of health care delivery system, organization and management of primary, secondary and tertiary care health services setup. Payment and reimbursement systems and methodology—DRG assignment. APGs, RBRVs.
7.	Information technology I (computer science)	IT-101	Introduction to the microcomputers, word processing, spreadsheets, presentation of graph, data versus information, database concepts. Basic concepts of development of computer applications (software)–special reference to health information
8.	English language II	El-102	Developing spoken language skills, hints development, letter and essay writing. Advanced communication skills related to health field.
9.	Health information management (HIM) II	MR-102	Medical record standards, general policies, legal aspects of medical records, legislative process, court system, patient rights/advocacy, advance directives, primary versus secondary records, retention procedure, security and confidentiality, release of information. Monitor change in regulations and accreditation standards on release. Retention of patient records

Contd...

COURSE DESCRIPTION *(Contd...)*

S. No	*Subject*	*Code*	*Syllabus*
10.	Basic and allied sciences-II	AS-102	Fundaments of general and clinicalpathology, biochemistry, microbiology, radio-diagnosis, pharmacology, and forensic medicine. Introduction to sociology and psychology. Role of different types of social worker, general psychology—study of the society and the social problems, general and medical ethics, health education. Health and wellness
11.	General statistics and biostatistics I	HI-102	Collection, compilation, analysis and interpretation of routine institutional (hospital) data—outpatient, inpatient, accident and emergency department, morbidity and mortality and vital statistics. Descriptive statistics, methods of presentation of data. Reliability and validity of data, knowledge based/library research technique, data search and access.
12.	Anatomy and physiology II	AP-102	To develop understanding of the clinical knowledge base through study of the structure and function of the healthy human body: Nervous, sensory, genitourinary, reproductive, endocrine, and lymphatic systems.
13.	Medical terminology I	MT-102	History of medical terminology—definitions and constructions of medical terms through analysis of word structure. Prefix, suffix, and roots.
14.	Health information management (HIM) III	MR-201	Organization needs of medical records department—determine equipment and supply needs for the department. Medical record systems—numbering filing, color coding, movement of records, medical record procedures. Methods of developing quality procedures to monitor accuracy of documentation of patient records, coding abstracting and transcription services.
15.	Hospital organization and management I (including business administration, principle of economics and HR)	OM-201	Concept of business administration including principles of economics. Development of department policies for employees operations and conduct, job descriptions. Orient and provide in-service and continuing education, participate in institutional committees/projects principles of human resources management, man power development, job descriptions, duties and responsibilities, professional categories. Assign projects to appropriate personnel, collect and report on employee and their productivity, perform job analysis. Ergonomics. Ergonomics equipment section, marketing HIM services. Utilization and resource management
16.	Medical terminology II	MT-201	Symptoms, diagnostic and operative medical terms related to various systems of human body
17.	Information technology II (computer science)	IT-201	Structured problem solving methods in computer by developing algorithms, flowchart. Developing simple computer application (software) on hospital information system. Coordinate other relevant functions with appropriate departments, creating and handling database inventory of all data components, maintain integrity of patient numbering system. Document imaging, electronic record storage and backup. Concept and development of electronic medical records. Automatic identifications and voice recognition technology.

Contd...

COURSE DESCRIPTION *(Contd...)*			
S. No	*Subject*	*Code*	*Syllabus*
18.	International classification and indexing methods of diseases and procedures I	IC-201	General overview of nomenclature and classification systems with focus on coding, introduction to international classification of diseases-10th revision. Basic CPT coding and outpatient coding. Instructions in coding diagnosis and procedures, sequencing and coding conventions. Review of complications and morbidity.
19.	Health information management (HIM)-IV	MR-202	Organization and management of MRD in primary, secondary, specialty and long term care hospitals. Healthcare data sets, maintaining of registers and indexes. Develop plans, goals and objectives for those you supervise, communicate work-related change, design ergonomically sound work environment, and compare work performances to establish new standards. Clinical critical paths/care or case management accreditation and licensing quality improvement standards.
20.	International classification and indexing methods of diseases and procedures II	CI-202	Advanced classification and indexing methods. Other specialty classification systems ICD-10, ICD-9CM coding, CPT, HCPCSC, SNOMED-CT
21.	Hospital Organization and Management II (hospital departments medial legal ethics, insurance, reimbursement, Consumer Protection Act)	HO-202	Hospital budgeting, finance, health insurance, reimbursement, third party payers, billing, and insurance procedures. Explanation of benefits, peer review organizations, charges master description, managed care/capitation. Introduction to various departments of hospital—hospital administration, medical, nursing, dietary, laboratory, radiology. organization of OP, emergency, IP, OT, ICU, CCU, CCU, ward and units of the hospital and their function, ethics, medical legal, Consumer Protection Act.
22.	Quality assurance and research methodology	QA-202	Introduction to quality assessment and performance improvement and to develop knowledge, skills, attitudes and values needed to coordinate quality and resource management programs. Risk management through investigation, identification, assessment, and analysis. Problem solution. Collect, analyze, prepare and present data using QI tools and designing reports using database report generation. Medical auditing. Participate in institutional QI programs. JCHO Standards. Systematic investigation and study of data and source in order to establish facts with analytical results. Case mix analysis and indexes, severity of illness systems. Data quality.
23	Internship including seminar	IN-202	Clinical and directed practice in different sections of the MRD of different categories of hospital. Electives—undertaking project assignments and presenting seminars and workshops. Supervised clinical experience in performing actual tasks and responsibilities focused on release of information, assembling, analysis, information retention and retrieval, medical transcription, personnel administration, health statistics, coding and abstracting and quality assessment and improvement.

Facilities to be made available: Adequate space for administrative and faculty offices, classrooms, laboratories, equipment, teaching aids, supplies should be made available for diploma in health information management program. Laboratories should be equipped with adequate space for effective demonstration of Health Record Systems to provide opportunities for student's participation in skill learning and group projects. There should be well equipped library facilities in the institute of health information management should be made available in addition to online library facilities.

The whole atmosphere of the HIM program should be conducive for learning and lesson preparation and privacy for counseling and dealing with confidential matters.

Faculty: It is strongly suggested to ensure that the number of faculty planned for the program to be always there. In any case, a minimum HIM faculty determined should be available at any time of semester.

Full Time Faculty

- Dean 1
- Assistant professor 1
- Lecturer 2
- Senior clinical instructor 2
- Clinical instructor 1
- Computer instructor 1S
- English language teacher 1 (part time)
- Curriculum assistant developer 1
- Office boy/assistant 2

Guest lecturers: Guest lecturers from medical, surgical, obstetrics, gynecology, pediatrics, and other discipline, nursing, paramedical and administrative departments in case the institute does not have the facilities of the above specialties.

Out of 1200 lecture hours related to medical records, medical terminology and hospital Information, full-time faculty covers around 800 hours and rest 400 hours lectures will be covered by Part-time lectures. The guest lecturers will cover around 50 hours related to other subjects.

Equipment: Besides the space and other furniture, the HIM should be equipped with sophisticated audio-visual equipment, computers with internet facilities, books and periodicals, on-line library connections and office equipment and mock HIM library in order to give lively training to the students.

Diploma in Health Information Management (Sample structure program)

Introduction

Objectives of the course: To develop competent health information management professionals capable of performing the tasks that is prescribed for HIM technicians.

Eligibility for admission: A minimum of higher secondary education (10 + 2) or equivalent qualifications recognized by any Indian or overseas universities and any gender to be eligible, however, he/she should be physically fit and mentally sound to get admitted.

Duration of the course: 2 years including; theory, laboratory and practical classes.

Medium of instruction: English language

Attendance: Minimum of 80% attendance is required to appear any university examination during the period of study, i.e. for each semester period. Or the rules and regulations prescribed for attendance by the university will be applicable.

Suggested subjects, hours in each semester, credit hours in each semester, minimum percentage (%) marks required to be successful in the examination:

S. No	*Subject*	*Total hours of study in each semester*	*Total credits in each semester*	*Total exam marks*	*Minimum passing marks*
1	Anatomy and physiology				
2	Medical terminology				
3	Health information management (HIM)				
4	English language including communication skills				
5	Basic allied health sciences: Clinical pathology, biochemistry, microbiology laboratories, radio-diagnosis, pharmacology and forensic medicine. Blood bank, sociology, psychology and general and medical education, health and wellness				
6	Information technology–computer skills–electronic health records and health systems				
7	International classification of diseases (ICD-10 and ICD-9CM, CPT and SNOMED-CT and other classification systems, etc.				
8	National health care delivery system including public health				
9	Hospital organization and management encompassing, finance, billing, insurance, medical ethics and legal aspects.				
10	General mathematics, biology, physics and chemistry. Introduction to general statistics, and biostatistics				
11	Medical audits, patient care evaluations, quality improvements quality assurance and research methodology				
12	Organization and management business administration, principle of economics				
13	Organization and management human resources management				
14	Special lectures on leadership, motivation, team-building, health economics and patient satisfaction measures and community service				
15	Health information laboratory practices in HIM department				
16	Hospital and health institution internship practice including seminars, workshops, brainstorm sessions, group-discussions and presentations, symposia and conferences.				
17	Overall behavior, attitude, involvement and commitment to the program learning activities				
	Total				

Contd…

COURSE DESCRIPTION

S. No	*Subject*	*Code*	*Syllabus*
1	Anatomy and physiology		**Fundamentals of anatomy and physiology:** To develop understanding of the clinical knowledge through study of the structure and function of the healthy human body. Cell, skeletal system, muscular system, respiratory system and digestive system, cardiovascular system. To develop understanding of the clinical knowledge base through study of the structure and function of the healthy human body: Nervous, sensory, genito-urinary, reproductive, endocrine, and lymphatic systems
2	Medical terminology		**History of medical terminology:** Definitions and constructions of medical terms through analysis of word structure. Prefix, suffix, and roots. Symptoms, diagnostic and operative medical terms related to various systems of human body and related medical abbreviations
3	Health information management (HIM)		History of medical records, concept of medical records, role of medical records in health care delivery, development of medical record forms. Medical record standards, general policies, legal aspects of medical records, legislative process, court system, patient rights/advocacy, advance directives, primary versus secondary records, retention procedure, security and confidentiality, release of information. Monitor change in regulations and accreditation standards, release of information, retention and preservation of patient records organization needs of medical records department—determine equipment and supply needs for the department. Medical record systems—numbering filing, color coding, movement of records, medical record procedures. Methods of developing quality procedures to monitor accuracy of documentation of patient records, coding abstracting and transcription services.
4	English language and communication skills		Fundamentals of english language, including grammar. Various methods of communication systems including oral, written, non-verbal and body language. Reading, speaking, listening, conversation including telephonic skills and developing spoken language skills, hints development, letter and essay writing. Advanced communication skills related to health field.
5	**Basic allied health sciences:** Clinical pathology, biochemistry, microbiology laboratories, radio-diagnosis, pharmacology and forensic medicine. Blood bank, sociology, psychology and general and medical education, health and wellness		Fundaments of general and clinical pathology, biochemistry, microbiology laboratories, radio-diagnosis, pharmacology, and forensic medicine. Blood bank, introduction to sociology and psychology. Role of different types of social worker, general psychology-study of the society and the social problems, general and medical ethics, health education. Health and wellness
6	Information technology–computer skills—electronic health records and eHealth systems		Introduction to the microcomputers, word processing, spreadsheets, presentation of graph. Data versus information. Database concepts. Basic concepts of development of computer applications (software)—special reference to

Contd...

Contd...

S. No	*Subject*	*Code*	*Syllabus*
			health informationstructured problem solving methods in computer by developing algorithms, and flowchart. Developing simple computer application (software) on hospital information system. Coordinate other relevant functions with appropriate departments, creating and handling database inventory of all data components, maintain integrity of patient numbering system. Document imaging, electronic record storage and backup. Concept and development of electronic medical records. Automatic identifications and voice recognition technology
7	International classification of diseases (ICD - 10 and ICD-9CM, CPT and SNOMED-CT and other classification systems, etc.		Advanced classification and indexing methods. Other specialty classification systems including international classification of diseases (ICD -10 and ICD-9CM, CPT and SNOMED-CT and other classification systems, etc. Knowledge and use of built-in automatic computerized coding system
8	National health care delivery system including public health		Structure of health care delivery system, organization and management of primary, secondary and tertiary care health services setup. Public health and environmental heath including communicable diseases, control of epidemics and endemics, and continuing monitoring of morbidity and mortality reports including infant mortality
9	Hospital organization and management encompassing finance, billing, insurance, medical ethics and legal aspects.		Hospital budgeting, finance, health insurance, reimbursement, third party payers, billing, and insurance procedures. Explanation of benefits peer review organizations, charge master description, managed care/capitation. Introduction to various departments of the hospital: Hospital administration, medical, nursing, dietary, laboratory, radiology. Payment and reimbursement systems and methodology drg assignment. Need to have clear policies dealing with legal issues in general and electronic health records in particular; information generated by computer system including privacy, security and confidentiality and data exchange and release of information to authorized and so, on. Principles of law applied to the health field with emphasis on central, state and local laws; automated information acceptance and computer generated signature acceptance in the court of law, etc.
10	General mathematics, biology, physics and chemistry. Introduction to general statistics, and biostatistics		Basic mathematics including, algebra, geometry, trigonometry, calculus. Introduction to biology, physics and chemistry. Introduction to general statistics, collection and presentation of data. central tendency—mean, median, mode, standard deviation, ratios, range, rates collection, compilation, analysis and interpretation of routine institutional (hospital) data—outpatient, inpatient, accident andemergency department, morbidity and mortality and vital statistics. Descriptive statistics, methods of presentation of data. Reliability and validity of data, knowledge based/library research technique, data search and access

Contd...

Contd...

S. No	Subject	Code	Syllabus
11	Medical audits, patient care evaluations, quality improvements quality assurance and research methodology		Introduction to quality assessment and performance improvement and to develop knowledge, skills, attitudes and values needed to coordinate quality and resource management programs. Risk management through investigation, identification, assessment, and analysis. Problem solution. Collect, analyze, prepare and present data using QI tools and designing reports using database report generation. Medical auditing. Participate in institutional QI programs. JCHO standards. Systematic investigation and study of data and source in order to establish facts with analytical results. Case mix analysis and indexes, severity of illness systems. Data quality.
12	Organization and management business administration, principle of economics		Concept of business administration including principles of economics. Development of department policies for employees operations and conduct, job descriptions. Orient and provide in-service and continuing education, participate in institutional committees/projects
13	Organization and management human resources management		Principles of human resources management, man power development, job descriptions, duties and responsibilities, professional categories. Assign projects to appropriate personnel, collect and report on employee and their productivity, perform job analysis. Ergonomics. Ergonomics equipment section, marketing HIM services, utilization and resource management
14	Special lectures on leadership, motivation, team building, health economics, patient satisfaction measures and community service		Expert speakers on the following subjects to be invited in accordance with the scheduled program. The students should be asked to do their homework to actively participate in the deliberations to gain adequate knowledge, skills and positive attitude. Topics to be covered are: Leadership, motivation, team-building, health economics, patient satisfaction and community service
15	Health information laboratory practices in HIM department		HIM department should develop a mock-laboratory with all the practical experience "Hands-on" on HIM functions. HIM students prior to expose to the hospital or HIM departments will have an understanding the type of work is being carried out by HIM department. This experience makes them more confident in understanding the virtual working system with getting clarification/answers to their doubtful queries. There are many institutions does not have adequate and well established HIM departments. This mock laboratory facility would be a great boon to the institution and to the students.
16	Hospital and health institution internship practice including seminars, workshops, brainstorm sessions, group-discussions and presentations, symposia and conferences		Clinical and directed practice in different sections of the MRD/HIM department of different categories of hospitals. Electives—undertaking project assignments and presenting seminars and workshops. Supervised clinical experience in performing actual tasks and responsibilities focused on release of information, assembling, analysis, information retention and retrieval, medical transcription, personnel

Contd...

Contd...

S. No	*Subject*	*Code*	*Syllabus*
			administration, health statistics, coding and abstracting and quality assessment and improvement. Periodical seminars, brainstorming sessions, workshops, group-discussions and presentation and participating in conferences will benefit enormously
17	Overall behavior, attitude, involvement and commitment to the program in learning activities		There should be a mechanism of to recording behavior, attitude, involvement and commitment to the program in learning activities by student. The faculty should develop a mechanism with the cooperation and coordination of different faculty members and the students to determine criteria as to measure in one to ten scales or any other appropriate method so as to get near to accurate valuation without any personal bias. The objective of this process is to address promptly, if there is any problem or deviation from normal ways so that required counseling or any other corrective action can be taken instantly

Chapter 11

Bachelor's Degree in Health Information Management

INTRODUCTION

The healthcare industry continues to evolve in the midst of great change. Changes caused by patient demographics, spiraling costs, and advancement in technology present substantial challenges to healthcare industry. There is widespread adoption of interoperable electronic health records in the technologically advanced countries. Many countries are contemplating to implement electronic health records in their health institutions. In the next 10 years entire world be moving towards implementing the electronic health records and the demand for Health Information Management (HIM) professionals will grow dramatically. Better and more effective use of information promises to make the healthcare system more effective. The ability to organize and turn data into information and knowledge includes being able to determine who needs what information, when and where; how information is defined; how information accuracy and consistency is verified; and how information is explained. The need for more information and better data requires a concentrated movement toward processes that place value on how the data is defined, understood, analyzed, and interpreted.

Health information management is a vital field for the healthcare institutions to manage efficiently. The HIM professionals are managers: Experts in processing, analyzing and reporting information vital to the health care industry, respected staff members who interact daily with the clinical and administrative staff, all of whom depend on health information to perform their jobs. HIM professionals have a tremendous role in initiating and maintaining documentation in manual or electronic that will support in the clinical care, e.g. to be precise, efficient patient care, helps the physician in his clinical management, hospital depends on health information to monitor performance of all the professionals quantitatively and qualitatively, the national health or public health depends on controlling morbidity and mortality and eradicate the communicable disease. The International Organization such as the World Health Organization too depends on national health information. The medical record is the mother of health information.

Health Information Management (HIM) professionals play a key role in the design, development and management of health information within interconnected, community-wide health data exchanges and regional networks which are vital foundations of a national health information network. HIM professionals at the graduate levels of the academic framework reflect core knowledge in health information management coupled with applied informatics skill sets to ensure quality health information and system interoperability for all healthcare settings and organizations that create and use it.

The e-HIM vision for the future statement emphasizes that core HIM function become more crucial as healthcare moves further into the information age.

Health information management is the body of knowledge and practice that assures the availability of health information to facilitate to real-time healthcare delivery and critical health-related decision making for multiple purposes across diverse organizations, settings, and disciplines.

Dramatic change in health information management demands new thinking, about how we educate tomorrow's professionals. Redefining roles, competencies, and educational progression should be the foundation of College of HIM Education. When tomorrow's graduates enter the HIM workplace, they will be ready for the e-HIM environment.

II. Program Vision

To provide adequate fitting HIM professionals who can contribute effectively and meet the needs of ever changing healthcare system of the nation in the 21 century.

III. Program Mission

The mission of bachelor's degree curriculum in HIM is to prepare confident, innovative and contributing professionals who can design, identify and use a variety of information resources and technologies to accomplish the information management objectives of diverse practice environment.

Educate adequate highly qualified HIM professionals to meet the national requirements in providing effective health care delivery to the citizens and residents of India.

The goal: The goal is to prepare a bachelor's degree curriculum in HIM program under able faculty, to generate confident, innovative and contributing professionals who can design identify and use a variety of information resources and technologies to accomplish the information management objectives of diverse practice environments that benefit community through healthcare institutions.

IV. Objectives

The objective is to develop curriculum that would meet the HIM professional who after successfully completing the bachelor's degree in HIM should be able to:

- Endow with knowledge and skills necessary to become self-directed learners.
- Solve problems by critical thinking
- Attain informatics skills, communication and interpersonal skills.
- Instill a commitment to life-long learning, and important ethical values.
- Foster the acquisition of leadership abilities.
- Adapt careers within changing healthcare environment.
- Serve society and the profession through collaborative practice.
- Provide innovative teaching by generating and application of new knowledge
- Conduct research devoted to HIM in an electronic environment
- Carry-out activities that are focused on evolving the strategic and operational relevance and robustness of clinical information resources of healthcare industry and public health sector.

- Participate actively in quality and performance improvement management
- Collaborate and cooperate with Information Technology department in developing electronic health records

V. Role of HIM Bachelors' Degree Graduates

The individual holding a bachelors' degree in health information management is engaged in executive level, enterprise-wide administrative, research activities. These activities are focused on evolving the strategic and operational relevance and robustness of clinical information resources of the healthcare industry and public health sectors. Graduates may perform research that advances the body of knowledge and standards associated with the management of health information in electronic health environment. Suggested roles for graduates may include:

- Academic faculty
- Applied health information researcher
- Chief executive officer
- Chief information officer
- Chief compliance officer
- Chief privacy officer
- Corporate health information manager/officer
- Data analytics/data mining engineer
- Data sets, nomenclature and classification standards developer
- Health information applications developer
- Health information management specialized practice consultant
- Public health information officer

VI. Student Population

The curriculum should be designed to attract individuals from a verity of educational backgrounds and disciplines. These back ground and disciplines may include individuals with prior coursework at an undergraduate level in HIM or those with a baccalaureate or advanced degrees in another area of study. Students who do not have a prior background in HIM may need to take additional prerequisite and/or requisite course content as defined by the academic program in line with the goals of the program and expertise of the faculty. Providing identified curriculum pathways with prerequisites and required courses based on entering students' education, experience and skill sets, will assist with appropriate student advisement and guidance in their career direction.

The program of study should meet established qualifications and educational standards. However, it is imperative that the graduate program clearly state that focus of the program in all marketing literature so that the incoming student is made aware of the nature of the program to which they are applying. The program must also meet 'best practice' criteria as established by University College or institute.

Several factors make approval valuable including

1. Identified for the public specialized programs at the bachelor's level that meet established standards of educational quality.
2. Stimulates improvement of educational standards by involving faculty and staff in self-evaluation and planning.
3. Promotes a better understanding of the goals of health information management at the graduate level.

4. Allows students in approved bachelor's level programs to quality for student membership in the professional association as stipulated in the AHIMA by laws.
5. Assist graduate programs in achieving their objectives.

Program Mission and Goals

A. The HIM program is established as a core concentration or specialized track within graduate level program of study; culminates with bachelor's degree.

The HIM graduate program is design in concert with the institutional mission and the goals of the college division or department in which it is located.

A program evaluation plan exists for systematic evaluation of the mission, goals and objectives of the HIM program.

The program uses the results of evaluation and assessment to identify improvements and to modify program objectives.

Expectation of future postgraduates in supporting future healthcare: HIM professionals have a varieties scope to work besides the hospitals and health institutions. They work for accounting firms, insurance companies, information systems vendors, government agencies, pharmaceutical research companies, and others. Wide varieties of employers actively recruit health information managers. According to the department of labor, employment opportunities for Health Information Management (HIM) professionals continue to grow much faster that the average for all occupations. They may look for career choices not only in acute-care settings, but in all types of alternative care settings, as well as in education, business, and legal settings. Services provided in these areas range from technical to administrative, with emphasis being placed on the latter. As a vital member of the healthcare team, the health information manager is responsible for managing health information systems. This professional plans and develops health information systems that meet standards of accrediting and regulatory agencies. They also design health information systems appropriate for various sizes and types of healthcare facilities. A postgraduate serves as an advocate for privacy and confidentiality of health information and plans and offers in service educational programs for healthcare personnel.

There are multiple job opportunities available to HIM graduates. The job opportunities are not limited to the following settings:

Traditional settings		
S. No	*Job positions*	*Job responsibilities*
1	Management, HIM (medical records)	Responsible for the day-to-day operations of an HIM department, maintains a budget, oversees staff, and interacts with other hospital departments, plans for the department
2	Tumor registry	Reviews, abstracts, and codes clinical cancer information in order to comply with government regulations. Maintains a database. Also provides data for physicians and research studies
3	Coding	Reviews medical documentation and assigns appropriate diagnosis and/or procedure codes in order for billing to occur
4	Trauma registry (ER)	Collects, codes, and maintains data unique to trauma registry, maintains a database. Assists with research projects, performance improvement, and administrative planning
5	Transcription	Responsible for providing accurate and timely reports for patient care, documentation and billing

Contd...

Traditional settings *(Contd...)*		
S. No	*Job positions*	*Job responsibilities*
6	Quality improvement	Collect and summarize performance data, identify opportunities for improvement, and present data to other clinicians and administrative staff
7	Release of information	Track, process, and evaluate requests for release of medical information. Requires knowledge of central and state laws and regulations
8	Patient admissions	Responsible for patient admission, insurance verification, database maintenance. Oversees a staff, maintains a budget, and communicates with other hospital departments
9	Compliance auditor	Responsible for conducting chart audits, preparing reports, and reporting data. Also, develops policies and procedures for staff training
10	Physician accreditation	Maintains databases with physician information in order to provide data to administrative staff for physician accreditation.
11	Risk management	Collects, evaluates, and maintains data concerning patient injuries, claims, worker's compensation, etc. Reports data to administrative staff and makes changes to policies and procedures as needed
12	Physician offices	Manages day-to-day operations of a physician office, including scheduling, billing, staffing, budgeting, and record keeping, and reporting
13	Utilization review	Works closely with clinicians to analyze patient records in order to determine admission criteria and use of resources for length of stay. Must be knowledgeable of insurance requirements

Non-traditional settings		
1	Government agencies	Possible job opportunities involve working with state and central government agencies
2	Law firms	Provide HIM expertise to areas within health law, central and state regulations concerning health care
3	Correctional facilities	Maintain health records, perform quality reviews and assist in research studies
4	Insurance companies	Work with various providers in order to negotiate contracts, assist clients with claims
5	Extended care facilities	Maintain health records to provide a continuum of care, comply with central and state regulations, conduct quality reviews, and maintain accreditation requirements
6	Consulting firms	Works with various clients to provide HIM expertise
7	Information technology system analyst project manager data manager	Works with software vendors to design clinical software, provides training to end-user staff, assists with system installations, provides system support
8	Medical software companies software designer software tester	Designs and develops databases, performs various software testing, assists clients with system installations
10	Pharmaceutical research statistician, clinical trials coordinator, data manager	Provides data management services in order to meet customer needs. Manages projects, staff, and timelines.

VII. Curriculum

1. Health data management (HDM)
   - Health date structure, content and standards
   - Healthcare information requirement and standards
   - Clinical classification
   - Reimbursement methodologies
2. Health statistics, biomedical research and quality management
   - Healthcare statistics and research
   - Quality management and performance improvement
3. Domain—health services organization and delivery
   - Healthcare delivery
   - Healthcare privacy, confidentiality, legal, and ethical
4. Domain—information technology and systems
   - Information and communication technologies
   - Data information and file structure
   - Data storage and retrieval
   - Data security
   - Healthcare information system
5. Domain—organization and management
   - Human resource management
   - Financial and resource management
   - Strategic planning and organization development
   - Project and operation management

VIII. Faculty

There should be full time professionally qualified faculty supported by part-time and guest lecturers to provide quality teaching, advisement, research and service, as reflected in the college mission.

The Minimum Required Faculty

Full time faculty

1. Professor of HIM—1
2. Assistant professors (HIM-1, IT-1)—2
3. Assistant professor-IT—1
4. Clinical instructor or demonstrators—2
5. Secretary—1
6. Administrator—1

Part-time faculty

1. Health information statistics—1
2. Healthcare organization and management—1

Guest lecturers

There should be guest lecturers from medical, surgical, obstetrics, gynecology, pediatrics and other discipline, nursing, paramedical and administrative departments.

Solution to Solve the Faculty Requirements

Student Support and Advices

Prerequisites

- Program ensures that students maintain an awareness of academic and career opportunities through advising and mentoring by faculty and preceptors.
- Career paths of graduates are monitored, documented and used in program evaluation.
- Instructional resources, technology, reference/library resources needed to fulfill the requirements of the curriculum, are available and accessible to all students.
- The sponsoring educational institutions support for the program and the financial resources available to the program are sufficient to provide an environment in which the program can achieve its objectives.
- Program leadership has authority commensurate with responsibility for program management can achieve evaluation.
- The program maintains sufficient relationships with a variety of health related organizations and agencies to support its teaching, research and service goals.

IX. Scope of Application for Bachelor's Degree

In view of huge demand for health information management professionals throughout globe in general and India in particular, there would be many applicants for admissions, not only from within the country but also from other neighboring countries. There would be high demand for admissions; hence, we have to make provision to accommodate and rendering service to other sister countries.

X. Duration

The course is of four years includes one year practical. The course will consist of six semesters and one year practical which includes project work too, the first from September, and second from February as per the university program.

XI. Commencement of the Course

First or second week of September, every year.

XII. Number of Admissions

Principally, depends on the infrastructure and facilities, initially, a total of 30 to 40 candidates, male and female candidates could be admitted every year. If the demand is more, the intake could be increased gradually.

XIII. Pre-requisites

The bachelor's degree level of Health Information Management education acknowledges that certain prerequisite and requisite course work may be necessary to support advanced course content that institutional prerogatives must be considered in implementing any academic curriculum. The model serves as guide while supporting the individuality of program curriculum design and implementation.

XIV. Selection Procedure

Applications to the course will be invited by the college as done in other courses. An ad hoc selection committee will have to select the candidates purely on merit basis as per the criteria laid down. If the demand from other countries increases, appropriate selection criteria have to be developed and followed.

Evaluation: Continuous periodical written tests will be conducted in each subject monthly or in each chapter of study. Assignments, research work, project work and performance in seminars, *viva voce* will have greater impact in the evaluation process. At the end of each semester, final written tests, followed by lab/practical assignment evaluation will be carried out.

a. Credits: The credit ratios are set at:

15 hours theory = 1 credit

30 hours laboratory = 1 credit

45 hours directed practice at the hospital = 1 credit

b. Grade points:

Grade	*Percentage of marks*	*Reported as*	*Points*
A	>90% (>95% = A +; >90% = A)	Excellent	4
B	>80% (>85% = B +; >80% = B)	Verygood	3
C	>70% (>75% = C +; >70% = C)	Good	2
D	>60% (>65% = D +; >60% = D)	Pass	1
E	<60%	Fail	0

c. Grade points are calculated as follows

Grade points = Credit hours × points

d. Grade point average is calculated as follows

Total grade points earned

Total credits attempted

e. Pass

A candidate will be deemed to have been passed in each subject, if he secures not less than 50% internal and as well as external examinations with an aggregate of not less than 60%.

The internal assessment marks are based on overall performance of the candidates in theoretical and practical assessment.

f. Location of the program

All theoretical classes and laboratory will be conducted at the college site, directed professional practice; project work, etc. will be carried out at different hospitals/health institution sites.

Attendance: Each candidate should put in attendance at least of 85%.

Discipline: Each candidate shall observe discipline according to rules and regulations laid down by the department of HIM or university. Any violation of discipline the candidate may run the risk of removal from the program.

Eligibility for admission:

Pass in any 10 + 2 or equivalent program with minimum aggregate of 50% marks in any science/commerce/arts/group.

Provision for lateral entry or direct entry

The lateral or direct entry for diploma in HIM with 50% of aggregate marks, are eligible. They are eligible for lateral entry to third semester. Those who have completed 6 months of internship only are eligible for lateral entry.

Selection procedure

Admission to Bachelor's degree in HIM (Health Information Management) course shall be made on the basis of eligibility and an entrance test to be conducted for the purpose. No candidate will be admitted on any ground unless he/she has appeared in the admission test and interview.

Successful candidates on the basis of written test will be called for the interview and shall have faced an interview board. The interview board will include the Head of the Department of Health Information Management and Head of the Institution, or anyone who is nominated for the purpose, whose recommendations shall be final for selection of students.

Students will be given counseling and seats will be allotted as per the merit of the candidates. All the selected candidates have to undergo medical examination on the notified dates. The college rules prescribed for the purpose of admission and their minimum attendance required will be applicable.

Duration of the course

The duration of certified study of the bachelor's degree in HIM course shall extend over a period of 4 (two) academic years/8 semesters including 7th and 8th semester will be allotted for practical and projects.

Medium of instruction

English shall be the medium of instruction for all the subjects of study and for examination of the course.

- Assessment
- Marks qualifying for a pass

A candidate shall be declared to have passed the examination if he or she obtains the following qualifying marks: 50% marks in the university examination and 50% marks in internal assessment evaluated by the department with the total aggregate average marks of 60%.

Practical examination and 50% aggregate in practical and 50% internal evaluation marks evaluated by the department with the total aggregate average marks of 60%.

Evaluation and crading system criteria

Evaluation and grading (manual relative grading) of students shall be based on GPA (grade point average) and CGPA (cumulative grade point average).

4-YEAR DEGREE IN HEALTH INFORMATION MANAGEMENT (HIM)

SEMESTER 1						
Subject	*Code*	*Lectures*	*Lab*	*Practical*	*Total hr.*	*Credit hrs. prerequisite*
English language and communication skills	ELC-101	1	2		75	3
Anatomy and physiology	AP-101	1	1		45	2
Medical terminology	MT-101	1	1		45	2

Contd...

SEMESTER 1 *(Contd…)*						
Subject	*Code*	*Lectures*	*Lab*	*Practical*	*Total hr.*	*Credit hrs. prerequisite*
Health care delivery system (pH and community healthcare)	HCD-101	2			30	2
Basic allied health sciences (mathematics, introduction to biology, physics, chemistry	AHS-101	3	1		75	4
Health information management (HIM)-I (medical law and ethics)	HIM-101	1	1		45	2
Information technology (basic computers)	IT-101	1	1		45	2
Total		**10**	**7**		**360**	**17**

SEMESTER 2						
Subject	*Code*	*Lectures*	*Lab*	*Practical*	*Total hr*	*Credit hrs prerequisite*
English language and communication skills	ELC-102	1	2		75	3
Anatomy and physiology	AP-102	1	1		45	2
Medical terminology	MT-102	1	1		45	2
Basic allied health sciences (pathology, biochemistry, microbiology, radio-diagnosis, forensic medicine, pharmacology sociology, psychology, health education)	AHS-102	4			60	4
General statistics and biostatistics and research methodology	GSB-102	1	2		75	3
Health information management (HIM)-II	HIM-102	1	1		45	2
IT (computer applications, database management system)	IT-102	1	1		45	2
Total		**10**	**8**		**360**	**18**

SEMESTER 3						
Subject	*Code*	*Lectures*	*Lab*	*Practical*	*Total hr*	*Credit hrs Prerequisite*
Hospital organization and management—introduction to various departments of hospital	HOM-201	3			45	3
International classification and indexing methods of diseases and procedures I	ICD-201	2	3		120	5
Quality assurance and quality management, research and performance management	QAR-201	2			30	2
Health information management III MR, quality management, medical legal	HIM-201	1	2		75	3
Information technology	IT-201	1	2		75	3
General statistics and biostatistics	GSB-102	1	1		45	2
Total		**10**	**8**		**390**	**18**

Contd…

SEMESTER 4 *(Contd...)*						
Subject	*Code*	*Lectures*	*Lab*	*Practical*	*Total hr*	*Credit hrs prerequisite*
Hospital organization and management-medical law and ethics, consumer protect act; healthcare policies and standards	HOM-202	3			45	3
Overview of health data management	HDM-202	2	2		90	4
Hospital information system (HIS) electronic health records	HIS-202	2	2		90	4
Health information management-IV	HIM-202	1	2		75	3
Principles of organizing and management-POM-1 (HR management, financial and resource management	POM-202	3	1		75	4
Total		**11**	**7**		**375**	**18**

SEMESTER 5						
Subject	*Code*	*Lectures*	*Lab*	*Practical*	*Total hr*	*Credit hrs prerequisite*
Health date management (HDM)-health data structure, content and standards	HDM-301	2	2		90	4
HDM-healthcare information requirements and standards	HDM-301	1	1		45	2
HDM-clinical classification systems	HDM-301	2	2		90	4
Reimbursement methodologies	RM-301	1	1		15	1
IT systems—information and communication technologies	ITS-301	1	1		45	2
IT systems-data, information, file structures, data storage and retrieval, data security, and healthcare information systems	ITS-301	1	1		45	2
HIM (healthcare privacy, confidentiality, legal, and ethical issues)	HIM-301	1	1		45	2
Total		**9**	**9**		**375**	**17**

SEMESTER 6						
Subject	*Code*	*Lectures*	*Lab*	*Practical*	*Total hr.*	*Credit hrs. prerequisite*
GS-biostatistics (healthcare statistics, biomedical research)	GSB-302	2	2		90	4
Quality assurance and quality management and performance improvement	QAR-302	2	2		90	4
Healthcare delivery systems–HCD-II	HCD-302	2			30	2
Health information management (HIM)-medical transcription, telemedicine, application of HIM in non-traditional settings	HIM-302	2	1		60	3

Contd...

SEMESTER 6 (*Contd...*)						
Subject	*Code*	*Lectures*	*Lab*	*Practical*	*Total hr.*	*Credit hrs. prerequisite*
Principles of organizing and management (POM) II (strategic planning and organizational development, project and operation management	POM-302	3	1		60	3
Total		**11**	**6**			**17**

SEMESTER 7						
Subject	*Code*	*Lectures*	*Lab*	*Practical*	*Total hr*	*Credit hrs prerequisite*
Practical training at hospitals						
Total						

SEMESTER 8						
Subject	*Code*	*Lectures*	*Lab*	*Practical*	*Total hr.*	*Credit hrs. prerequisite*
Project for implementation and improvement						
Total						

HIM BACCALAUREATE DEGREE COURSE CONTENT	
Subject	*Syllabus*
Anatomy and physiology	Fundamentals of anatomy and physiology—to develop understanding of the clinical knowledge through study of the structure and function of the healthy human body. Cell, skeletal system, muscular system, respiratory system and digestive system, cardiovascular system. To develop understanding of the clinical knowledge base through study of the structure and function of the healthy human body—nervous, sensory, genito-urinary, reproductive, endocrine, and lymphatic systems
Medical terminology	History of medical terminology—definitions and constructions of medical terms through analysis of word structure. Prefix, suffix, and roots. symptoms, diagnostic and operative medical terms related to various systems of human body and related medical abbreviations
Health information management (HIM)	History of medical records, concept of medical records, role of medical records in healthcare delivery, development of medical record forms. Medical record standards, general policies, legal aspects of medical records, legislative process, court system, patient rights/advocacy, advance directives, primary versus secondary records, retention procedure, security and confidentiality, release of information. Monitor change in regulations and accreditation standards, release of information, retention and preservation

Contd...

HIM BACCALAUREATE DEGREE COURSE CONTENT *(Contd...)*

Subject	*Syllabus*
	of patient records organization needs of medical records department—determine equipment and supply needs for the department. Medical record systems—numbering filing, color coding, movement of records, medical record procedures. Methods of developing quality procedures to monitor accuracy of documentation of patient records, coding abstracting and transcription services
English language andcommunication skills	Fundamentals of English language, including grammar. Various methods of communication systems including oral, written, non-verbal and body language. Reading, speaking, listening, conversation including telephonic skills and developing spoken language skills, hints development, letter and essay writing. Advanced communication skills related to health field
Basic allied health sciences—clinical pathology, biochemistry, microbiology laboratories, radio-diagnosis, pharmacology and forensic medicine. Blood bank, sociology, psychology and general and medical education, health and wellness	Fundaments of general and clinical pathology, biochemistry, microbiology laboratories, radio-diagnosis, pharmacology, and forensic medicine. Blood bank, introduction to sociology and psychology. Role of different types of social worker, general psychology—study of the society and the social problems, general and medical ethics, health education. Health and wellness
Information technology—computer skills—electronic health records and eHealth systems	Introduction to the microcomputers, microsoft word (basics, formatting, tables, page design, mail merges and creating documents), MS-PowerPoint (toolbars, drawing palette, working with slides), MS-Excel (introduction cell formatting, charts and graphic objects, database, pivot table, data validation, dynamic data range and controls, file protection, what if analysis and templates), presentation of graph. Data versus information. Database concepts. Basic concepts of development of computer applications (software)—special reference to health information structured problem solving methods in computer by developing algorithms, and flowchart. Developing simple computer application (software) on hospital information system. Coordinate other relevant functions with appropriate departments, creating and handling database inventory of all data components, maintain integrity of patient numbering system. Document imaging, electronic record storage and backup. Concept and development of electronic medical records. Automatic identifications and voice recognition technology
International classification of diseases (ICD-10 and ICD-9CM, CPT and SNOMED-CT and other classification systems, etc.	Advanced classification and indexing methods. Other specialty classification systems including international classification of diseases (ICD-10 and ICD-9CM, CPT and SNOMED-CT (and other classification systems, etc.) Knowledge and use of built-in automatic computerized coding system

Contd...

HIM BACCALAUREATE DEGREE COURSE CONTENT *(Contd...)*	
Subject	*Syllabus*
General statistics and bio-statistics	Advanced statistical techniques building on existing knowledge of descriptive statistics and fundamental inferential statistics as applied in the field of health information; biostatistics, methods of health data collection, analysis, and interpretation, including descriptive statistics, probability, and hypothesis—testing and confidence interval estimation for normally distributed data; tools in using data to make informed management decisions; use of data from clinical information systems in performing clinical effectiveness research, including the strengths and limitations of these data
HOM—medical law and ethics, consumer act, health care policies and standards	History and development—various code of ethics in medical and medical records practice—atreya anushasana, charaka samhita, sushruta samhita, Hippocratic oath, international code of medical ethics, code of ethics for biomedical research, code of conduct for halth information professionals. Genetics, right to life, sex pre-selection, female feticide and infanticide, care of terminally ill patient, euthanasia, quality of life. Malpractice and negligence, irrational use of drug, autonomy of patient vs paternalism, informed consent, confidentiality, sophisticated drug and technology, research, clinical trial, human experimentation, organ transplantation. Right to health, health policy, distributive justice in health care. Medico-legal case—definition, types, handling medico-legal case in hospital. Regulatory framework in Indian context—Indian Penal Code, Consumer Protection Act.
Hospital organization and management encompassing finance, billing, insurance, medical ethics and legal aspects	Hospital budgeting, finance, health insurance, reimbursement, third party payers, billing, and insurance procedures. Explanation of benefits peer review organizations, charge master description, managed care/capitation. Introduction to various departments of hospital. Hospital administration, medical, nursing, dietary, laboratory, radiology. Payment and reimbursement systems and methodology—DRG assignment. Need to have clear policies dealing with legal issues in general and electronic health records in particular; information generated by computer system including privacy, security and confidentiality and data exchange and release of information to authorized and so son. Principles of law applied to the health field with emphasis on central, state and local laws; automated information acceptance and computer generated signature acceptance in the court of law, etc.
General mathematics, biology, physics and chemistry. Introduction to general statistics, and biostatistics	Basic mathematics including, algebra, geometry, trigonometry, calculus. Introduction to biology, physics and chemistry. Introduction to general statistics, collection and presentation of data. Central tendency—mean, median, mode, standard deviation, ratios, range, rates collection, compilation, analysis and interpretation of routine

Contd...

HIM BACCALAUREATE DEGREE COURSE CONTENT *(Contd...)*

Subject	*Syllabus*
	institutional (hospital) data—outpatient, inpatient, accident and emergency department, morbidity and mortality and vital statistics. Descriptive statistics, methods of presentation of data. Reliability and validity of data, knowledge based/ library research technique, data search and access.
Medical audits, patient care evaluations, quality improvements quality assurance and research methodology	Introduction to quality assessment and performance improvement and to develop knowledge, skills, attitudes and values needed to coordinate quality and resource management programs. Risk management through investigation, identification, assessment, and analysis. Problem solution. Collect, analyze, prepare and present data using QI tools and designing reports using database report generation. Medical Auditing. Participate in institutional QI programs. JCHO standards. Systematic investigation and study of data and source in order to establish facts with analytical results. Case mix analysis and indexes, severity of illness systems. Data quality.
Organization and management business administration, principle of economics	Concept of business administration including principles of economics. Development of department policies for employees operations and conduct, job descriptions. Orient and provide in-service and continuing education, participate in institutional committees/projects
Organization and management human resources management	Principles of human resources management, man power development, job descriptions, duties and responsibilities, professional categories. Assign projects to appropriate personnel, collect and report on employee and their productivity, perform job analysis. Ergonomics. Ergonomics equipment section, marketing HIM services. Utilization and resource management.
Special lectures on leadership, motivation, team building, health economics, patient satisfaction measures and community service	Expert speakers on the following subjects to be invited in accordance with the scheduled program. The students should be asked to do their homework to actively participate in the deliberations to gain adequate knowledge, skills and positive attitude. Topics to be covered are: Leadership, motivation, team-building, health economics, patient satisfaction and community service
Health information laboratory practices in HIM department	HIM department should develop a mock-laboratory with all the practical experience "Hands-on" on HIM functions. HIM students prior to expose to the hospital or HIM departments will have an understanding the type of work is being carried out by HIM department. This experience makes them more confident in understanding the virtual working system with getting clarification/answers to their doubtful queries. There are many institutions does not have adequate and well established HIM departments. This mock laboratory facility would be a great boon to the institution and to the students.

Contd...

HIM BACCALAUREATE DEGREE COURSE CONTENT *(Contd...)*	
Subject	*Syllabus*
Hospital and health institution internship practice including seminars, workshops, brainstorm sessions, group-discussions and presentations, symposia and conferences,	Clinical and directed practice in different sections of the MRD/HIM department of different categories of hospitals. Electives—undertaking project assignments and presenting seminars and workshops. Supervised clinical experience in performing actual tasks and responsibilities focused on release of information, assembling, analysis, information retention and retrieval, medical transcription, personnel administration, health statistics, coding and abstracting and quality assessment and improvement.Periodical seminars, brainstorming sessions, workshops, group-discussions and presentation and participating in conferences will benefit enormously
Overall behavior, attitude, involvement and commitment to the program in learning activities	There should be a mechanism of to recording behavior, attitude, involvement and commitment to the program in learning activities by student. The faculty should develop a mechanism with the cooperation and coordination of different faculty members and the students to determine criteria as to measure in one to ten scales or any other appropriate method so as to get near to accurate valuation without any personal bias.The objective of this process is to address promptly, if there is any problem or deviation from normal ways so that required counseling or any other corrective action can be taken instantly
I. **Domain:** Health data management A. Sub-domain: Health data structure, content and standards 1. Manage health data (such as data elements, data sets and databases). 2. Ensure that documentation in the health record supports the diagnosis and reflects the patient's progress, clinical findings and discharge status. 3. Maintain processes, policies and procedures to ensure the accuracy of coded data. 4. Monitor use of clinical vocabularies and terminologies used in the organization's health information systems.	• Health data structure, content, and standards • Structure and use of health information • Individual, comparative aggregate (5) • Health information media (paper, electronic/computer-based; e-health-personal, web-based) (5) • Type and content of health record (paper, electronic, computer-based e-health personal, web based) (5) • Data quality assessment and integrity (5) • Secondary data sources (registries and indexes; databases—such as MEDPAR, NPDB, HCUP (4) • Health information archival systems (5) • National healthcare information infrastructure (NHII) (5) • Data collection tools (such as forms, computer input screens, other health record documentation tools) (5)
B. Sub-domain: Healthcare information Requirements and standards 1. Develop organization-wide health record documentation guidelines 2. Maintain organizational compliance with regulations and standards. 3. Ensure organizational survey readiness for accreditation licensing and/or certification processes.	Healthcare information requirements and standards and regulations for documentation (such as JCAHO, CARF, COP, AAAHC, AOA) (5) Health information standards (such as HIPAA, ANSI, ASTM, LOINC, UMLS, MESH, Arden Syntax, HL-7) (5)

Contd...

HIM BACCALAUREATE DEGREE COURSE CONTENT *(Contd...)*	
Subject	*Syllabus*
C. Sub-domain: Clinical classification systems 1. Select electronic applications for clinical classification and coding. 2. Two implement and manage applications and processes for clinical classification and coding	**Clinical classification systems:** • Healthcare taxonomies, clinical vocabularies, terminologies/nomenclatures (such as ICD-9-CM, ICD-10, CPT, SNOMED-Ct, DSM-IV 94) • Severity of illness systems (4) • Biomedical sciences • Anatomy (3) • Physiology (3) • Medical terminology (5) • Pathophysiology (4) • Pharmacology (4)
D. Sub-domain: Reimbursement methodologies 1. Manage the use of clinical data required in prospective payment systems (PPS) in healthcare delivery. 2. Manage the use of clinical data required in other reimbursement systems in healthcare delivery. 3. Participate in selection and development of applications and processes for charge master and claims management. 4. Implement and manage processes for compliance and reporting such as the National Correct Coding Initiative.	**Reimbursement methodologies:** • Clinical data and reimbursement management (5) • Compliance strategies and reporting (e.g. national correct coding initiative) (4) • Charge-master management (4) • Casemix management (4) • Audit process such as compliance and reimbursement (5) • Payment systems (such as PPS, DRGs, APCs, RBRVS, RUGs) (4) • Commercial care and federal insurance plans (4)
II. Domain: Health statistics, biomedical research and quality management A. Sub-domain: Healthcare statistics and research 1. Manage clinical indices/databases/registries. 2. Analyze and present data for quality management, utilization management, risk management, and other patient care related studies 3. Utilize statistical software. 4. Ensure adherence to institutional review board (IRB) processes and policies.	**Healthcare statistics, biomedical research and quality management-healthcare statistics and research:** • Statistical analysis on healthcare data (5) • Descriptive statistics (such as means, standard deviations, frequencies, ranges, percentiles) (5) • Inferential statistics (such as t-tests, ANOVAs, regression analysis, statistical process control, reliability, validity) (5) • Vital statistics (5) • Epidemiology (4) • Data reporting and presentation techniques (5) • Computerized statistical packages (5) • Research design/methods (such as quantitative, qualitative, evaluative, outcomes) (5) • Knowledge-based research techniques (such as medline, CMS, libraries, websites) (5) • National guidelines regarding human subjects' research (4) • Institutional review board process (5) • Research protocol data management (4)
B. Sub-domain: Quality management and performance improvement 1. Organize and coordinate facility—wide quality management and performance improvement programs.	**Quality management and performance improvement:** • Quality assessment and management tools (such as benchmarking, ORYX, SQC) (5) • Utilization and resource management (4) • Risk management (4)

Contd...

HIM BACCALAUREATE DEGREE COURSE CONTENT *(Contd...)*	
Subject	*Syllabus*
2. Analyze clinical dat to identify trends. 3. Analyze and present data for healthcare decision-making (such as demonstrating quality, safety and effectiveness of healthcare).	• Disease management process (such as case management, critical paths) (4) • Outcomes measurement (such as patient, customer satisfaction, disease specific) (5)
III. Domain: Health services organization and delivery A. Sub-domain: Healthcare delivery systems 1. Monitor the impact of national health information initiatives on the healthcare delivery system for application to information to system policies and procedures 2. Interpret, communicate, and apply current laws, accreditation, licensure and certification standards related to health information initiatives at the national, state, local and facility levels. 3. Analyze and respond to the information needs of internal and external customers throughout the continuum of healthcare services. 4. Revise policies and procedures to comply with the changing health information regulations. 5. Translate and interpret health information for consumers and their caregivers. B. Sub-dodmain: Healthcare privacy, confidentiality, legal, and ethical issues 1. Coordinate the implementation of legal and regulatory requirements related to the health information infrastructure. 2. Manage access and disclosure of personal health information. 3. Develop and implement organization-wide confidentiality policies and procedures 4. Develop and implant privacy training programs. 5. Resolve privacy issues/problems. 6. Apply and promote ethical standards of practice.	**Health services organization and delivery:** • Organization of healthcare systems (5) • Components and operation of healthcare organizations including e-health delivery (5) • Accreditation standards (such as JCAHO, AOA, NCQA, CARF, CHAP, URAC) (5) • Regulatory and licensure requirements (such as COP, state health departments) (5)
IV. Domain information technology systems	• Healthcare privacy, confidentiality, legal and ethical issues

Contd...

HIM BACCALAUREATE DEGREE COURSE CONTENT *(Contd...)*	
Subject	*Syllabus*
A. Sub-domain: Information and communication technologies 1. Implement and manage use of ensure data collection, storage, technology, including hardware and software, to and analysis and reporting of information. 2. Contribute to the development of networks, including intranet and internet applications to facilitate the electronic health record (PHR), public health, and other administrative applications. 3. Interpret the derivation and use of standards to achieve interoperability of healthcare information systems.	• Legislative and legal system (4) • Privacy, confidentiality, security principles and procedures (5) • Health information laws, regulations, and standards (such as HIPAA, e-health, JCAHO, state laws) (5) • Elements of compliance programs (5) • Professional and practice related ethical issues (5) • Information technology and systems • Computer concepts (hardware components, systems, architectures, operating systems and languages, and software packages and tools) (4) • Communications technologies (networks—LANS, WANS, VPNs; data interchange standards—NIST, HL-7) (4) • Internet technologies (Intranet, WBG-based systems, standards—SGML, XML) (4)
B. Sub-domain: Data, information, and file structures 1. Apply knowledge of data base architecture and design (such as data dictionary, data modeling, data warehousing and so on) to meet or ganizational needs.	**Data, information and file structures (data administration) data:** • Data, information and file structures (data administration, data definitions, data dictionary, data modeling, data structures, data warehousing, database management systems) (5) • Data storage and retrieval (storage media, query tools/ applications, data mining, report design, search engineers) (5) Data security (protection methods-physical, technical, managerial, risk assessment, audit and control program, contingency planning data recovery, Internet, web-based and e-Health security) (5)
C. Sub-domain: Data storage and retrieval 1. Apply appropriate electronic or imaging technology for data/ record storage. 2. Apply knowledge of database querying and data mining techniques to facilitate information retrieval. 3. Implement and manage knowledge-based applications to meet end-user information requirements. 4. Design and generate administrative report using appropriate software D. Sub-domain: Data security 1. Enforce confidentiality and security measures to protect electronic health information. 2. Protect data integrity and validity using software or hardware technology.	

Contd...

HIM BACCALAUREATE DEGREE COURSE CONTENT *(Contd…)*	
Subject	*Syllabus*
3. Implement and monitor department and organizational data and information system security policies. 4. Recommend elements than must be included in the design of audit trail and data quality monitoring programs. 5. Recommend elements that should be included in the design and implementation of risk assessment, contingency planning, and data recovery procedures.	
E. Sub-domain: Healthcare information systems 1. Compared and contrast the various clinical, administrative, and specialty service applications used in healthcare organizations. 2. Apply appropriate systems life cycle concepts, including systems analysis, design implementation, evaluation, and maintenance to selection of healthcare information systems. 3. Facilitate project management by integrating work efforts and planning and executing project tasks and activities. 4. Formulate the planning, design, selection, implementation, integration, testing evaluation and support for organization—wide information systems. 5. Apply ergonomic and human factors in interface design.	**Applied health informatics:** • Leading development of health information resource and systems (4) • Brokering of information services (5) • Clinical, business and specialty system applications administrative, clinical decision support systems, electronic health record and computer-based health record systems, nursing, ancillary service systems, patient numbering systems at master and enterprise levels) (5) • Systems development (planning, analysis and design, customization, selection/procurement, implementation, integration, support, testing and evaluation, auditing and monitoring) (5) • Human factor and user interface design (4) • Systems life cycle (systems analysis, design implementation, evaluation, and maintenance) (5)
V. Domain: Organization and management	**Organization and management:** • Principles of management (5) • Negotiation techniques (4) • Communication and interpersonal skills (5) • Team/consensus building (5) • Professional development for self and staff (4) • Problem solving and decision-making process (5)
A. Sub-domain: Human resource management 1. Manage human resources of acilities staff recruitment, retention, and supervision. 2. Ensure compliance with employment laws. 3. Develop and implement new staff orientation and training programs. 4. Develop and implement continuing education programs.	**Human resources management:** • Employment laws (4) • Principles of human resources management (recruitment, supervision, retention, counseling, disciplinary action) (5) • Workforce education and training (4) • Performance standards (5)

Contd…

HIM BACCALAUREATE DEGREE COURSE CONTENT *(Contd...)*

Subject	*Syllabus*
5. Develop productivity standards for health information functions. 6. Monitor staffing levels and productivity and provide feedback to staff regarding performance. 7. Benchmark staff performance data. 8. Develop, motivate and support work teams.	
B. Sub-domain: Financial and resource Management 1. Demonstrate knowledge of financial management and accountings principles. 2. Prepare and monitor budgets and contracts 3. Demonstrate and apply knowledge of cost-benefit analysis techniques to justify resource needs. 4. Manage organization—wide coding and revenue cycle processes	**Financial and resource management:** • Health finance (payer mix, bond rating, investment, capitalization) (3) • Accounting principles (4) • Budget process (capital and operating) (5) • Cost/benefit analysis (5)
C. Sub-domain: Strategic planning and organizational development 1. Develop strategic and operational plans for facility—wide information systems. 2. Assess organization—wide information needs. 3. Facilitate retrieval, interpretation, and presentation of date/information appropriate to user needs. 4. Demonstrate and apply principles of organization behavior to facilitate team building, negotiation, and change management.	**Strategic planning and organizational development:** • Strategic leadership, management and planning (4) • Organizational behavior (4) • Business building (entrepreneurialism-building your own business; intrapreneurialism—championing best practices, processes, services within your organization) (3) • Change management (4) • Organizational assessment and benchmarking (4)
D. Sub-domain: Project and operations management 1. Apply general principles of management in the administration of health information services. 2. Assign projects and tasks to appropriate staff 3. Implement process engineering and project management techniques to ensure efficient workflow and appropriate outcomes.	**Project operations management:** • Process reengineering and work redesign (4) • Project management (5)

KEY: Learning Competency Levels

1. Awareness—introductory recall and recognition
2. Literacy—knowledge of framework and content
3. Concept—comprehension, translation, extrapolation and interpretation of meaning
4. Detailed understanding—appropriate application of knowledge in a structured or controlled context
5. Skilled use—application using analysis, synthesis, and evaluation in new situations

Chapter 12

Master's Degree in Health Information Management

INTRODUCTION

The healthcare industry continues to evolve in the midst of great change. Changes caused by patient demographics, spiraling costs, and advancement in technology present substantial challenges to healthcare industry. There is widespread adoption of interoperable electronic health records in the technologically advanced countries. Many countries are contemplating to implement electronic health records in their health institutions. In the next ten years entire world be moving towards implementing the electronic health records and the demand for Health Information Management (HIM) professionals will grow dramatically. Better and more effective use of information promises to make the healthcare system more effective. The ability to organize and turn data into information and knowledge includes being able to determine who needs what information, when and where; how information is defined; how information accuracy and consistency is verified; and how information is explained. The need for more information and better data requires a concentrated movement toward processes that place value on how the data is defined, understood, analyzed, and interpreted.

Health information management is a vital field for the healthcare institutions to manage efficiently. The HIM professionals are managers: Experts in processing, analyzing and reporting information vital to the healthcare industry, respected staff members who interact daily with the clinical and administrative staff, all of whom depend on health information to perform their jobs. HIM professionals have a tremendous role in initiating and maintaining documentation in manual or electronic that will support in the clinical care, e.g. to be precise, efficient patient care, helps the physician in his clinical management, hospital depends on health information to monitor performance of all the professionals quantitatively and qualitatively, the national health or public health depends on controlling morbidity and mortality and eradicate the communicable disease. The International Organization such as the World Health Organization too depends on national health information. The medical record is the mother of health information.

Health information management (HIM) professionals play a key role in the design, development and management of health information within interconnected, community-wide health data exchanges and regional networks which are vital foundations of a national health information network. HIM professionals at the graduate levels of the academic framework reflect core knowledge in health information management coupled with applied informatics skill sets to ensure quality health information and system interoperability for all healthcare settings and organizations that create and use it.

The e-HIM Vision for the future statement emphasizes that core HIM function become more crucial as healthcare moves further into the information age.

Health information management is the body of knowledge and practice that assures the availability of health information to facilitate to real-time healthcare delivery and critical health-related decision making for multiple purposes across diverse organizations, settings, and disciplines.

Dramatic change in health information management demands new thinking, about how we educate tomorrow's professionals. Redefining roles, competencies, and educational progression should be the foundation of college of HIM education. When tomorrow's graduates enter the HIM workplace, they will be ready for the e-HIM environment.

Program Vision

To provide adequate fitting HIM professionals who can contribute effectively and meet the needs of ever changing healthcare system of the nation in the 21 century.

Program Mission

The mission of master's degree curriculum in HIM is to prepare confident, innovative and contributing professionals who can design, identify and use a variety of information resources and technologies to accomplish the information management objectives of diverse practice environment.

Educate adequate highly qualified HIM professionals to meet the national requirements in providing effective health care delivery to the citizens and residents of India.

The goal: The goal is to prepare a master's degree curriculum in HIM program under able faculty, to generate confident, innovative and contributing professionals who can design identify and use a variety of information resources and technologies to accomplish the information management objectives of diverse practice environments that benefit community through healthcare institutions.

Objectives

The objective is to develop curriculum that would meet the HIM professional who after successfully completing the master's degree in HIM should be able to:

- Endow with knowledge and skills necessary to become self-directed learners.
- Solve problems by critical thinking
- Attain informatics skills, communication and interpersonal skills.
- Instill a commitment to life-long learning, and important ethical values.
- Foster the acquisition of leadership abilities.
- Adapt careers within changing healthcare environment.
- Serve society and the profession through collaborative practice.
- Provide innovative teaching by generating and application of new knowledge
- Conduct research devoted to HIM in an electronic environment

- Carry-out activities that are focused on evolving the strategic and operational relevance and robustness of clinical information resources of healthcare industry and public health sector.
- Participate actively in quality and performance improvement management
- Collaborate and cooperate with information technology department in developing electronic health records

Role of HM Master's Degree Graduates

The individual holding a master's degree in health information management is engaged in executive level, enterprise-wide administrative, research activities. These activities are focused on evolving the strategic and operational relevance and robustness of clinical information resources of the healthcare industry and public health sectors. Graduates may perform research that advances the body of knowledge and standards associated with the management of health information in electronic health environment. Suggested roles for graduates may include:

- Academic faculty
- Applied health information researcher
- Chief executive officer
- Chief information officer
- Chief compliance officer
- Chief privacy officer
- Corporate health information manager/officer
- Data analytics/data mining engineer
- Data sets, nomenclature and classification standards developer
- Health information applications developer
- Health information management specialized practice consultant
- Public health information officer.

Student Population

The curriculum should be designed to attract individuals from a verity of educational backgrounds and disciplines. These back ground and disciplines may include individuals with prior coursework at an undergraduate level in HIM or those with a baccalaureate or advanced degrees in another area of study. Students who do not have a prior background in HIM may need to take additional prerequisite and/or requisite course content as defined by the academic program in line with the goals of the program and expertise of the faculty. Providing identified curriculum pathways with prerequisites and required courses based on entering students' education, experience and skill sets, will assist with appropriate student advisement and guidance in their career direction.

The program of study should meet established qualifications and educational standards. However, it is imperative that the graduate program clearly state that focus of the program in all marketing literature so that the incoming student is made aware of the nature of the program to which they are applying. The program must also meet 'best practice' criteria as established by university college or institute.

Several Factors Make Approval Valuable Including

1. Identified for the public specialized programs at the masters' level that meet established standards of educational quality.

2. Stimulates improvement of educational standards by involving faculty and staff in self-evaluation and planning.
3. Promotes a better understanding of the goals of health information management at the graduate level.
4. Allows students in approved masters' Level programs to quality for student membership in the professional association as stipulated in the AHIMA by laws.
5. Assist graduate programs in achieving their objectives.

Program Mission and Goals

A. The HIM program is established as a core concentration or specialized track within graduate level program of study; culminates with master's degree.

The HIM graduate program is design in concert with the institutional mission and the goals of the college division or department in which it is located.

A program evaluation plan exists for systematic evaluation of the mission, goals and objectives of the HIM program.

The program uses the results of evaluation and assessment to identify improvements and to modify program objectives.

Expectation of future postgraduates in supporting future healthcare: HIM professionals have a varieties scope to work besides the hospitals and health institutions. They work for accounting firms, insurance companies, information systems vendors, government agencies, pharmaceutical research companies, and others. Wide varieties of employers actively recruit health information managers. According to the department of labor, employment opportunities for Health Information Management (HIM) professionals continue to grow much faster that the average for all occupations. They may look for career choices not only in acute-care settings, but in all types of alternative care settings, as well as in education, business, and legal settings. Services provided in these areas range from technical to administrative, with emphasis being placed on the latter. As a vital member of the health care team, the health information manager is responsible for managing health information systems. This professional plans and develops health information systems that meet standards of accrediting and regulatory agencies. They also design health information systems appropriate for various sizes and types of health care facilities. A postgraduate serves as an advocate for privacy and confidentiality of health information and plans and offers in-service educational programs for health care personnel.

There are multiple job opportunities available to HIM graduates. The job opportunities are not limited to the following settings:

Traditional settings		
S. No	*Job positions*	*Job responsibilities*
1	Management, HIM (medical records)	Responsible for the day-to-day operations of an HIM department, maintains a budget, oversees staff, and interacts with other hospital departments, plans for the department
2	Tumor registry	Reviews, abstracts, and codes clinical cancer information in order to comply with government regulations. Maintains a database. Also provides data for physicians and research studies
3	Coding	Reviews medical documentation and assigns appropriate diagnosis and/or procedure codes in order for billing to occur.

Contd...

Traditional settings *(Contd...)*		
S. No	*Job positions*	*Job responsibilities*
4	Trauma registry (ER)	Collects, codes, and maintains data unique to trauma registry, maintains a database. Assists with research projects, performance improvement, and administrative planning
5	Transcription	Responsible for providing accurate and timely reports for patient care, documentation and billing
6	Quality improvement	Collect and summarize performance data, identify opportunities for improvement, and present data to other clinicians and administrative staff
7	Release of information	Track, process, and evaluate requests for release of medical information. Requires knowledge of central and state laws and regulations
8	Patient admissions	Responsible for patient admission, insurance verification, database maintenance. Oversees a staff, maintains a budget, and communicates with other hospital departments
9	Compliance auditor	Responsible for conducting chart audits, preparing reports, and reporting data. Also, develops policies and procedures for staff training
10	Physician accreditation	Maintains databases with physician information in order to provide data to administrative staff for physician accreditation
11	Risk management	Collects, evaluates, and maintains data concerning patient injuries, claims, worker's compensation, etc. Reports data to administrative staff and makes changes to policies and procedures as needed
12	Physician offices	Manages day-to-day operations of a physician office, including scheduling, billing, staffing, budgeting, and record keeping, and reporting
13	Utilization review	Works closely with clinicians to analyze patient records in order to determine admission criteria and use of resources for length of stay. Must be knowledgeable of insurance requirements

Curriculum

1. Health data management (HDM)
   - Health date structure, content and standards
   - Healthcare information requirement and standards
   - Clinical classification
   - Reimbursement methodologies
2. Health statistics, biomedical research and quality management
   - Healthcare statistics and research
   - Quality management and performance improvement
3. Domain—health services organization and delivery
   - Healthcare delivery
   - Healthcare privacy, confidentiality, legal, and ethical

4. Domain—information technology and systems
   - Information and communication technologies
   - Data information and file structure
   - Data storage and retrieval
   - Data security
   - Healthcare information system
5. Domain—organization and management
   - Human resource management
   - Financial and resource management
   - Strategic planning and organization development
   - Project and operation management

Faculty

There should be full time professionally qualified faculty supported by part-time and guest lecturers to provide quality teaching, advisement, research and service, as reflected in the college mission.

The Minimum Required Faculty

Full time faculty

1. Professor of HIM—1
2. Assistant professors (HIM-1, IT-1)—2
3. Assistant professor-IT—1
4. Clinical instructor or demonstrators—2
5. Secretary—1
6. Administrator—1

Part-time faculty

1. Health information statistics—1
2. Healthcare organization and management—1

Guest Lectures

Guest lecturers from medical, surgical, obstetrics, gynecology, pediatrics and other discipline, nursing, paramedical and administrative departments.

Solution to solve the faculty requirements

The following suggestions are made; the appropriate one may be selected:

1. Master degree students to be provided with scholarship during their period of degree course so that we can utilize their services in the laboratories and other places, they would be future potential teaching staff.
2. Students will have to work under the supervision and guidance of faculty as assistants that will provide an opportunity for the students to gain learning and teaching methods.

3. Qualified master degree students to be recruited in the university attached hospitals as HIM officers cum clinical instructors to gain managerial and teaching experience.
4. The best outgoing HIM undergraduate students should also be considered to be posted in the university attached hospitals where HIM students getting directed professional practice.
5. There should be a proposal to start doctoral degree in HIM field. The students selected for doctoral degree would be full-time student/staff.
6. A special teaching allowances to be created and paid to staff those who deal with our university HIM program.

   Student support and advisement:

7. Prerequisites:
   - Program ensures that students maintain an awareness of academic and career opportunities through advising and mentoring by faculty and preceptors.
   - Career paths of graduates are monitored, documented and used in program evaluation.
   - Instructional resources, technology, reference/library resources needed to fulfill the requirements of the curriculum, are available and accessible to all students.
   - The sponsoring educational institutions support for the program and the financial resources available to the program are sufficient to provide an environment in which the program can achieve its objectives.
   - Program leadership has authority commensurate with responsibility for program management can achieve evaluation.
   - The program maintains sufficient relationships with a variety of health related organizations and agencies to support its teaching, research and service goals.

Scope of Application for Master's Degree

In view of huge demand for Health Information Management professionals throughout globe in general and India in particular, there would be many applicants for admissions, not only from within the country but also from other neighboring countries. There would be high demand for admissions; hence, we have to make provision to accommodate and rendering service to other sister countries.

Duration

The course is of two years. The course will consist of four semesters, the first from September, and second from February as per the university program.

Commencement of the Course

First or second week of september, every year

Number of Admissions

Principally, depends on the infrastructure and facilities, initially, a total of 10 to 12 candidates, male and female candidates could be admitted every year. If the demand is more, the intake could be increased gradually.

Pre-requisites

The masters degree level of Health Information Management education acknowledges that certain prerequisite and requisite course work may be necessary to support advanced course content that institutional prerogatives must be considered in implementing any academic curriculum. The model serves as guide while supporting the individuality of program curriculum design and implementation.

Selection Procedure

Applications to the course will be invited by the college as done in other courses. An ad hoc selection committee will have to select the candidates purely on merit basis as per the criteria laid down. If the demand from other countries increases, appropriate selection criteria have to be developed and followed.

Evaluation: Continuous periodical written tests will be conducted in each subject monthly or in each chapter of study. Assignments, research work, project work and performance in seminars, viva voce will have greater impact in the evaluation process. At the end of each semester, final written tests, followed by lab/practical assignment evaluation will be carried out.

a. Credits: The credit ratios are set at:

15 hours theory = 1 credit

30 hours laboratory = 1 credit

45 hours directed practice at the hospital = 1 credit

b. Grade points:

Grade	*Percentage of marks*	*Reported as*	*Points*
A	>90% (>95% = A +; >90% = A)	Excellent	4
B	>80% (>85% = B +; >80% = B)	Verygood	3
C	>70% (>75% = C +; >70% = C)	Good	2
D	>60% (>65% = D +; >60% = D)	Pass	1
E	<60%	Fail	0

c. Grade points are calculated as follows:

$$\text{Grade points} = \text{Credit hours} \times \text{Points}$$

d. Grade point average is calculated as follows:

$$\frac{\text{Total grade points earned}}{\text{Total credits attempted}}$$

e. Pass

A candidate will be deemed to have been passed in each subject, if he secures not less than 50% internal and as well as external examinations with an aggregate of not less than 60%. The internal assessment marks are based on overall performance of the candidates in theoretical and practical assessment.

f. Location of the program

All theoretical classes and laboratory will be conducted at the college site, directed professional practice; project work, etc. will be carried out at different hospitals/health institution sites.

Attendance: Each candidate should put in attendance at least of 85%.

Discipline: Each candidate shall observe discipline according to rules and regulations laid down by the department of HIM or university. Any violation of discipline the candidate may run the risk of removal from the program.

Eligibility for admission:

Bachelor degree or equivalent program with minimum aggregate of 50% marks in any science/commerce/arts/group. Preference for BS in HIM field.

Selection procedure:

Admission to master's degree in HIM (health information management) course shall be made on the basis of eligibility and an entrance test to be conducted for the purpose. No candidate will be admitted on any ground unless he/she has appeared in the admission test and interview.

Successful candidates on the basis of written test will be called for the interview and shall have faced an interview board. The interview board will include the Head of the Department of Health Information Management and Head of the Institution, or anyone who is nominated for the purpose, whose recommendations shall be final for selection of students.

Students will be given counselling and seats will be allotted as per the merit of the candidates. All the selected candidates have to undergo medical examination on the notified dates. The college rules prescribed for the purpose of admission and their minimum attendance required will be applicable.

Duration of the course

Duration of certified study of the master's degree in HIM course shall extend over a period of 2 (two) academic years/4 semesters including 3rd and 4th semesters will be allotted for practical and projects

Medium of instruction

English shall be the medium of instruction for all the subjects of study and for examination of the course.

Assessment

Marks qualifying for a pass

A candidate shall be declared to have passed the examination if he or she obtains the following qualifying marks: 50% marks in the university examination and 50% marks in internal assessment evaluated by the department with the total aggregate average marks of 60%.

Practical examination and 50% aggregate in practical and 50% internal evaluation marks evaluated by the department with the total aggregate average marks of 60%.

Evaluation and grading system criteria

Evaluation and grading (manual relative grading) of students shall be based on GPA (Grade point average) and CGPA (cumulative grade point average).

2-YEAR MASTER DEGREE IN HEALTH INFORMATION MANAGEMENT (HIM)

SEMESTER 1							
Subject	*Code*	*Lectures*	*Lab*	*Practical*	*Total hr*	*Credit hr*	*Prerequisite*
English language and communication skills	ELC-101	1	1		45	2	
Health data management (HDM)—classification: Anatomy and physiology	HDMAP-101	1	1		45	2	
Health data management (HDM)—classification: Medical terminology	HDMMT-101	1	1		45	2	
Health data management (HDM)—classification: Mathematics, introduction to biology, physics, chemistry	HDMCL-101	1	1		45	2	
Health statistics, biomedical research and quality management (SRQM)—healthcare statistics and research	SRQM-101	2	2		90	4	
Health information management (HIM)-1	HIM-101	1	1		45	2	
Information technology (IT)—fundamentals of computer applications	IT-101	1	1		45	2	
Health data management (HDM)—classification: ICD-10, ICD-9CM-CPT, SNOMED	HDMC-101	1	1		45	2	
Total		**9**	**9**		**405**	**18**	

2-YEAR MASTER'S DEGREE IN HEALTH INFORMATION MANAGEMENT (HIM)

SEMESTER 2							
Subject	*Code*	*Lectures*	*Lab*	*Practical*	*Total hr*	*Credit hr*	*Prerequisite*
English language and communication	ELC-102	1	1		45	2	
skills	HDMAP-102	1	1		45	2	
	HDMMT-102	1	1		45	2	
Health data management (HDM)-health data structure, content and standards	HDMDS-102	1	1		45	2	
Health data management (HDM)—healthcare information requirements and standards	HDMHI-102	1	1		45	2	
Health data management (HDM)—classification: Pathology, biochemistry, microbiology, radio-diagnosis, forensic medicine, pharmacology sociology, psychology, health education)	HDMC-102 HDMC-102	4 1	 1		60 45	4 2	
Health information management (HIM)-2	HIM-102	1	1		45	2	
Total		**11**	**7**		**375**	**18**	

2- YEAR MASTER'S DEGREE IN HEALTH INFORMATION MANAGEMENT (HIM)

SEMESTER 3							
Subject	*Code*	*Lectures*	*Lab*	*Practical*	*Total hr*	*Credit hr*	*Prerequisite*
Health date management (HDM)—reimbursement methodologies	HDMRM-201	1	1		45	2	
Health services organization and delivery (HSOD)—healthcare delivery	HSOD-201	1	1		45	2	
Health services organization and delivery (HSOD)—healthcare privacy, confidentiality, legal and ethical	HSOD-201	1	1		45	2	
Information technology system (ITS)—information and communication and technologies	ITSIC-201	1	1		45	2	
Information technology system (ITS)—data information and file structure, data storage and retrieval, data security and health information system	ITSDI-201	2	2		90	4	
Organization and management (OM)—HRM, financial and resource management, strategic planning and organization development, project operation management	OMHF-201	2	2		90	4	
Healthcare information management	ITS-301	1	1		45	2	
Total		**9**	**9**		**405**	**18**	

2-YEAR MASTER DEGREE IN HEALTH INFORMATION MANAGEMENT (HIM)

SEMESTER-4							
Subject	*Code*	*Lectures*	*Lab*	*Practical*	*Total hr.*	*Credit hrs.*	*Prerequisite*
GS-biostatistics (healthcare statistics, biomedical research)	GSB-302	2	2		90	4	
Quality assurance and quality management and performance improvement	QAR-302	2	2		90	4	
Healthcare delivery systems—HCD-II	HCD-302	2			30	2	
Health information management (HIM)—medical transcription, telemedicine, application of HIM in non-traditional settings	HIM-302	2	1		60	3	
Principles of organizing and management-POM-II (strategic planning and organizational development, project and operation management	POM-302	3	1		60	4	
Total		**11**	**6**		**330**	**16**	

HIM Master degree Course Content	
Subject code	*Syllabus*
Domain: Health data management A. Sub-domain: Health data structure, content and standards	• Health data structure, content, and standards • Structure and use of health information (Individual, comparative aggregate) (5) • Health information media (paper, electronic/computer-based; e-health-personal, web-based) (5) • Type and content of health record (paper, electronic computer-based e-health personal, web based) (5) • Data quality assessment and integrity (5) • Secondary data sources (registries and indexes) • Databases such as MEDPAR, NPDB, HCUP (4) • Health information archival systems (5) • National Healthcare Information Infrastructure (NHII) (5) • Data collection tools (such as forms, computer • Input screens, other health record documentation tools) (5) – Manage health data (such as data elements, data sets and databases). – Ensure that documentation in the health record supports the diagnosis and reflects the patient's progress, clinical findings and discharge status. – Maintain processes, policies and procedures to ensure the accuracy of coded data. – Monitor use of clinical vocabularies and terminologies used in the organization's health information systems.
B. Sub-domain: Healthcare information requirements and standards	Healthcare information requirements and standards and regulations for documentation (such as JCAHO, CARF, COP, AAAHC, AOA) (5) Health information standards (such as HIPAA, ANSI, ASTM, LOINC, UMLS, MESH, Arden Syntax, HL-7) (5) • Develop organization-wide health record documentation guidelines • Maintain organizational compliance with regulations and standards. • Ensure organizational survey readiness for accreditation licensing and/or certification processes.
C. Sub-domain: Clinical classification systems	**Clinical classification systems** • Healthcare taxonomies, clinical vocabularies, • Terminologies/nomenclatures (such as ICD-9-CM, • ICD-10, CPT, SNOMED-Ct, DSM-IV 94) • Severity of illness systems (4) • Biomedical sciences • Anatomy (3) • Physiology (3) • Medical terminology (5) • Pathophysiology (4) • Pharmacology (4) – Select electronic applications for clinicalclassification and coding. – Implement and manage applications and processes for clinical classification and coding

Contd...

HIM Master degree Course Content *(Contd…)*

Subject code	*Syllabus*
D. Sub-domain: Reimbursement methodologies	**Reimbursement methodologies** • Clinical data and reimbursement management (5) • Compliance strategies and reporting (e.g. national correct coding initiative) (4) • Charge-master management (4) • Case-mix management (4) • Audit process such as compliance and • Reimbursement (5) • Payment systems (such as PPS, DRGs • APCs, RBRVS, RUGs) (4) • Commercial care and federal insurance plans (4) – Manage the use of clinical data required in prospective payment systems (PPS) in healthcare delivery. • Manage the use of clinical data required in other reimbursement systems in healthcare delivery. – Participate in selection and development of applications and processes for charge master and claims management. – Implement and manage processes for compliance and reporting such as the National Correct Coding Initiative.
II. Domain: Health statistics, biomedical research and quality management	Healthcare statistics, biomedical research and quality management.
A. Sub-domain: Healthcare statistics and research	• Statistical analysis on healthcare data (5) • Descriptive statistics (such as means, standard deviations, frequencies, ranges, percentiles) (5) • Inferential statistics (such as t-tests, ANOVAs, • Regression analysis, statistical process control, • Reliability, validity) (5) • Vital statistics (5) • Epidemiology (4) • Data reporting and presentation techniques (5) • Computerized statistical packages (5) • Research design/methods (such as quantitative, qualitative, evaluative, outcomes) (5) • Knowledge-based research techniques (such as medline, CMS, libraries, websites) (5) • National guidelines regarding human subjects' research (4) • Institutional review board process (5) • Research protocol data management (4) – Manage clinical indices/databases/registries. – Analyze and present data for quality management, utilization management, risk management, and other patient care related studies – Utilize statistical software. – Ensure adherence to institutional review board (IRB) processes and policies
B. Sub-domain: Quality management and performance improvement	**Quality management and performance improvement** • Quality assessment and management tools (such as benchmarking, ORYX, SQC) (5)

Contd…

HIM Master degree Course Content *(Contd...)*	
Subject code	*Syllabus*
	• Utilization and resource management (4) • Risk management (4) • Disease management process (such as case management, critical paths) (4) • Outcomes measurement (such as patient, customer satisfaction, disease specific) (5) – Organize and coordinate facility—wide quality management and performance improvement programs. – Analyze clinical data to identify trends. – Analyze and present data for healthcare decision-making (such as demonstrating quality, safety and effectiveness of healthcare).
III. Domain: Health services organization and delivery A. Sub-domain: Healthcare delivery systems	**Health services organization and delivery** • Organization of healthcare systems (5) • Components and operation of healthcare organizations including e-health delivery (5) • Accreditation standards (such as JCAHO, AOA, NCQA, CARF, CHAP, URAC) (5) • Regulatory and licensure requirements (such as COP, state health departments) (5) – Monitor the impact of national health information initiatives on the healthcare delivery system for application to information to system policies and procedures – Interpret, communicate, and apply current laws, accreditation, licensure and certification standards related to health information initiatives at the national, state, local and facility levels. – Analyze and respond to the information needs of internal and external customers throughout the continuum of healthcare services. – Revise policies and procedures to comply with the changing health information regulations. – Translate and interpret health information for consumers and their caregivers.
B. Sub-domain: Healthcare privacy, confidentiality, legal, and ethical issues	• Healthcare privacy, confidentiality legal and ethical issues • Legislative and legal system (4) • Privacy, confidentiality, security principles and procedures (5) • Health information laws, regulations and standards (such as HIPAA, e-health, JCAHO, state laws) (5) • Elements of compliance programs (5) • Professional and practice related ethical issues (5) – Coordinate the implementation of legal and regulatory requirements related to the health information infrastructure – Manage access and disclosure of personal health information

Contd...

HIM Master degree Course Content *(Contd...)*	
Subject code	*Syllabus*
	– Develop and implement organization—wide confidentiality policies and procedures – Develop and implant privacy training programs – Resolve privacy issues/problems – Apply and promote ethical standards of practice
IV. Domain information technology systems A. Sub-domain: Information and communication technologies	• Information technology and systems • Computer concepts (hardware components, systems architectures, operating systems and languages, and software packages and tools) (4) • Communications technologies (networks—LANS, WANS, VPNs; data interchange standards—NIST, HL-7) (4) • Internet technologies (intranet, WBG-based systems, standards—SGML, XML) (4)
B. Sub-domain: Data, information, and file structures	• Data, information and file structures (data administration, data definitions, data dictionary, data modeling, data structures, data warehousing, database management systems) (5) • Data storage and retrieval (storage media, query tools/applications, data mining, report design, search engineers) (5) • Data security (protection methods—physical, technical, managerial, risk assessment, audit and control program, contingency planning • Data recovery, internet, web-based and e-health security) (5) – Implement and manage use of ensure data collection, storage, technology, including hardware and software, to and analysis and reporting of information. – Contribute to the development of networks, including internet and internet applications to facilitate the electronic health record (PHR), public health, and other administrative applications. Interpret the derivation and use of standards to achieve interoperability of healthcare information systems.
C. Sub-domain: Data storage and retrieval	• Apply appropriate electronic or imaging technology for data/record storage. • Apply knowledge of database querying and data mining techniques to facilitate information retrieval. • Implement and manage knowledge-based applications to meet end—user information requirements. • Design and generate administrative report using appropriate software
D. Sub-domain: Data security	• Enforce confidentiality and security measures to protect electronic health information. • Protect data integrity and validity using software or hardware technology.

Contd...

HIM Master degree Course Content *(Contd...)*	
Subject code	*Syllabus*
	• Implement and monitor department and organizational data and information system security policies. • Recommend elements than must be included in the design of audit trail and data quality monitoring programs. • Recommend elements that should be included in the design and implementation of risk assessment, contingency planning, and data recovery procedures.
E. Sub-domain: Healthcare information systems	**Applied health informatics** • Leading development of health information resource and systems (4) • Brokering of information services (5) • Clinical, business and specialty system applications administrative, clinical decision support systems, electronic health record and computer-based health record systems, nursing, ancillary service systems, patient numbering systems at master and enterprise levels) (5) • Systems development (planning, analysis and design, customization selection/procurement implementation, integration, support testing and evaluation, auditing and monitoring) (5) • Human factor and user interface design (4) • Systems life cycle (systems analysis design implementation, evaluation, and maintenance) (5) – Apply knowledge of data base architecture and design (such as data dictionary, data modeling, data warehousing and so on) to meet organizational needs. – Apply appropriate electronic or imaging technology for data/record storage. – Apply knowledge of database querying and data mining techniques to facilitate information retrieval. – Implement and manage knowledge-based applications to meet end—user information requirements. □ Design and generate administrative report using appropriate software
V. Domain: Organization and management	**Organization and management** • Principles of management (5) • Negotiation techniques (4) • Communication and interpersonal skills (5) • Team/consensus building (5) • Professional development for self and staff (4) • Problem solving and decision making process (5)

Contd...

HIM Master degree Course Content *(Contd...)*	
Subject code	*Syllabus*
A. Sub-domain: Human resource management	**Human resources management** • Employment laws (4) • Principles of human resources management (recruitment, supervision, retention counseling, disciplinary action) (5) • Workforce education and training (4) **Performance standards (5)** • Manage human resources o facilities staff recruitment, retention, and supervision. • Ensure compliance with employment laws. • Develop and implement new staff orientation and training programs. • Develop and implement continuing education programs. • Develop productivity standards for health information functions. • Monitor staffing levels and productivity and provide feedback to staff regarding performance. • Benchmark staff performance data. • Develop, motivate and support work teams.
B. Sub-domain: Financial and resource management	**Financial and resource management** • Health finance (payer mix, bond rating, investment, capitalization) (3) • Accounting principles (4) • Budget process (capital and operating) (5) • Cost/benefit analysis (5) • Demonstrate knowledge of financial management and accountings principles. • Prepare and monitor budgets and contracts • Demonstrate and apply knowledge of cost-benefit analysis techniques to justify resource needs. • Organization-wide coding for disease classification; and revenue cycle management.
C. Sub-domain: Strategic planning and organizational development	**Strategic planning and organizational development** • Strategic leadership, management and planning (4) • Organizational behavior (4) • Business building (building your own business; championing best practices, processes, services within your organization) (3) • Change management (4) • Organizational assessment and benchmarking (4) • Develop strategic and operational plans for facility—wide information systems. • Assess organization—wide information needs. • Facilitate retrieval, interpretation, and presentation of date/information appropriate to user needs.

Contd...

HIM Master degree Course Content *(Contd...)*

Subject code	*Syllabus*
	• Demonstrate and apply principles of organization behavior to facilitate team building, negotiation, and change management.
D. Sub-domain: Project and operations management	**Project operations management** • Process reengineering and work redesign (4) • Project management (5) – Apply general principles of management in the administration of health information services. – Assign projects and tasks to appropriate staff – Implement process engineering and project management techniques to ensure efficient workflow and appropriate outcomes

KEY: Learning competency levels

1. Awareness—introductory recall and recognition
2. Literacy—knowledge of framework and content
3. Concept—comprehension, translation, extrapolation and interpretation of meaning
4. Detailed understanding—appropriate application of knowledge in a structured or controlled context
5. Skilled use—application using analysis, synthesis, and evaluation in new situations

Chapter 13

Directed Professional Practice Internship and Project Assignment

INTRODUCTION

The **Directed Professional Practice Internship and Project Handbook** has been prepared at par with the United States of American Universities standards with an objective to help the students/interns, mentor or supervisor or adviser and the hospital or health institution where the intern gets the directed practice under the authorized supervisor/s the required practice. The professional practice is designed to offer experience in a medical record department (or health information department) that develop the student/intern's cognitive, affective and psychomotor skills to produce a qualified Health Information Management & Technology professional. The MRD/HIM is a hub of hospital organization; has many sections; the work performed by different categories of staff; some are operational, supervisory and managerial levels. The students have to expose to all the sections without fail as each section/division has some important functions to carry out. During the directed professional internship practice, they will absorb and learn with ease. This exposure will give them the opportunity to critically exam and learn the systems, methods, and procedures that are followed in the institution.

In order to have comprehensive assimilation of practical knowledge, required skills and right attitude to perform given tasks, students/interns have to be placed initially in the "Mock-up medical record laboratory (MR simulation lab) and later in the medical record or health information management departments of hospitals or health institutions to have practical "hands on" experience. This experience will not only make the student a competent HIM worker but also an efficient manager. Generally, students can be posted to "Mock-up" lab from 3rd year onwards and to hospital from 4th year. With this mechanism, the students will have clear idea about the sections and type of work they are going to do and learn in the hospitals. First of all they will be too curious and critical to analyze the system practiced in the hospital with their theoretical knowledge and exposure to "mock-up" lab. This will motivate the students to be involved with the system effectively.

The Project handbook contains directed professional practice for students/interns and project program. The Directed Practice Program has been divided into four parts:

Part I: Related to practical working experience in the mock-up (simulation) medical record laboratory at the university or institute.

Part II: Related to directed professional practice at the hospital/health institution-environment.

Part III: Related to internship program

Part IV: Related to project work

The Directed Professional Practice has been further divided into two sections:

a. The first section is related to 4th year students.
b. The second section related to interns; when they are posted for directed practice, other than the project work, they need to observe guidelines as suggested for directed practice for 4th year students.

Directed Practice Time Schedule

There should be a clear time schedule for entire directed practice and project program for students/interns so that each student/intern gets motivated to complete all the topics required to learn in the Health Information Management and Technology program. Therefore, the need for specifying comprehensive list of all the functions and ensure that each and every function has been covered by each student/intern during his/her hospital/health institution postings. A sample Directed Practice Time Schedule is furnished in the Part II section.

The handbook will serve as unified guidelines to all the teaching and learning participants and useful for the smooth carrying out of the Directed Professional Practice in general and the Internship and Project Program in particular. Therefore, this handbook should be updated whenever changes are made in the program and meticulously observed by all in order to get the student/intern optimum benefit of the hospital directed experience in all the fields so as to equip themselves with modern knowledge, skills, techniques and right attitude to become worthy HIM and T graduate.

I am extremely grateful to all those with whom I was associated in developing HIM educational/training programs, in this process, my special gratitude for their guidance and encouragement in bringing out this handbook.

Last but not the least, all the teaching staff of Health Information Management and Technology Program to cooperate in effective utilization of the handbook and give their valuable suggestions for achieving the goal of effective running of the directed professional practice and project program.

The Mission and Philosophy of the Health Information Management and Technology (HIM AND T) University Colleges Or Institutes

The mission and philosophy of the college of HIM should be consistent with the mission of the university/national health programs and addresses these four major objectives:

- To create undergraduate and graduate education of the highest quality in liberal and professional disciplines.
- To provide best possible facilities for carrying out the undergraduate and graduate programs at par with international standards
- To examine the moral and ethical foundations of their thought and action and to develop personal values and ethical commitment.
- To participate in result oriented dialogue opens to all beliefs.
- To extend educational opportunities to those with special financial, educational, and physical needs.

The philosophy of the HIM and T should be in accordance with the educational philosophy and objectives of the university. Students in the HIM and T are to be exposed to a broad liberal education with emphasis on understanding the scientific/theoretical/theological constructs in the world. The academic programs focus on the scientific theories of the various professions coupled with a strong appreciation and understanding of human values.

The mission of the HIM&T is to educate students who are excellent clinical practitioners, who can assume positions of leadership, who understand the unique individual qualities of those with whom they work, and who have concern for the general welfare. Moral and ethical values support the scientific underpinning of the academic programs, which provide a comprehensive background for advanced graduate education, research, and scholarship. Graduates are prepared for successful careers in Health Information Management and Technology; professionals who graduate from HIM and T possess expertise, initiative, responsibility, and a profound moral and ethical respect for their patients, the profession, and the community.

This mission of the Department of Health Information Management and Technology at the University College or Institute is to combine the disciplines of the health information management, information technology, and clinical medicine to create an environment that utilizes current university resources and serves to:

- Educate students and currently practicing professional in the art of applying information technology including electronic health records maintenance, patient care information to reengineer processes within the healthcare delivery system that promote the highest quality and most cost effective healthcare.
- Promote research into methods of delivery and utilization health information, and the promotion of a patient-oriented continuous quality improvement culture through the use of information technology.
- Provide health information expertise in efficient healthcare delivery system of the nation.
- Develop new methods and techniques with required infrastructure to meet the needs of the nation in the field of health information management and technology expertise and manpower.

Agreement for Internship Program for HIM and T Students

The Ministry of Health should have to some sort of collaboration and cooperation with the state and private universities for effective utilization of HIM and T students the hospital environment for optimal gaining the knowledge, skills and positive attitude towards the healthcare management system.

The placement site provided should be capable for learning experiences and recognizes the professional responsibility of assisting in teaching of university students and its interest in providing assistance to the university in its curricula including practical learning experience in the health institutions. The following to be agreed mutually.

1. University shall coordinate plans with placement site to make learning experiences available to their students.
2. University acknowledges that its students shall be expected to comply with all current policies and procedures of placement site.
3. University shall, as mutually agreeable to the parties, provide by the beginning of each term: (a) Number of students and the dates and hours which they will be assigned; (b) the expected level experience to which they will be assigned; and (c) the expected learning objectives of its students.

4. University shall provide a faculty member who will serve as liaison with placement site field instructors when necessary.
5. University shall provide and maintain the records and reports—manual or electronically required by placement site for conducing clinical learning experience of its students under this agreement.
6. Placement site shall provide learning experiences to students enrolled in the college of HIM and T. The number of students and their program of education within the placement site and scheduling of their education at the placement site shall be determined by mutual agreement between the placement site's coordinator for clinical education and the University's academic coordinator for clinical education or their representatives.
7. Placement site shall provide learning experiences under the supervision of qualified personnel, which meet the experience standards of recognized professional accrediting agencies or state agencies and the stated objectives of the educational program.
8. Placement site shall, in its patient units, clinics, laboratories, classrooms, and other selected departments, provide opportunities for observations practical experience, conducive to the learning process of the student and to the meeting of the stated learning objectives.
9. Placement site shall provide orientation for the appropriate university faculty and students to the physical facilities, policies and procedures of the placement site, and where appropriate, to the needs of individuals and/or groups with which they will be working.
10. Placement site shall provide available time, when possible, to field instructors for attending management and clinical supervisors meetings and conferences called by the university as part of educational program.
11. Placement site shall provide, whenever necessary, available conference rooms, dressing rooms, and locker space for university students participating this program.
12. Placement site shall recommend to university the withdrawal of a program student if: (1) the achievement, progress, adjustment or health of the student does not warrant continuation at placement site, or (2) the behavior of the student fails to conform to the applicable regulations of placement site. Placement site shall assist university in implementing these recommendations. Placement site reserves right, exercisable in its discretion after consultation with university, to exclude any student form its premises in the event that such student's conduct or state of health is deemed objectionable or detrimental to the proper administration of placement site.
13. Placement site shall provide and maintain records and reports and access to health information required by the university for conducting the educational program.
14. Placement site shall provide notification to relevant non-acute care facilities that a student will be provided with a learning experience at the facility. The university shall contact separately with such facilities if requested to do so by the placement site or the facility.
15. University students shall be required to carry professional liability insurance and health insurance in accordance with the university's prevailing policies. (This paragraph, if applicable to be retained; otherwise to be deleted.)
16. University agrees to indemnify and hold harmless, the placement site, its officers, directors, agents, and employees from and against any and all claims, demands, and liabilities for personal injuries, deaths, or damaged property arising out of any act or omission of any faculty member or student.

17. University and placement site shall not discriminate against anyone applying to or enrolled in the program contemplated under this agreement or employed by either party because of race, color, creed, age, sex or national or tribe origin.
18. University and placement site agree that they shall abide by all applicable national, regional and local laws, rules, regulations and executive orders in effect as of the date of the agreement, and as they may change or be amended from time to time.
19. This agreement is of indefinite duration, however, can be terminated by either party at the end of any academic term of the university upon thirty (30) days written notice to the other delivered by registered mail. Such termination shall not affect students affiliated with the placement site at the time of notice is given.
20. This agreement shall not be assigned or transferred by either party without written approval of the other.
21. This agreement constitutes the entire agreement between the parties. No change or addition shall be made without written consent of both the parties. This agreement, when fully executed, shall supersede any and all prior or existing agreements, either oral or in writing with respect to the subject matter thereof.
22. This contract shall be governed by, construed and interpreted in accordance with the laws of the Government of India.
23. Any notices required to be sent under this agreement, except a termination notice pursuant to point 19, shall be sent by regular official mail to the following addresses:

If the Place or Site	**If the University**
	Coordinator, clinical contracts
Ministry of Health	College of the university or institute
PO Box ____________	of HIM and T
Name of other organizations	

24. Any dispute concerning a question of fact arising under this contract which is not disposed by agreement shall be decided by the Dean of the College or Chief of HIM and and coordinator of the placement site.

Directed Practice Program

Directed Practice Program can be divided into Four Parts

Part I: Related to practical working experience in the mock-up (simulation) medical record laboratory at the university students will be posted in the mock-up MR. Laboratory from the 3rd year onwards as part of practical experience. This is prior to posting in the hospital medical record (HIM) departments.

Part II: Related to directed professional practice at the hospital/health institution environment.

The directed professional practice can further be divided into two sections:

a. The first section is related to 4th year students.
b. The second section related to interns; when they are posted for directed practice, other than the project work, they need to observe all the guidelines as suggested for directed practice for 4th year students.

Part III: Related to internship program (internship posting in hospitals)

Part IV: Related to project work (project assignments)

PART I

MOCK-UP MR LABORATORY

I. Introduction

The mock-up (simulation) medical record laboratory is essentially required to provide the student the real life experience in the areas of maintain and managing medical records (health information) department. The student will have clear concept of hospital medical record system; they will have better understanding when their hands-on different sections of medical record department. They will be able to absorb and learn with ease. This exposure will give them the opportunity to critical exam and learn the systems, methods, and procedures that are followed.

Medical record department is a hub of hospital organization; has many sections; the work performed by different categories of staff; some are operational, supervisory and managerial levels. The students have to expose to all the sections without fail as each section/division has some important function to carry out. However, the duration of field training vary. Therefore, prior to posting to hospital field work, the exposure in mock-up lab will allow spending more time on important sections in MRD.

II. Upon Completion of Directed Practice at Mock-up Lab and at Hospitals/Health Institution

The Student should be able to:

- Demonstrate the role of medical records in healthcare delivery concept and importance of medical records and standards
- Demonstrate the uses and values of medical records
- Understand the organization and functions of medical record department
- Recognize all medical record forms, contents and their importance.
- Assemble and analyze the medical records
- Design medical record forms and develop forms control methods
- Understand and carry out medical record systems—numbering, filing, color coding system, movement of A/E, OP and IP records, policies and procedures observed
- Select appropriate equipment and furniture for MRD
- Write rules and regulations for patient record control
- Identify the deficiencies in the record and Importance of completion of records
- Understand the legal requirement, confidentiality, and release of information
- Classify the records by coding of diagnoses and surgical procedures as per the international classification of diseases and operations
- Understand primary and secondary records and active and inactive record system
- Carry out the functions in registration, admission and other sections of MRD.
- Operate computers and able to feed and retrieve information
- Prepare duty roster for the staff and make arrangements in proper posting of staff
- Manage the section effectively.

The students are posted in all the sections of laboratory with dates and time schedule to cover all the functions under the supervision of clinical instructor or demonstrator. During the postings and rotation, the student should maintain a log that will gauge the effectiveness of laboratory practice.

Annexure I

DAILY TIME SCHEDULE LABORATORY LOG

Student's Name: .... ID No: ....

Year Semester: ....

Section/functions	*Date*	*Time*		*Activities carried out*	*Clinical Instructors Remarks*
		From	*To*		

The student should maintain the log on daily basis and submit to the clinical instructor every week end and obtain his comments. The log will give comprehensive picture of the functions covered. Overall assessment will be done on the basis of completion of laboratory work.

III. Mock-up Lab Layout

a. General Rules and Guidelines

- Each session held would consist of a lecture and practical training that would follows. There should always be time for discussion.
- Each PC would have program installed on it as well as other window programs
- Each student is to write reflective essays about each days work and assignments.
- There should be a "problems and solutions" session to see students' reactions to them and their response.
- Each procedure no matter how simple should be implemented in the training program
- Retrospective teaching sessions should be implemented where a student

  Would explain to fellow student's procedures of performing a given task.

b. Topics to be Covered

- MR specific topics such as registration, appointment, admission, etc. and importance of MRD (HIM) in the facility and its weight.
- Management topics to ensure good people management as well the time and self management. Management topic should include peoples' skills.
- Communication topics to emphasize the importance of the latter in the smoothness of work in MRD.
- Importance of continuous education process.
- English language and medical terms to be the hot topic.

c. Areas of Concentration

- Record assembly and consistence of all patients' records.
- Critical analysis of incomplete records
- Typing (word processing) classes and spelling session
- Quality assurance and CQI
- Team work importance; should assign team projects.

d. General Overview

- Healthcare in India
- Administration and other department issues
- Flow of command in the facility
- Specific hospital policies and procedures as well as job descriptions
- Lenience is some extent is good but too much; will lead to indiscipline
- Seriousness is very essential for effective learning, penalty measures should be taken if needed for the benefit of student

IV. Requirements for Medical Record Mock-up Laboratory

The most important requirement is a place located near the HIM lecture classes. A hall with minimum of 150 Sq. M space (15 M × 10 M) would help in organizing the mock-up medical record laboratory. The other needs are as follows:

1. Medical Record Folders (empty or unused) ... 10, 000
2. Medical Records of discharged patients or outpatient records which are meant to be destroyed ... 20,000
3. Steel filing shelves (2M × 1M) seven dividers making six compartments 30
4. Pigeon hole rack with 100 compartments with the length 1 and half meter...1
5. Medical record forms used in different hospitals (sample forms) five sets
6. 12 (single person sitting) cubicles
7. Working table round or square (2M × 2M)
8. Armless movable chairs 30
9. Color coding labels (10 colors) 100 pockets
10. PC with all accessories...one
11. LCD...one
12. Overhead projector...one
13. Bar code instrument...one
14. Screen...one
15. Books shelves...two
16. Stationary, e.g. staplers, punching machines, stapler pins, scissors, cutting machines, glue, stapler pins, stapler removers, color strips, color writing pens, transparencies, rulers, white correctors, pens and pencils .... .

PART II

DIRECTED PROFESSIONAL PRACTICE

The second part of directed professional practice will be carried out at the hospital site.

Introduction

The professional practice is designed to offer experience in a medical record department or (health information department) that develop the student's cognitive, affective and psychomotor skills to produce a qualified Health Information Management and technology student.

In order to have comprehensive assimilation of practical knowledge, required skills and right attitude to perform given tasks, students have to be placed initially in the "Mock-up medical record laboratory (MR simulation lab) and later in the medical record departments of hospitals or health institutions to have practical "hands on" experience. This experience will not only make the student a competent HIM worker but also an efficient manager. Generally, students can be posted to "Mock-up" lab from 3rd year onwards and to hospital from 4th year. With this mechanism, the students will have clear idea about the sections and type of work they are going to do and learn in the hospitals. First of all they will be too curious and critical to analyze the system practiced in the hospital with their theoretical knowledge and exposure to "mock-up" lab. This will motivate the students to be involved with the system effectively.

Upon completion of hospital directed professional practice the student should be able to carry out the following specific tasks with 90% competency.

- Develop an understanding the role of HIM department in enhancing the organization wise performance program
- Develop a mission and vision statement specific for the HIM department aligned with that of the organization.
- Develop a plan specifically for the HIM department
- Participate in organization's ongoing medical record review process
- Understand the type of work carried out by each section, e.g. registration and appointment, census, assembling, deficiency check, coding, incomplete and complete record control, discharge analysis, filing and retrieving and release of information including confidentiality, privacy and security of information.
- Develop MR policies and procedures required to maintain medical records
- Understand the objectives of the Joint Commission on Accreditation of Health Organizations (JCACHO) required measures.
- Understand the importance of continuous quality improvement
- Identify different medical record forms and understand the importance of each form.

The students have to observe the following instructions during their directed professional practice:

Instructions for Completion of Clinical Experience Log

Purpose

This log is to be completed by the students on a daily basis giving detailed outlines of all the activities/procedures performed step by step, in order that the clinical instructor can evaluate the level of knowledge and performance of the student. The log is an important document for evaluation of the student in clinical experience.

Part A

1. The student must complete the identification section giving full name, student number.
2. Course title and course number.
3. Year and the semester number
3. Write the name of the hospital and name of the assigned section

Part B

This form has to be filled to reflect the different activities on a daily basis.

1. **Date:** Write the date in the date column daily.
2. **Time:** State the starting and ending time of each function.
   a. Times used for other activities which are not related to said function, i.e. for coffee break, telephone call and in activity time.

3. **Activities:** The detailed step by step report on the clinical experiences has to be written.
4. **Return of log:** This log has to be returned by the student to the clinical instructor on a weekly basis.
5. **Clinical instructor:** To write comments and signed and should discuss with faculty members the student progress before returning to the student.
6. **Faculty:** The faculty members at the completion of each section shall discuss with the students the performance to a competence level. The faculty members shall also be responsible for any and all problems arising from the students, clinical instructor and hospital. A sample example is furnished below:

Annexure II

STUDENT/INTERN DAILY HOSPITAL DIRECTED PROFESSIONAL PRACTICE LOG

Part A

Student's Name: .... ID No: ....
Course Title: .... Course Number: ....
Year: .... Semester: ....
Hospital Name: ....
Section: ....

Part B

Date	*Time*		*Activities*
	From	*To*	

Annexure III

CLINICAL INSTRUCTOR—STUDENT PROGRESS REPORT

Student Name: .... ID No. ....
Hospital Name: .... Section ....
Instructions: ....

For clinical instructor—to be based on observation and activities log:

Part-I Tasks Performed	*Acceptable*	*Needs more practice*	*Not performed*

Comments: Signature:

Annexure IV

LAB AND CLINICAL PRACTICE EVALUATION

Student Name: .... ID No ....

Area of clinical instruction: ....

Sub area: ....

1. Quality of work:
   Comment: ....
   ....
2. Application to work:
   Comment: ....
   ....
3. Understanding of assigned tasks:
   Comments: ....
   ....
4. Knowledge of medical record principles:
   Comments: ....
   ....
5. Understanding where assigned area fits into flow of department:
   Comments: ....
   ....
6. Professionalism (attitude)
   Cmments:..
   ....
7. Initiative:
   Comments: ....
   ....

Grading Points

Grade	*Percentage of marks*	*Reported as*	*Points*
A	>90% (>95% = A+; >90% = A)	Excellent	4
B	>80% (>85% = B+; >80% = B)	Very good	3
C	>70 % (>75% = C+; >70% = C)	Good	2
D	>60%) (>65% = D+; >60% = D)	Pass	1
F	< 60%	Fail	0
I	Incomplete (a temporary grade given by an instructor when; neither passing nor failing grade can be determined because of incomplete course work. Unless the missed examination or required assignment is made up by the date specified by the instructor and student standing committee, the "I" becomes a permanent "F" grade.		

Grading is based on the following:

1. Assessment sheet
2. Written reports by student
3. Student log
4. Observation of a job duties explanation
5. Written test based on above

Signature of:

I. Clinical instructor
II. Faculty member

GUIDELINES FOR EVALUATING STUDENTS

The following points have to be taken into consideration while evaluating the students.

Quality of Work

Considering the students degree of familiarity with the facility procedure and the assigned task, does the student produce a technically accurate product? Complete product?

Application to Work

Was student attentive?
Willing to work?
Show enthusiasm in the learning task?

Understanding of the assigned tools:

Does complete task with full understanding? or Unsure.
Does student pose pertinent questions?

Knowledge of medical record principles:

Does the student relate or display knowledge of medical record principles and apply them in their proper context?

Understanding where assigned area fits work into flow of department

This is an integral part of "pulling I it all together" and makes a clinical experience much more meaningful. Your reinforcement in this area will identify the relationship of the assigned task to the overall facility health information system.

Professionalism

Did the student exhibit tact and discretion interacting with other professionals, peers, and area personnel? Was the student considered so as not to disrupt the workflow of the department? Was the student neat in appearance?

Initiative:

Does the student ask for other work when assigned task has been completed? Do not downgrade the student on this point, it will only be considered a plus if present, not a minus if absent.

Directed Practice Time Schedule

There should be a clear time schedule for entire Directed Practice and Project Program for students/interns so that each student will have completed all the topics required to learn in the Health Information Management and Technology program. Therefore, the need for specifying comprehensive list of all the functions and ensure that each and every function has been covered by the student/intern during their hospital/health institution postings. A sample Directed Practice Time Schedule is furnished below:

Annexure V

DIRECTED PRACTICE IN A HOSPITAL WITH TOPIC WISE TIME SCHEDULE FOR STUDENT/INTERN

Name of Student/Intern: .... ID#: ....

Name of Hospital: .... Intern Supervisor: ....

Duration: From Date: .... To Date: ....

Topic/activity	*Name of the unit /section*	*Date*		*Name of site supervisor*	*Remarks*
		From	*To*		
Numbering control and registration of new and old cases					
Appointment section					
Preparation of new folders					
Admission and discharge section					
Daily census					
Assembling or records					
Investigation report sorting and mounting					
Deficiency check and incomplete record control					
ICD-coding and indexing					
Quantitative and qualitative analysis					
Medical transcription					
Completion of records by medical staff and others					
Filing, retrieving storing and retention of records					
Quality management and performance improvement					
Release of information and legal issues					
Supply of records for medical education and research					

Preparation of general and special reports				
Medical record form design and control				
Information technology department				
Other department				

Annexure VI

DIRECTED PRACTICE COMPLETE COVERAGE IN DIFFERENT HOSPITALS WITH TOPICS AND TIME SCHEDULE

Name of Student/Intern: .... ID No: ....
Duration: From Date: .... To Date: ....

Topic/Activity	*Hospital name Date:*		*Hospital name Date*		*Hospital name Date*		*Hospital name Date*		*Hospital name Date*	
	From	*To*	*From*	*To*	*From*	*To*	*From*	*To*	*From*	*To*
Numbering control and registration of new and old cases										
Appointment section										
Preparation of new folders										
Admission and discharge section										
Daily census assembling or records										
Investigation report sorting and mounting										
Deficiency check and incomplete record control										
ICD-coding and indexing										
Quantitative and qualitative analysis										
Medical transcription										

Completion of records by medical staff and others					
Filing, retrieving storing and retention of records					
Quality management and performance improvement					
Release of information and legal issues					
Supply of records for medical education and research					
Preparation of general and special reports					
Medical record form design and control					
Information technology department					
Other department					

Annexure VII

TOPICWISE DIRECTED PRACTICE FOR STUDENT/INTERN WITH HOSPITAL, SECTION/UNIT AND TIME SCHEDULE

Topic/activity	*Student/intern number 1* *Hospital Name Section/Unit Date: From/To*	*Student/intern number 2* *Hospital Name Section/Unit Date From/To*	*Student/intern number 3* *Hospital Name Section/Unit Date: From/To*	*Student/intern number 4* *Hospital Name Section/Unit Date: From/To*
Numbering control and registration of cases new and old				
Appointment section				

Preparation of new folders				
Admission and discharge section				
Daily census				
Assembling or records				
Investigation report sorting and mounting				
Deficiency check and incomplete record control				
ICD—coding and indexing				
Quantitative and qualitative analysis				
Medical transcription				
Completion of records by medical staff and others				
Filing, retrieving storing and retention of records				

Quality management and performance improvement				
Release of information and legal issues				
Supply of records for medical education and research				
Preparation of general and special reports				
Medical record form design and control				
Information technology department				
Other department				

PART III

INTERNSHIP POSTINGS IN HOSPITALS

Internship Postings are also Divided into three Sections

Section 1: Related to health information management department

Section 2: Related to quality management (QM) and performance improvement (PI).

Section 3: Related to information technology

Note: When the interns are posted for directed professional practice, other than the project work, they need to observe all the guidelines as suggested for directed practice for 4th year students.

Section 1: Internship in Health Information Management (HIM) Department

Overview

This professionalpractice experience is designed to provide the intern with real life experience in the areas of health information management (HIM) specific emphasis is placed on the role of establishing, organizing and management of HIM department in the hospital or health institutions.

Objectives

Upon completion of directed practice, the intern should be able to:

- Demonstrate the role of medical records in healthcare delivery concept and importance of medical records and standards
- Organize and effectively manage medical record department
- Prepare medical records standards, policies and procedures
- Develop a mission and vision statement specific for the HIM and T department aligned with that of the organization
- Design and develop medical record forms in accordance with the requirement of the hospital.
- Prepare the deployment of staff for HIM department according to the type and load of work.
- Provide orientation to the staff for performing their duties and responsibilities effectively and efficiently.
- Accomplish intra- and inter-departmental relationship for efficient coordination and cooperation.
- Prepare job descriptions for different categories of HIM department.
- Introduces appropriate numbering, color coding and filing system.
- Manage efficiently the MR services of A/E, OP and inpatient departments
- Select appropriate equipment and furniture for MRD
- Understand and effectively impose legal requirement, security, confidentiality, and release of information
- Classify the records by coding of diagnoses and surgical procedures. As per the international classification of diseases and operations
- Understand and have clear idea about insurance policies related to patient care and billing methods
- Understand primary and secondary records and active and inactive record system
- Introduce computerization in all the sections of MRD and coordinate and cooperate with IT department in introducing electronic health records in the hospital.
- Assist in medical education and research programs and to other departments in MR issues and administration in providing required information
- Develop appropriate information collection, compilation, interpretation and reporting system
- Participate in policy making and management meetings
- Develop an understanding of the role of the HIM and T department aligned with that of the organization wide quality and performance improvement program
- Develop a professional practice plan specifically for the HIM&T department.
- Participate in the organization's ongoing medical record review process
- Develop standards that meet the joint commission requirement.

Section 2: Internship in Quality Management (QM) and Performance Improvement (PI) Department

Interns spend considerable time in quality management department besides HIM department.

Upon completion of the directed practice in the QM and PI department, the intern should be able to:

1. Understand the role of performance improvement and quality management in the HIM department.
2. Understand the joint commission requirements for the ongoing medical records review process
3. Understand the PI model utilized by the HIM department for making continuous improvements.
4. Develop an understanding of the HIM mission/vision statement and how it aligns with that of the organization's mission and vision statement.
5. Develop an understanding of the team approach utilized by HIM department for making improvements.
6. Develop an underrating of the HIM department monthly deficiency rate and PI mechanisms utilized to impact this process.
7. Benchmark the performance of the HIM department with that of external organizations.
8. Assess and evaluate the performance of the HIM department using PI data overtime.
9. Translate PI data into information that impacts the performance of the department.
10. Assist with the identification of opportunities for improvements as indicated PI data.
11. Develop an understanding to the HIM department strategies for continued readiness and compliance with joint commission.
12. Assess with the development of a corrective action plan (CAP) that would impact improvement opportunities and the performance of the department.
13. Assist, where possible, with the implementation and monitoring of the corrective action plan.
14. Articulate the defined and documented plans with employees of the department.

Teaching Methods

1. Written assignment related to the supervised activity at the professional practice site.
   a. Weekly reports should be typed and a copy submitted to the coordinator. The original should be placed in the intern's notebook.
   b. Activity logs and schedules should be maintained. Documents should be signed by your directed practice supervisor and placed in your notebook.
2. Interns are encouraged to share their experience during class periods and schedule meetings with the coordinator to discuss critical issues relative to their field experience if necessary.

Evaluation

1. The professional practice supervisor upon completion of the directed practice will evaluate interns individually.
2. Questions and answers, weekly reports, activity logs and daily schedule forms must be typed and placed in the student's notebook.

3. All questions/forms are due at least two weeks prior to the end of the term.
4. Near the end of the semester the professional practices supervisor and/or instructor will discuss your directed practice experience with you.
5. Interns will receive a satisfactory grade if they have:
   - Completed the minimum hours required (40) and completed an activity log/daily schedule and obtained appropriate signatures
   - Complete and submit in typed weekly reports as directed
   - Demonstrated an understanding of their experience based on:
   - Notebook with typed questions and answers, weekly reports and forms
   - Evaluation completed by the directed practice supervisor.
   - Satisfactory completion assigned tasks as noted on your evaluation by your supervisor.
   - Your ability to discuss procedures, processes and data outcomes during class periods and with your instructor
6. Interns who have not received a satisfactory evaluation by the supervisor will be re-evaluated by the coordinator and provided an opportunity to master the skills in which they are deficient.
7. Intern who are unable to complete the required assigned hours due to illness or unavailability of professional practice sits will receive an incomplete grade. If he or she is ill, he/she must present a doctor's note in order to receive an incomplete grade. It is the student's responsibility to complete the hours and turn in all required assignments in order to receive a grade. Interns who refuse to submit in required assignments will receive an automatic "F" grade. Student must make the necessary arrangements with their current manager to complete the hours during the same semester as registered.

Grading procedure: Grades will be either pass (P) or fail (F).

University HIM College or Institute—Student Badge

Interns should wear their ID badge at all times. ID badge (panther ID card) and clip can be obtained from photo ID office at the university college or institute. Interns who fail to follow or do not wear ID badge risk the possibility of being sent home.

Dress Code

Interns are required to dress professionally and in accordance with the healthcare facility's dress code.

Code of Conduct

Seniors will

- Conduct themselves in a professional manner at all times
- Adhere to the organization's code of ethics as related to the assigned department (s)
- Adhere to the organization's code of conduct
- Abide by the organization's rules and regulations, policies and procedures
- Maintain patient confidentiality at all times
- Submit to all other professional and educational requirements as defined by clinical supervisor.

Assignment One

Complete the following as related to the organization to which you have been assigned:

1. What is the mission of the organization?
2. What is the vision of the organization?
3. What is the mission of the HIM department?
4. What is the vision of the HIM department?
5. How does the mission and vision of the HIM department align with that of the organization?
6. Is there an ongoing process for review of open and closed medical record? Yes or No (If yes, describe the process?)
7. Review the data for the part—6 months to 1 year and summarize the outcomes? You may wish to graph if appropriate.
8. Is there improvements noted, if not what was done to correct the opportunities identified?
9. Was there a corrective action plan developed?
10. What is the organization's current medical record deficiency rate?
11. How does the delinquency rate compare with that of other healthcare organizations?
12. Is the consistent with the expectations of the Joint Commission? Yes or No (If not, what is being done to impact and correct the problem?
13. Is there a PI plan developed for the HIM department? If so please secure a copy for your notebook. (Briefly explain in five lines)
14. Is there an organization-wise PI plan? Secure a copy for your notebook.

Upon completion of directed practice in the QM and PI department, the intern should be able to:

- Describe the integrated multidisciplinary, collaborative approach to quality management and performance improvement as applied to a healthcare setting.
- Develop an understanding of the role of the HIM and T department aligned with that of the organization wide performance program.
- Develop a mission and vision statement specific for the HIM and T department aligned with that of the organization.
- Develop a professional practice plan specifically for the HIM and T department.
- Participate in the organization's ongoing medical record review process.
- Identify the role of the customer in quality management and performance improvement.
- Identify the role of the various organizational committees in enhancing quality management.
- Articulate the organization professional practice reporting structure.
- Discuss the role of the medical staff in performance improvement.
- Discuss the role of the environment of care (EOC) committee in ensuring patient safety.
- Understand the objectives of the JCAHO required measures.
- Understand the importance of continuous quality improvement.
- Understand the importance of ongoing monitoring, assessment, measurements and evaluation.
- Discuss the role of board of directors in professional practice.
- Discuss the role of executive management in professional practice.
- Discuss the role of the middle managers.
- Discuss the role of line staff.
- Understand the JCAHO accreditation process.

Expectations

During the practicum, the student should be informed of and participate as many of the following activities as possible:

1. Become familiar with the organization-wide quality/PI plan and specifically that of the health information management department
2. Participate in the HIM department accreditation preparation process if possible.
3. Develop an understanding of the PI model utilized by the department for making improvements.
4. Assist with the ongoing medical record review process.
5. Assist with the collection, management, analysis and interpenetration PI data.
6. Attend the management of information committee meetings.
7. Participate in HIM department PI team meetings.
8. Observe the role of the PI director and quality manager
9. Attend the performance improvement council committee meetings.
10. Participate in the HIM department PI/quality management studies as applicable.

Assignment Two

Complete the following as related to the organization to which you have been assigned.

1. What is the PI model adapted by the organization for making improvement?
2. What performance improvement priorities have been established for the HIM department for the year 2014?
3. Are there functional PI teams established in the HIM department?
4. Describe the goals/objectives of a function of this committee?
5. Is there management of information committee? Yes or No.
   If yes, describe the role and the function of this committee; If No, how is it managed?
6. Who are the members?
7. How often does it meet?
8. How successful the committee has been to date?
9. Describe the challenges and opportunities identified by the committee.
10. Describe the PI reporting structure of the organization to which you have been assigned?
11. Who is ultimately responsible for PI and QM within the organization?

Assignment Three

1. Each of the following categories describes their role in performance improvement specific to the organization to which you have been assigned:
   a. Performance improvement council
   b. Board of directors
   c. Medical staff
   d. Executive management
   e. Middle management
   f. Quality management department
3. Discuss the role of environment of care committee (EOC) in ensuring patient safety.
4. Review the joint commission required measures and determine the process for monitoring the same at the organization to which you have been assigned.
5. Review and discuss the role of the PI director or quality manager.
6. Describe the process utilized by the organization to ensure multidisciplinary collaboration?

Section 3: Internship Program in Information Technology (IT) Department

Interns should have a good working knowledge of computers including windows (latest version or NT) environment and Microsoft office software. Additionally, interns should be able to use internet resources to access information and to communicate electronically.

It is expected that all interns obtain a personal university college or institute computer account, which will give them access to a personal e-mail box and web-publishing environment. If you do not have one yet, please secure one. Once you obtain an email address, send the instructor an e-mail to include in the class distribution list.

Theoretical Background

With the theoretical knowledge of the concept of software, hardware and internet, operating system, programming languages, compilers, different types of memories, input and output devices architecture, parallel processing, issues and common applications of software such as word processing, spreadsheets, computerized presentations, operating systems and internet.

Current strategies of system analysis, data gathering techniques, analyze model information system, system design and implementation, knowledge of basic SQL skills and programming using access. The system architecture design user interface design, data design, project management, documentation, testing and evaluation. CASE tools will be used to specify the requirement and the design of the system. Principles of computer networks with emphasis on internet, the structure and components of computer networks, network classifications, data transmission media, local area networks, network layers, TCP/IP, error control, congestion control.

Upon completion of directed practice in the HIM and associated departments with information technology (IT) related field, the student, should be able to:

- Interact with the computer, that is, generate input to the computer and interpret output from the computer
- Identify major elements of computer hardware (memory, processor, and input/output devices)
- Identify major elements of computer software (operating systems, programming languages, and application software)

  Demonstrate reasonable proficiency with: M
- Know the tools, design and function of the systems analysts.
- Use systems analysis models to document the information system requirements of a real organization.
- Work in teams to specify, analyze and model the requirements of an information system.
- Introduction to systems design and implementation.
- Describe the essentials of systems design
- Use system design models and CASE tools to specify the requirements, and
- Design of an information system
- Design systems input, output and a graphical user interface
- Work in teams to design an information system
- Understand the concepts of networks and protocols
- Identify the components of a computer networks
- Describe the ISO/OSI application model and understand the functions of different layers
- Understand the characteristics of different types of cables

- Differentiate between physical topology and logical topology of a network
- Identify the concepts of internet-working and internet protocols
- Specify a project topic and individual learning activities
- Develop a project time-line, project and implement
- Present project to the health information management faculty and students
- Participate with the IT personnel in developing patient care information
- Understand and use the electronic medical record system
- Design HIM and related computer screens for collecting information
- Understand the back up storage mechanisms and computer downtime
- Associate with the computer (information technology) department in designing and programming new screens for MR related subjects.
- Orient new staff on computerization medical record system
- Evaluate concurrently the clinical information such as history, physical exam, investigation reports, progress reports, diagnoses, surgical procedures, for the attention of medical, nursing other concerned staff.
- Code and classify disease and operation information.
- Collect and compile various types of information maintained and stored.
- Use intra- and internet system for the benefit of patient care information
- Concurrent completion of patient records
- Transcribe medical reports, surgical procedures, discharge and other certificates
- Prepare HIM department employee data base for management purpose
- Ensure the computer system is functioning effectively

Seminars and Workshops for Internship Program

There should be regular seminars/workshops to be conducted for the benefit of internship program.

Number of seminars: At least one seminar every month and minimum of three in a semester.

Topics to be presented: Generally, related to the clinical directed practice during the semester period.

Number of workshops: At least two workshops in a semester.

Topics: Should be most important topic that will benefit all the students including 3rd year onwards.

Topics for Directed Practice

- Number control and registration new and repeat cases
- Appointment bookings
- Preparation of new folders or preventing duplication of registration
- Admission and discharge of patients
- Daily census collection, compilation and presentation
- Assembling patient records in a standard prescribed order
- Investigation report sorting and mounting
- Deficiency check and incomplete record control
- ICD-coding and indexing of diagnostic and operations
- Quality and quantity analysis including discharge analysis; collection of statistics

- Transcription of medical reports, history notes, operation notes, discharge summary and certificates.
- Completion of records by medical and other staff
- Filing and retrieving, storing and retention of records,
- Quality improvement; performance improvement, etc
- Release of information (birth, death, attendance, admission and discharge certificates, legal issues
- Supply of records for medical education and research
- Preparation of general repots as required by the hospital administration and others.
- Participation in medical, continuous education and research programs
- Medical record forms design, control
- Coordination and cooperation with other departments in relation to the work
- Preparation of special reports as and when needed by the administration
- Human resource management.

PART IV

PROJECT ASSIGNMENTS

The faculty of the department of health information management (HIM) believes the project opportunity to be the crucial of the HIM curriculum.

In a formal partnership within the organization and outside healthcare organizations, HIM faculty, healthcare representatives and interns come together to challenge, educate and train students in the transition to professional careers.

The project opportunities intended to:

- Encourage students to complete, at the outset, the required field of specialty to fulfill the course outline requirement of the curriculum.
- Encourage students to consider and explore particular career interests that exist within the broad scope of HIM opportunities.
- Encourage students to develop skills of professionalism in behavior and communication.
- Aid students in the development of project management skills.
- Aid students in the development of problem solving skills that typically involve the utilization of information technology.
- Assist students in the development of formal presentation

The project sequence of the curriculum is considered and planned well in advance of the actual semester in which it is performed. Healthcare organization representatives are encouraged to communicate future opportunities as they arise and students are encouraged to begin discussions with HIM faculty advisers/supervisors at the onset of their junior year.

GUIDELINES TO STUDENTS ON INTERNSHIP PROGRAM

Introduction

You are starting on a wonderful adventure. This will take you, beyond the confines of the classroom and into the world of real work. This invaluable experience is your project, a vital component of the Health Information Management and Technology curriculum. Here, you will attain the building blocks necessary to start your career and smooth your transition into the workplace.

The work environment is vastly different from the one found at school or college class-room. You will encounter many new situations for which you are not prepared. This hand book will act as a guide to help you negotiate your way around these situations. It contains useful tips on acting in a professional manner.

This handbook offers practical advice on how to manage your time more efficiently as you try to juggle the demands of college and work. There is also information on project requirements and grading as well as the forms necessary to complete this assignment.

These hands on experience will give you the tools that will help you during your working life. You will learn to work within guidelines and to meet deadlines and acquired the basic skills necessary to work with other people. You will have the opportunity to meet people, make friends, and develop contacts. These contacts are very important in building career. The experience will be meaningful and can become part of your resume.

This is an experience of a lifetime. If you follow the instructions in this guide, it will be one that is profitable for both you and people at your project site.

PROJECT REQUIREMENTS

The following guide will help you understand what is required for a successful project. It includes duration, objectives, faculty meetings, grading, evaluation, and final presentations. There is also a prescribed form that can be used for submitting a project proposal.

Project Proposal due Dates

Students must submit project proposals according to the following schedule:

Semester project	Proposal due by
First semester	January 1
Second semester	May 1

Contractual Agreement

Once a student commits to a particular project and site, the department of health information and management will notify the office of the dean to assure that a formal contractual agreement exists with the selected facility. If one does not exist, the office of the dean will issue the contract to the site. The student may not begin the project until the signed contract has been returned.

Project Duration

The semester begins in september or february and ends at the completion of allocated hours. Total on site hours are 450–480 hours in each semester.

The project extends for the length of the semester for which it is proposed. This means a minimum of 15 weeks. For a 4-credit project, there is a minimum of 30 hours weekly at the project site in first semester/second semester. Total site hours are 450 though it is appropriate for homework to be assigned beyond the on-site requirement, for a 6-credit project, the total is 600 hours, typically 40 hours per week.

Project Allocation

Objectives: Based upon the preliminary goals, one significant project or a series of small projects will be issued by the site. It is the responsibility of the student, and the site supervisor to develop specific, measurable objectives for each project. This is the basis of evaluating performance and grade assignment. Please note that objectives must be specific, measurable, achievable, and faculty approved. To aid in the design of objectives, consider the following: "What do I want as a final product; in what format; by when." Or, "What service is I am expecting this student to provide; what end product would be considered based on the following grades.

Grading

- Grade will be based on the scope of the project, the achievement of the predetermined objectives, and attendance.
- The project must be meaningful to get a desired grade as determined by the faculty.

The following is the officially recognized method of grading course work and rating the academic performance of students in the professional phase

Grading Points

Grade	*Percentage of marks*	*Reported as*	*Points*
A	>90% (>95% = A+; >90% = A)	Excellent	4
B	>80% (>85% = B+; >80% = B)	Very good	3
C	>70 % (>75% = C+; >70% = C)	Good	2
D	>60%) (>65% = D+; >60% = D)	Pass	1
F	<60%	Fail	0
I	Incomplete (a temporary grade given by an instructor when either a neither passing nor failing grade can be determined because of incomplete course work. Unless the missed examination or required assignment is made up by the date specified by the instructor and student standing committee, the "I" becomes a permanent "F" grade.		
W	Official withdrawal (used on student's permanent record to indicate termination of attendance in courses under conditions of official withdrawal.)		
NG	No grade reported (used on student's grade report only.) Students in certain programs (e.g. health information management and technology) may be participating in projects for course credit which span more than a single semester. In such cases, the student may receive a NG until the project work is completed at which point the grade will be converted to a later.		

Student—Faculty Meetings

During the course of the semester, you will be expected to meet as required with your faculty adviser for project updates. You will be alerted to the schedule. The purpose is to asses your progress and to troubleshoot current projects and problems. If you feel additional meetings are needed, please consult with your faculty advisor.

There should be a regular communication between the faculty and the site supervisor and mentor (college/institute coordinator). The telephone; mobile numbers and e-mails of all concerned to be given for effective communications.

Evaluation

At the conclusion of each significant, objective-driven project or at the end of the semester, an evaluation is due. Two types of evaluations have been included. The first evaluates professional dimensions. The second evaluates specific project performance. Several project evaluations may be issued.

A grade based upon compliance with objectives will be recommended.

A face to face evaluation with the student is strongly encouraged.

Evaluation forms for both the students and the project site supervisor are included in this package. This allows both parties of the project to give input into the end results of this exercise. Please review these forms so that you will have an understanding as to what will be evaluated.

Annexure VIII

INTERNSHIP—WEEKLY TIME SHEET

Student Name .... ID No: ....

Internship Site: ....

Week #	*Day*	*Time: 9.00 am to 3.00 pm (6 hours) (specify site)*	*Total hours worked*	*Remarks*
1	Monday			
	Tuesday			
	Wednesday			
	Thursday			
	Friday			
	Total hours for week			
	Total cumulative hours			
	Mentor approval (initials)			
2	*Day*	*Time: 9.00 am to 3.00 pm (6 hours) (specify site)*	*Total hours worked*	*Remarks*
	Monday			
	Tuesday			
	Wednesday			
	Thursday			
	Friday			
	Total hours for week			
	Total cumulative hours			
	Mentor approval (initials)			

FINALIZING AND PRESENTING THE PROJECT

At the end of your project, you will be responsible to:

- Submit a written description of what you felt you gained during the project. This evaluation is in this package.
- Submit a one to two page summary of the project to be used as a guide for future students.
- Submit attendance records, objective updates and other materials such as logs, journals and project management tools.
- Submit a copy of any deliverable outlined in the objectives.
- Submit any presentation-related material.

You will also be expected to give an oral presentation of your project. When a team is involved in a project, all members of the team are expected to present. No exceptions will be made.

The presentation should consist of:

- The name of the organization.
- A description of the project
- The objectives of he project
- How you reached these objectives
- Any problems encountered
- Knowledge gained
- Your assessment of the project including recommendations

The oral presentation should be done in a professional manner and creative manner. This includes speaking and addressing as a professional. The presentation should be enhanced by professional audio-visual tools.

DRESS CODES

It is expected to observe dress code strictly if recommended by the college/institute. However, in other parts of the world, the organizations have different dress codes. It is wise to dress professionally the first day of your project. For men, this should be a suit and tie. For women, a business style suit or dress. If the organization for which you are doing the project has a relaxed dress.

The following internship instructions are to be observed for effective practical (field work training):

If there are no directions in the matter of dress, always be neat and well groomed. Ensure to wear socks, or in the case of women, stockings, and clean shoes. You are representing the University/institute and should dress in a manner that will give a favorable impression.

To create a favorable impression does not wear:

1. Dirty, unkempt worn, unconventional, torn or cutoff clothing
2. Clothing with obscene, profane, or suggestive words, pictures, or symbols
3. Clothing with advertisements of drugs or tobacco products
4. Excessive jewelry
5. Sandals or any other material that creates unfavorable impression

ATTENDANCE AND TARDINESS

Attendance: A minimum of 40 hours are required to be worked on a weekly schedule as determined by the program and site student. The site supervisor should document this attendance requirement. A sample "weekly time sheet" is provided though any similar format that can be returned to the college is appropriate.

1. All health information management and technology students are required to attend pre-planned projects site days and all related classes regularly on time.
2. Each student is permitted one explained (illness, personal business) missed day during each semester.
3. All students are expected to be prompt for each visit to their site.
4. If a student is more than 15 minutes late at the project site, it will be the project supervisor's decision to accept and 'count" the student's attendance for that day. If this is a one time occurrence, leniency may be considered; however, if this happens more than one, then the student should be reprimanded by either dismissing them for the day as soon as they arrive (not letting them work that day) or letting them work that day, but not counting it as an attendance.
5. If this becomes a chronic problem (more than 3 occurrences), that student should be removed from the project.
6. It is the right of the project supervisor to dismiss the student whom "show up" on time, but not do their work during their time. That student Will not be permitted to claim project experience hours, even through they were there. Just "showing up" is not a project experience. If this activity is repeated more than three times, the outcome will be the same as those who are chronically late.

CONFIDENTIALITY

The following policy statement regarding professional conduct and confidentiality will be adhered to strictly by all health information management students while participating in the project as part of the curriculum of the HIM. Any one failing to adhere to this policy will fail the project and will be required to repeat this portion of the curriculum.

As a HIM student, you have an obligation to yourself, your colleagues, your supervisor', and to the university college/institute to withhold from anyone, other than your immediate supervisors, any information you acquire professionally or socially which is considered professionally confidential. This includes information about the facility in which you are placed or any medical information about any patient, which is considered to be non-public information. Any professional rapport you establish with your colleagues is tainted by your lack of discretion and violation of this code of ethics. The following is the specimen copy of the "student confidentiality agreement".

Annexure IX

STUDENT CONFIDENTIALITY AGREEMENT

I .... ID NO: ....

aware of the ethical and legal implications regarding the confidentiality of medical/health records and information as well as being aware of an individual's absolute right to privacy, hereby sign this form. I understand and agree that I will not in any way (verbally, written, electronically or otherwise) divulge any information whatsoever regarding any person whose health record I may come in contact with in conjunction with my directed professional practice or internship/education except to authorized, in accordance with hospital policies. I am also well aware, that violation of the confidentiality policy will result in disciplinary action. I also acknowledge that I have received a copy of this document.

Student/Intern Signature Date: ....

....

Witness (Name and Signature) Date: ....

....

PROFESSIONAL CONDUCT

You are about to enter a profession. Even through you are undertaking a project as a student, you should act in a manner befitting a member of that profession.

A professional is a person who projects the qualities of one who follows a certain set of professional standards. This means that a professional is a person who abides by the rules and regulations of that profession. He or she learns these and applied them to everyday working life, and respects the rules of his or her employer.

Above all, a professional places the good of the employer, project, and co-workers above personal feeling. This person realizes that little good comes from undermining any endeavor due to a personal prejudice.

Annexure X

STUDENT/INTERNSHIP CONTACT INFORMATION

Student/intern information	*Project information*
Name:	Site Name:
ID Number:	Mentor/Supervisor Name:
Address:	Title:
	Address:
Phone #:	Phone #:
	Fax #:
Email:	Email:

Note: Whenever the original contact delegates the mentoring function to another individual, the change information has to be informed to update the changed information.

Annexure XI

PROJECT PROPOSAL FORM

(To be compiled and reviewed in conjunction with a hospital/health institution and presented to the HIMS faculty for review and approval prior to the project semester)

Name of the Hospital/Health Institution: ....

Address of the Hospital: ....

Division: ....

Department: ....

Project Site Contact: ....

Telephone Number: ....

Fax Number: ....

Name of Proposed Project: ....

Detailed Description of Project Objectives: ....

Scope of Project: ....

Outline of Activities: ....

Total Hours Required: ....

Number of Students Required: ....

Skill and Experience Required: ....

Benefits to Project Site: ....

Benefits to Students: ....

General Remarks: ....

Annexure XII

PROJECT EVALUATION

(To be completed by the project coordinator, discussed in person with the student and delivered to the HIM division one week prior to the completion of the semester).

Organization: ....

Project coordinator: ....

Student: .... ID# ....

Project: ....

PROJECT TIME FRAME

1. Describe the nature and objectives of the project.
2. What were the anticipated outcomes of the project?
3. What is your overall assessment of the final product?
4. Describe the student's strengths in achieving the goals of the project.
5. Describe the student's weaknesses in achieving the goals of the project.
6. Identify areas of knowledge deficits in student's ability to perform.
7. What grade would you assign to the student for the project?
8. General remarks:

Annexure XIII

PERFORMANCE ASSESSMENT CRITERIA

(To be completed by the project coordinator, discussed in person with the student and delivered to the HIM Division one week prior to the completion of the Semester)

Student: .... ID# ....

Project partner: ....

Communication: Student demonstrates ability to verbally convey information, in both a formal and informal setting, in a manner which is clear, concise, organized and appropriate.

Poor Average Good

Comments:

Professionalism: Student demonstrates courtesy, respect, and maturity in all interactions. Dress is appropriate to situation.

Poor Average Good

Comments:

Participation: Student practices good listening skills and gets involved in course discussions through appropriate questions and comments.

Poor Average Good

Comments:

Attendance/punctuality: Unless extenuating circumstances are communicated in advance, student is expected to attend every class, arrive on time, participate until the conclusion and meet all assignment time frames.

....

Poor Average Good

Comments: ....

....

....

....

....

....

....

....

Preparedness/work timeliness: Student demonstrates, through communication and participation, that assignment has been completed prior to class and student is prepared with appropriate tools to actively participate in class.

....

Poor Average Good

Comments: ....

....

....

....

....

....

....

Partner relationships: Student works with partner to define relationship that encourages professional growth and development.

....

Poor Average Good

Comments: ....

....

....

....

....

....

....

Self-learning/current events: Student institutes a systematic and opportunistic course of self-study to acquire knowledge and skills beyond curricular requirements.

Poor Average Good

Comments:

Writing skills: In every written document, student demonstrates communications skills in business and technical writing, which reflects relevance, logic, correct grammar, and spelling and appropriate style.

Poor Average Good

Comments:

Critical thinking/analytical skills: Student exhibits independent initiative in finding, defining, and solving problems using a systematic approach that utilizes all available information resources.

Poor Average Good

Comments:

Technologic skills: Student understands and creatively utilizes information technology to manage and improve personal and organizational effectiveness and efficiency.

Poor Average Good

Comments: ....

....

Ethics: Student protects confidentiality of patient data and observes highest standards of academic integrity, and advocates high standards of conduct in relation to profession, patient, and self.

....

Poor Average Good

Comments: ....

....

....

....

....

Annexure XIV

STUDENT PROJECT EVALUATION

(To be completed by the student and delivered to the HIM division one week prior to the completion of the semester)

Student: .... ID ....

Organization: ....

Project coordinator: ....

Project: ....

Project time frame: ....

....

....

1. Describe the nature and objectives of this project.
2. What was the final product that you were asked to produce?
3. Describe the mechanisms and skills that you employed to produce the outcomes of the project.
4. Describe the organizational support that you received in accomplishing this project.
5. Describe the strengths of your educational background in performing this project.
6. Describe the weaknesses of your educational background in performing this project.
7. Describe how the final product met the initial goals and objectives.
8. Describe the organization's response to the final product.
9. How much time did you commit to this project?
10. Briefly summarize the significance of this learning experience.
11. What grade do you feel you deserve for this project?

SCOPE FOR PROJECT ASSIGNMENTS

1. Incomplete records—the document does not meet the requirement for patient care or other purposes
2. Length of stay (duration of patient in the hospital) according to disease/operation
3. Retention period for medical records (number of years, medical records to be retained permanently)
4. Legal issues related to patient care, and management
5. Computerization of medical records
6. Patient waiting time in different sections of outpatient clinics
7. Patient visit pattern to the hospital
8. Patient disease pattern
9. Admission pattern including repeated admissions
10. HIM management system
11. Management of HR of HIM department
12. Patient problems in different areas of hospital or clinic
13. Medical and nursing staff problems related to HIM
14. Role of HIM in medical education
15. Role of HIM in medical research
16. Development of software:
    a. ICD coding
    b. Registration
    c. Admissions
    d. Appointments
    e. Record tracking
    f. Medical transcription—medical reports
    g. Quality improvement in HCD
    h. Quality improvement in HIM and T
    i. Data storage, coordinating master patient index
    j. Online lab and other investigations
    k. HIM department HR management
    l. Online transmission of health information
    m. Healthcare cost
    n. Information security, privacy and confidentiality
    o. Analysis of diseases as per approved ICD
    p. Risk management
    q. Drug prescription and abuse
    r. Safety and back-up information
    s. Hospital disaster program
17. Missing and mismatching of investigation reports
18. Incomplete diagnoses and operations
19. Incomplete records
20. Quality improvement and assurance
21. Performance improvement
22. Accreditation requirements
23. Technology—hospital computerization system

24. Study of patient visit pattern
25. Evidence-based medical practice
26. Cost effectiveness in HIM and T department
27. Cost effectiveness in hospital as a whole
28. Human resource management in HIM and T department
29. Retention period
30. Legal issues in HCD
31. HIM department requirements
32. Infection control and HIM
33. Medical staff relationship with HIM in efficient maintenance of records
34. Nursing staff relationship with HIM in efficient maintenance of records.
35. Other department relationship with HIM such as lab, radiology, pharmacy and administration
36. Relationship with patients and their relatives or attendants
37. Development of electronic health records:
    - Administration records
    - Clinical records
    - Patient information (statistics)
    - Investigation; lab, X-ray and other allied departments.
    - Development of formats for registration; appointments, clinical visits, etc.
38. HIM education/training and curriculum setting
39. HIM student needs and their performance in HIM theoretical program.
40. HIM staff improvement (continuing education or any orientation)
41. Development of efficient relationship with the administration to ensure the HIM moves forward with utmost efficiency.
42. Economic measures suggestions through HIM department
43. Minimize patient waiting time in different sections of the hospital.
44. Transformation of health records from manual to electronic records
45. Risk management
46. Drug prescription and abuse
47. Safety and back-up information
48. Hospital disaster program

SUGGESTED PROJECT WORKS FOR HIM POSTGRADUATE STUDENTS

Introduction

As a part of completion of HIM postgraduation program, the students have to take up some project works and especially related to their future professional practice and management purpose. The HIM professionals have to be involved with many healthcare related matters, and implementation of electronic health records in the hospitals and health institutions has become a necessity. Currently the priority for our country is implementation of electronic health records; improve efficiency and quality of care along with containing the spiraling healthcare cost. With this view, collaborating with the IT and clinical professionals to select, design, implement, test, and train staff on new software, hardware and network system. With the help healthcare providers, need to prepare standards, policies and procedures.

In the study and practice of medicine and other allied paramedical fields, there is constant need for guiding principles, brief summaries of subjects related to the allied medical sciences, and explanations of techniques and procedures are require to learn. It is evident that any medical, nursing and paramedics cannot become proficient in their respective field without having a team work among all the medical, nursing and other allied health science professionals and also to be part of global development in the advancement of medicine.

Consequent to advent of information technology: The entire world especially healthcare institutions are shifting from manual to electronic records. The author felt the dire need of present day is the implementation of hospital electronic health records. Hospital electronic Health Records are to serve the persons, who are concerned with the direct and indirect patient care, allied and health related professionals. Now, it is right time, the program on hospital electronic health records to be initiated by all the medical colleges and schools of medicine, nursing and other allied health science branches so that the future healthcare providers are well conversant with the modern digital system used in healthcare institutions.

In the last few years, entire world is in the process of conversion of manual records into electronic due to great advantage of using technology. Although information technology has changed the life style of many, most of public services have benefited tremendously by embracing the technology. Nevertheless, the health field due to various issues such as cost, privacy, confidentiality and security of information has been slow in implementation. Having realized the immense role it can play in swift, safe, improved quality care, and bring out cost unit gradually; many nations have embarked upon shifting to electronic health records and started scheduling the period for complete electronic health records.

The project work should help in development of electronic health record for hospital services encompassing all important services, use of manual and electronic formats, hybrid from manual medical records into electronic records, computerization of medical record management system, electronic health records including strategic planning, challenges of adoption, limitations, function and standards, technology infrastructure, standardization of paperless medical records, medical record management professional endurance and tips for evaluation of electronic health record software.

The project should also focus on introduction to electronic nursing records which plays a essential role in day to day work in the hospital, international standards required to be maintained, quality assurance, virtual implementation process of electronic records in all vital departments of the hospital, e.g. accident and emergency, outpatient and inpatient services, intensive care units, OT, diagnostic laboratory, radiology, pharmacy and concluding chapter deals with the challenges in IT and networking design.

The project would be of immense value besides to medical and paramedical students, to all healthcare professionals especially all personnel involved with patient care, e.g. medical, nursing and paramedical teachers and students. The healthcare providers, e.g. doctors, nurses and paramedical, software developers, medico-legal personnel, insurance, etc. The organizers of electronic health records in the hospital, health information management units, information technologists, medical record departments, health directorates, ministries of health and healthcare involved software companies besides medical records and health information management educational and paramedical courses and research institutions will also be immensely benefited by this masterpiece.

Next most important objective is to assist overburden nursing staff with nursing and non-nursing duties coupled with extensive documentation responsibilities. The advent of technology has changed many fields and health is one of them. It is a matter of time; all the health institutions would have to be ehealth managed organizations. Nursing being the most overwhelmed with recording work need to embrace the electronic system that minimize the duplication, efforts and optimum output for the benefit of everyone especially the patient. Nursing professional as a change agent, need to promote the e-Health system including implementing electronic recording system that help nursing staff to provide best possible healthcare to the needy patients.

Project results should deal with healthcare delivery system including functions of primary, secondary and tertiary care hospitals including superspecialty services. Nursing profession is exceptional because their role is involved in all these services with the responsibility of maintaining certain documents related to patient care, administrative, finance and other works. Hence, it would be appropriate to know the main functions of each unit /service, so that suitable design of electronic digital formats could be prepared by the software vendors.

Further project studies should contain exclusively prepared nursing information technology educational program specially designed syllabus, course content with time schedule to suit for the very busy working nursing professionals who are hard pressed coupled with shortage of staff, who with so much work to perform, and hardly find time to be away from the busy daily program. The outcome of studies will be a handbook and boon for all nursing educational institutions and others professionals, e.g. medical, paramedical including laboratory, radiology, pharmacy, nutritionists, biomedical engineering and administrative and finance staff will also benefit from the outcome of this service. Besides all these, this material is extremely valuable for software companies developing hospital information system including electronic health and nursing records.

Skills needed for conducting project: In order to conduct project or to serve effectively on project teams, the team members need particular skills. The student will learn not only the skills required, but also needed techniques of project management.

The project: The project is considered to be an endeavor undertaken to study in depth to find the facts and come out with the results. The results could be completely different from the assumed hypothesis, the need is honest collection of data, compiling, interpreting and reporting with positive and negative information. The project report, if done in a right place at right time by right people with right methods can produce excellent results that would definitely benefit to the to the government or organizations to take policy decision accordingly. The objective of choosing a project is classified into three parts; placement, productivity and stability. Any new project to undertake is to invest, hence, one has to be sure the planned project is completed according to planned schedule with the expected outcome. The purpose of placement is to support the government's strategic goals and leads to complete the project in time. While selecting a project, the outcome should be advantages and productive. The project results to be stable to meet the set target, it is necessary to maintain the infrastructure, i.e. entire force of communications, transportations in dealing with obstacles and move forward for the progress.

HIM practice transformation: *The transition from paper-based health records to electronic health records (EHRs) is ushering in a new virtual HIM department. Every healthcare organization will need to study and address the effect of the EHR and its management on their organizations and the HIM department.*

The EHR's impact: The EHR and its management require HIM professionals in collaboration with other specialty leaders to develop a road map leading from a paper-based to a virtual HIM practice. The seriousness of involvement will require a new way of thinking and proceeding. Work process improvements, implementation techniques, and new information management practices will be essential to HIM practice transformation in almost all types of care settings. The sincerity of change and carful management are critical to the successful creation of the virtual HIM department.

The virtual HIM department: It is the endeavor of any government or organization endeavor is to accomplish the virtual HIM department that will have a digital portal (the

HIM portal) which allows access to individual, longitudinal digital health records by consumers, care providers and others concerned with patient care. Consumers will access their medical information online for their personal health records. They will schedule appointments and pay bills based on access to their EHR. Consumers will access the HIM portal to authorize disclosure of their personal health information to employers and schools. Required Kiosks will have to be strategically located within facilities to provide access to the HIM portal for consumer transactions. Consumers may also access the portal via the healthcare organization's secured internet access. HIM staff will remotely access the portal to ensure that the system performs essential functions. The traditional HIM function carried out to support the paper health record today will be re-engineered, not required records are eliminated in the new virtual health record setting. The government authorities and organizational executives or policy makers will need to actively and full heartedly support their HIM teams in achieving the transformation of paper records to paperless.

In order to transform paper to paperless, the process will encompass the following:

- To ensure that current state of the paper health record is maintained well and put intact.
- To transition stage, i.e., by scanning the paper records into electronic, a hybrid system that includes paper and electronic health records maintenance side by side.
- To ensure that entire patient care system is on electronic health records

Future tasks of HIM: It is visualized that future of HIM will have to deal with eHIM. The HIM professionals have to think the dynamism of information technology growth; the professionals have to be prepared to meet the transition that is going to be there. It needs to understand the work process and best features of technology that could be applied with creativity; the HIM leaders should beside adopting the traditional methods, to understand the principles of change management that could contribute in bringing new techniques while transition from HIM to eHIM.

New Future Roles of HIM Professionals

The way the technology is progressing, with the same speed, the HIM professionals will have to move forward with the new advances by enhanced or modified education system including the learning and teaching application techniques. The entire progress has to be related to evidence based medicine, that means, the healthcare provided and the technology applied should be compatible in a sense, the technology applied is on the basis of established evidence. The experts in the HIM field feel the new roles would be IT training specialist, EHR system manager, business process engineer, clinical vocabulary manager, workflow and data analyst, consumer advocate, clinical alerts and reminder manager, clinical research coordinator, privacy coordinator, enterprise application specialist and many more. This entails the HIM professionals have to continuous up gradation of their knowledge, skills, and expertise with positive attitude to keep pace being successful leaders in the new virtual HIM practice and also will give marvelous boost to HIM professionals in successfully EHR implementation and efficient management.

SAMPLE PROGRAM DESCRIPTION DESIGN

The HIM graduate program is structured to facilitate the career advancement of practicing Health Information Management professionals. The program emphasizes quality health care data as the foundation for organizational information and knowledge management systems.

The curriculum focuses on emerging frameworks for creating integrated healthcare information, data management and decision support systems. It is specifically designed to prepare professionals to thrive in a technology-supported and information-driven health care environment.

This advanced education prepares the HIM professional for responsibilities in areas such as health care data resources administration, health care data security oversight, strategic and operational information resource planning, clinical data analysis, information systems development and implementation.

Outcomes

Upon completion of the health information management program, the graduate will be able to:

- Integrate advanced knowledge and skills in health care data and information management
- Evaluate, select and implement information technologies to manage health care data resources
- Leverage health care information to drive integrated clinical and administrative decision-making, strategic planning and outcomes management
- Take the leadership role in establishing an organizational culture that embraces the ethical use of confidential information and information technologies
- Apply effective communication skills and strategies in interactions with multidisciplinary and multifacility professionals
- Assume increasingly challenging administrative and leadership positions in complex provider organizations and related entities in the health care arena
- Thrive professionally in a practice environment that is undergoing fundamental change.
- Initiate hybrid from manual to electronic
- Design, develop and management of information technology
- Associate in developing electronic health records system
- Implement HER system and effective maintenance
- Initiate for health economics or cost containment by using technology
- Endeavor to improve quality and safety of patient care
- Assist the administration in efficient management of health institution

The healthcare costs worldwide are at an all time high. There is enough evidence that information technology can reduce the costs of healthcare services and also minimize medical error, and manage healthcare services.

The nation facing the biggest challenge is finding skilled knowledgeable people who know how to use IT shortage of people and jobs are not easily available.

Minimum Master's degree in HIM is requirement to be of Head of HIM Department of a teaching or specialized or big hospital (>500 beds).

Curriculum for Future HIM Professionals

With the new challenges and roles HIM professionals are going to assume, a minimum of masters degree in health information administration would be appropriate for the managerial level in the specialized, teaching and big hospitals. The baccalaureate degree with any one of the specializations, such as HIM administration, computers, coding and data analysis, health costing and quality assurance, or privacy would be suitable for the supervisory personnel working in the second level of management in five different sections of the HIM department. Out of four years of study for the bachelor's of science HIM program, the first three years should cover all of the basic subjects required, and the fourth year should be exclusively allocated for specialization. The operational staff should possess a minimum of extended HIM technology program credential, as they will rotate in all different sections of HIM with the purpose of gaining multifaceted experience.

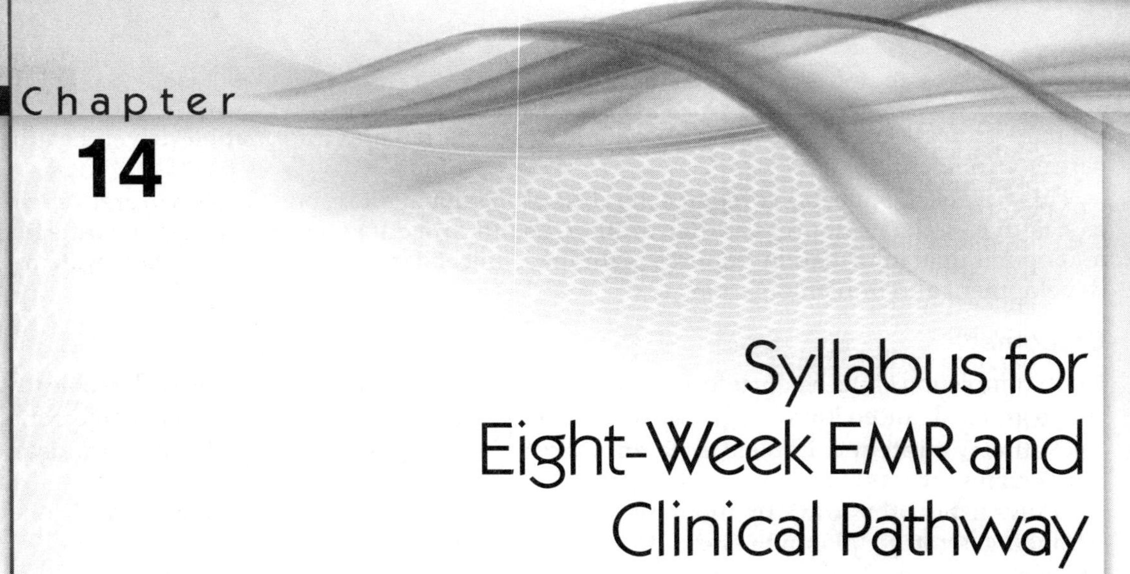

Chapter 14

Syllabus for Eight-Week EMR and Clinical Pathway

INTRODUCTION

Clinical pathways are multidisciplinary plan of care for best clinical practice for specified groups of patients with a particular diagnosis that aid in the coordination and delivery of high quality of care. They are a documented sequence of clinical interventions that help a patient with a specific condition or diagnosis move, progressively through a clinical experience to a desired outcome. They are management tools and clinical audit tool that are based on clinical information developed in other guidelines or parameters. They are specific to the institution using them. Originally critical pathways began with admission and ended with discharge from the hospital. Today, they are usually interdisciplinary in focus, merging the medical and nursing plans of care with those of other disciplines, such as physical therapy, nutrition, or mental health. They provide opportunities for collaborative practice and team approaches that can maximize the expertise of multiple disciplines. Clinical pathway is a medical team refers to doctors, nurses to work together to provide patients with best management practices. Clinical pathway deals with certain diagnosis and surgery to make the most appropriate, order and timing of the clinics plan to reduce the delay in rehabilitation and a waste of resources so that patient get the best quality of treatment.

1. Application of EMR and clinical pathway 5
   - Introduction to clinical pathway 2
     - Definition 1
     - Objective 1
   - EMR adaptive clinical pathway
     - Benefits
     - Barriers and problems
     - Complexity

   EMR functional requirements 1
2. Clinical pathway information management system 4
   - Introduction 1
   - Functions 2
     - Design pathway

- Executive pathway
- Statistical pathway

• Operating system 1

3. EMR software with built-in-clinical content and clinical pathways 12
   • Care plan integration
   • Care pathways
     - Background
     - Benefits
     - Barriers and problems
     - Novel approach
   • Pathway complexity 1
   • Pathway strategy 1
   • Technology requirements and solutions 1
   • Pulling patient into the pathway 1
   • Reporting from the application 1
   Costs 1
   Security and privacy 1
4. Electronic medical records (EMR) 22
   • Introduction 1
     - Computer-based patient record (CPR)
     - Electronic medical record (EMR)
     - Electronic health records (EHR)
   • The evolution of EMR early work 1
   • More recent development
   Setting computer-based patient medical records 5
   • Integrated delivery system 5
     - Ambulatory care 1
     - Emergency/urgent care 1
     - Long term care 1
     - Home care 1
     - Behavioral health 1
   Scope of electronic medical records 4
   • Computer architecture
   • Human interface
   • Operating system
   • Data management system
   • Application software
   • Networks
   The EMR pathway 1
   • The components of strategic planning
     - Preparation
     - Strategic analysis
     - Strategic direction
     - Process
   • Challenge of EMR adoption 5
     - Challenges and strategies to EMR adoption
       □ Lack of national information standards and code sets
       □ Lack of available funding
       □ Concern about physician usage
       □ Lack of interoperability

- EMR functional requirements 5
  - Administration requirements
  - Clinical decision requirements
  - Data export requirements
  - Clinical decision support
  - Prescribing requirements
  - Order management requirements
  - Privacy protection and security requirements

5. Implementation of EMR and other systems 21
- EMR implementation process 6
  - The paper-based medical record 1
  - Historical background
    - Introduction
    - Primitive medical records
    - Modern medicine
    - Medical records in western countries
    - Medical records in developing countries
- Role of medical records in healthcare delivery 1
  - Health care delivery system
  - Purposes of medical records
  - Importance of medical records
    - To the patient
    - To the physician
    - To the healthcare intuition
    - To the research team
    - To the teaching program
    - To the national health agencies
    - To the international organizations
  - Responsibility for medical records 1
    - Hospital administration
    - Healthcare providers
    - Medical records manager
- Standards for medical record services 1
  - Hospital must maintain adequate patient records
  - Outpatient records
    - Emergency records
    - Inpatient records
- Medical record must be secured confidentially assured
- Written policies and procedures for MR maintenance
- MR department must be adequately equipped
- Medical record policies
  - Introduction
- General rules and regulations for maintaining MR 2
  - Legal aspect of medical records
    - Medico-legal cases (MLC) registration
    - Patient consent
    - Security and privacy
    - Release of information

- Quality assurance
  - Quality control
  - Quantitative analysis
  - Qualitative analysis
  - Medical audit
  - Formation of medical record committee
- Hybrid medical record 1
  - Introduction
  - Definition of hybrid
- Transformation from paper (manual) to paperless (electronic)
- Hybrid health record policy
- EMR implementation process 4
  - An introduction to EMR systems 3
    - Software-vendor or tailor made
    - Hardware and enabling technologies
    - Choosing a successful EMR system
      - Technical features
        - Usage of CPOE and CDSS
        - Role in electronic research work
      - Event monitoring
      - Quality care and costs
    - Implementing EMR system
    - Technical standards
      - HL7
      - ANSI × 12 (ED)
      - CEN—CONTSYS (EN 13940)
      - CEN—EHRcom (EN 13606)
      - CEN—HISA (EN 12967)
      - DICOM
    - Regulatory compliance
      - HIPAA
      - HL7
      - DICOM
      - Title 21 CFR part 11
    - Legal issues
      - Introduction
      - Ownership of health information
      - Electronic medical records
        - Federal laws
        - State laws
      - Privacy, confidentiality and security
  - Checklist for readiness to implement EHER 1
- Other systems implementation 10
  - Personal health record (PHR) 2
      - Definition of PHR
      - Purpose of PHR
      - Implementation of PHR
      - PHR components
        - Patient ID format

- Health summary
- Immunization
- Self care
- Medication
- Investigations
- Obstetrics and gynecology
- Therapy
- Chronic disease record
- Dental

- Telemedicine and tele-health 2
  - Telemedicine 1
    - Introduction
    - Definition of telemedicine
    - Types of technology
    - Telemedicine concept
    - Telemedicine program support
    - Telemedicine challenges
  - Tele-health 1
    - Introduction
    - Clinical uses of technologies
    - Tele-health modes
      - Store-and-forward tele-health
      - Real time tele-health
      - Tele-cardiology
      - Tele-trauma
      - Tele-pharmacy
      - Tele-dentistry
      - Tele-radiology
      - Tele-pathology
      - Tele-nursing
- Remote patient monitoring
  - Home based-nocturnal dialysis
  - Cardiac and remote ICUs
  - Disease management
  - Mobile technology in healthcare 1
  - Smart cards, wireless, RFID 1
    - Introduction
    - History
    - Integrated circuits
    - Types of smart cards
      - Contact smart cards
      - Contact less smart cards
      - Combination smart cards
  - Standards
    - ISO 7816
    - ISO/IEC 14443
    - ETSI
    - EMV
    - JAVA card

- ◻ WHQL
- ◻ Applications of smart cards
- ◻ Identification
- ◻ Net work access
- ◻ Electronic purses
- ◻ Telecommunications
- ◻ Special applications

– Security with smart cards
- ◻ Standard security guards
  - ▪ Authentication
  - ▪ Confidentiality
  - ▪ Integrity
  - ▪ Non-repudiation

– Wireless 1
- ◻ Introduction
- ◻ Wireless services
- ◻ Wireless net works
- ◻ Modes
  - ▪ Radio
  - ▪ Microwave
  - ▪ Infrared

– Applications of wireless technology
- ◻ Mobile telephone
- ◻ Wireless data communications
  - ▪ Wi-Fi
  - ▪ Cellular data service
  - ▪ Mobile satellite communication
- ◻ Categories of wireless implementations
  - ▪ Devices standards
  - ▪ Radio
  - ▪ Broadcasting
  - ▪ Armature radio
  - ▪ Land mobile radio
  - ▪ Cordless telephone
  - ▪ Cellular networks
- ◻ Health information technology (HIT) 1
- ◻ Introduction
- ◻ Concept and definition
- ◻ Implementation of HIT
- ◻ Types of technology
  - ▪ HER
  - ▪ Clinical point of care technology–CPOE
- ◻ Financial: Revenue and expenditure 1
- ◻ Insurance and billing 1

– Health informatics professional's role 1
- ◻ Role
- ◻ Functions
- ◻ Key responsibilities

6. Preparations and assessment 16
7. Practical or fieldwork 40

COURSE DESCRIPTION

The course study encompasses the concept of clinical pathways, application of EMR and objectives of EMR adaption clinical pathway; benefits, barriers and problems, complexity. The study also covers clinical pathway management system with functions covering; design, executive and statistical pathways. System platform and operating system

The electronic medical records (EMR) software within built-in content and clinical pathways, care plan integration, with benefits, and barriers, and pathway complexity, pathway strategies, technology requirements, cost, security and privacy. The scope and challenges of EMR adoption and functional requirements, implementation of EMR and other system includes, paper-based medical records, role of medical records, standards, general rules and regulations for maintaining effective medical records. Hybrid system followed during implementation process, and implementation process including software—vendor and tailor-made, application of technical standards, legal issues, state laws, privacy, confidentiality and security. Other system implementation includes; personal health records, tele-medicine, tele-health, mobile technologies, and smart cards used in healthcare and role of health information management professional.

OBJECTIVES OF THE COURSE

Upon successful completion of the course, the students will be able to:

- Define clinical pathways
- Explain the EMR and clinical pathway objectives, benefits and barriers
- Specify the EMR functions and requirements
- Explain the clinical pathway information management system including functions and operating system
- Describe care plan integration, care pathways, pathway complexities, pathway strategy,
- Understand the difference between CPR, EMR and EHR
- Explain scope of EMR in clinical pathways
- Illustrate challenges of EMR adoption
- Describe EMR functions and implementation requirements
- Explain EMR implementation process including paper-based, hybrid and electronic
- Define PHR and the purpose of PHR and its utility to patient
- Explain tele-medicine and tele-health in healthcare delivery
- Elaborate mobile technology and its use in healthcare
- Stipulate healthcare information management professional role.

Chapter 15

Syllabus for Six-Month Diploma in Medical/Healthcare Informatics

INTRODUCTION

The health informatics could be conceived as the collection, storage, retrieval and organization of health related data, transformed into information and knowledge for effective management of healthcare organizations including medical and healthcare services. Prudent application of informatics tools, commonly known as information and communication technology (ICT) will result in efficient public health, biomedical and hospital operation system including medical education and research.

The diploma/certificate course in counseling include the areas of the study:

1. Introduction to healthcare information
   - Public health and biomedical — 10
     - Disease surveillance
     - Chronic disease management
     - Disease registries
     - Epidemiology
     - Health indicators
     - Statistical reporting
   - Hospital information — 12
     - Types of clinical/medical
     - Clinical or medical
     - Administrative including finance
     - Ancillary
     - Characteristics of useful management information — 4
     - Sources of health information — 2
     - Uses of health/hospital data — 2
     - Security and protection of data — 2
2. Healthcare data and quality
   - Data versus information — 2
   - Problems of poor quality data — 2

- Perspective: Documentation 6
- Ensuring the quality of data and information 4

3. Healthcare information regulations, laws and standards
   - Accreditation, licensure, and certification 3
   - ISO standards 1
   - JCAHO standards 2
   - HIPAA standards 2
   - Evidence-based medicine (EBM) 1
   - Health record as a legal document 3
   - Retention of health records 2
   - Security, privacy and confidentiality 2
   - Release of health information 2
4. Information technology and healthcare
   - Hardware 2
   - Software 2
     - Systems software
     - Applications software
   - Overview of networking 2
     - Intranets
     - Extranet
   - Internet services 1
5. Healthcare informatics and database knowledge management
   - History and evolution of health information systems 4
   - Database management 6
   - Information system 4
     - Hospital information systems 8
     - Clinic information systems 4
     - Laboratory information systems 1
     - Radiology information systems 1
     - Pharmacy information systems 1
     - Electronic medical record—EHR, HL7, XML 4
     - Computerized provider order entry (CPOE) 2
     - Clinical decision support system (CDSS) 2
     - Personal health record 2
     - Telemedicine and tele-health 2
     - Mobile in healthcare informatics 3
     - Smart cards, wireless, RFID 2
     - Administrative including HR information system 4
     - Financial: Revenue and expenditure 3
     - Insurance and billing 4
6. Introduction to human anatomy, physiology and medical terminology
   - Parts of a medical term 4
   - Prefixes, roots, and suffixes 4
   - Body systems 12
   - Medical abbreviations 2
   - Diagnostic procedures and therapeutic interventions 10
7. Introduction to international classification of diseases and surgical procedures
   - Coding and indexing guidelines 6

- Diagnostic coding and indexing procedures
  - Inpatient 16
  - Outpatient 4
- ICD 10 and ICD-9CM 4
- CPT coding system 2

8. Development and implementation of EMR
   - The paper-based medical record, hybrid medical records 8
   - EMR implementation process 10
9. Health informatics professional's role
   - With healthcare delivery, consumers, healthcare providers 2
   - Administrators and vendors 2
10. Standards for health informatics
    - Digital imaging and communications in medicine (DICOM) and packs 2
    - Health Insurance Portability and Accountability Act (HIPAA) 2
    - Health level seven (HL-7) 1
    - International Organization for Standardization (ISO) 1
    - American National Standard Institute (ANSI) 1
    - Standard nomenclature of medicine-clinical terms (SNOMED CT) 1
    - Logical observation identifier names and codes (LOINC) 2
11. Preparations and assessment (22) 22
12. English language (spoken and communication skills) (16) 16
13. Practical or field work 26

TOTAL: 288

COURSE DESCRIPTION

A study of the healthcare delivery services including medical, biomedical and public health and use of health information through healthcare processes by generation of documentation of encounters, application of required technology and regulations for obtaining quality information, and subsequent storage and access for the use of healthcare delivery.

With the emerging information technology, use of electronic medical record documents incorporating CPOE, CDSS in healthcare information systems and application of international medical informatics standards such as DICOM, HL-7, ISO, SNOMED CT, LOINC, and HIPAA in relation to healthcare, privacy, confidentiality, information security for effective, swift, safe and quality care.

A study of basic human anatomy, physiology and medical terminology to help in classification of diagnosis and surgical procedures by applying international prescribed numerical/alpha medical codes from ICD and CPT manual.

A study of the database knowledge management used in healthcare particularly in patient care, types of database management techniques, file and access techniques, query and update languages, data integrity, use of health record systems, and applications of databases to support the healthcare system for effective maintaining healthcare recording systems for generating quality information for efficient healthcare delivery to the customers.

OBJECTIVES OF THE COURSE

Upon successful completion of the course, the students will be able to:

- Explain the major types of healthcare services and information related to medical and public health

- Differentiate between data and information and explain good quality data
- Describe information flow through the healthcare process in the healthcare system
- Explain how technology that used for competitive advantage for the healthcare system
- Describe the security, privacy and confidentiality issues associated with healthcare
- State the healthcare regulations, laws and standards
- Explain how technology impacts implementation of EMR and its importance
- Understand the impact of technology on the healthcare system
- State the rules for building medical terms combing forms, prefixes, and suffixes
- Describe the purpose of codified and classification of health records
- Differentiate ICD-9-CM, ICD-10, CPT codes the use for each code
- Explain the advantages of computerized databases over manual record processing in healthcare system
- Describe effective management of healthcare information using a database
- Understand the use of technology standards in hospital information system.

Chapter 16

Syllabus for Twelve-Month Diploma in Medical/Healthcare Informatics

INTRODUCTION

The health informatics could be conceived as the collection, storage, retrieval and organization of health related data, transformed into information and knowledge for effective management of healthcare organizations including medical and healthcare services. Prudent application of informatics tools, commonly known as information and communication technology (ICT) will result in efficient public health, biomedical and hospital operation system including medical education and research.

The diploma/certificate course in counseling include the areas of the study:

1. Introduction to healthcare information	32	Doctor/PH
• Public health	13	
– The purpose and methods of epidemiology		
□ The purpose	4	
□ Planning and evaluating healthcare	1	
□ Identification of the determinants of disease	1	
□ Evaluation of methods of disease control	1	
□ Classification of disease	1	
• The methods of epidemiology	4	
– Descriptive studies	1	
– Analytical studies	1	
– Experimental studies	1	
– Disease surveillance	1	
• Chronic disease management	2	Doctor/PH
– Effectiveness of team care		
□ Population based care		
□ Treatment planning		
□ Evidence-based clinical management		
□ Self management support		
□ Effective consultation		

▫ Sustained follow-up		
▫ Team composition for effective chronic disease management		
• Disease registries	1	Doctor/PH
– Characteristics of disease register	1	
• Health indicators	1	Doctor/PH
– Basic health indicators including the UN	1	
▫ UN millennium development goals		
• Statistical reporting (written repots)	1	
– Basic principles of data		
▫ General purpose table		
▫ Special purpose table		
– Elements of table		
▫ Title		
▫ Unit of measurement		
▫ Captions and status		
▫ Interpretative aids		
– Classifications		
▫ Classification by space		
▫ Classification by attribute		
▫ Classification by time		
▫ Classification by size of observation		
• Presentation by graphs and diagrams		
• Time comparison		
• Space and attribute comparisons		
• Analysis of time series		
• Types of data		
– Categorical data		
– Numerical data		
– Data display		
– Tables		
– Graphs		
• Results		
• Discussion		
• Summary		
• Biomedical information	3	Doctor/Hosp
– Introduction to biomedical research	1	
– Integration of biomedical and clinical information	1	
– Role of IT in bioinformatics and its advantages	1	
• Hospital information	16	MRO/HIM
– Categories of information	2	
▫ Clinical or medical	1	
▫ Administrative	1	
▫ Finance and		
▫ Ancillary		
▫ Clinical or medical	6	
• Outpatient	1	
• Accident and emergency	1	
– Inpatient	2	
– Diagnostic and other	2	

Topic	Hours
• Administrative	4
– Human resource	1
– Financial	1
– Purchasing and inventory control	2
– Medical stores	
– General stores	
– Other	
• Ancillary (support)	4
– Engineering (civil, electrical, mechanical)	2
– Housing and maintenance of building	
– Water supply, drainage, fire extinguishers	
– Air-conditioning, central heating	
– Fire-extinguishers	
– Legal advice	1
– Consultant's advice	1
2. Healthcare data and quality	32
• Quality officer	
• Data characteristics and quality	16
• Data versus information	2
• Data	1
• Information	1
• Data characteristics	4
– Relevant	
– Sensitive	
– Unbiased	
– Comprehensive	
– Timely	
– Action oriented	
– Uniform	
– Performance targeted	
• Problems of poor quality data	5
– Estimation of institutional goals and objectives	1
– Demand estimate for service	1
– Resource allocate to meet demand	1
– Performance and quality control	1
– Evaluation of program impact	1
• Ensuring quality data	5
– Quality control	5
□ Operational control	2
□ Program control	2
□ Social control	1
• Perspective: Documentation	6
– Comprehensive document	6
– Complete	1
– Accurate	1
– Relevant and timely	1
– Authenticated	1
– Secured	1
– Privacy	1

• Health information characteristics	10	
– Sources of health information	2	
– Primary	1	
– Secondary	1	
– Uses of health/hospital data	6	
– Administrative	2	
– Medical	2	
▫ Health agencies	1	
– Accrediting agencies	1	
– Security and privacy of data	2	
– Security	1	
– Privacy	1	
3. Information technology and healthcare	32	Network Eng. IT
• Computer	20	
– Hardware	4	
– Software	10	
▫ Systems software	5	
▫ Applications software	5	
– Overview of networking	4	
▫ Intranets	2	
▫ Extranet	2	
– Internet services	2	
– History of information technology	4	
– Evolution of information technology	4	
– Phases of information technology	4	
4. The IT strategic plan	32	Comp. Eng. IT
• Technologies	4	
• Computing architectures	6	
• Human interface	4	
• Operating systems	6	
• Data management systems	6	
• Application software	4	
• Networks	2	
5. Introduction to anatomy, physiology and medical terminology	64	Doctor/Hosp
• Medical terminology	24	
– Chief source of medical words	2	
▫ Anglo-saxon (old english)		
▫ Greco-roman (Greek and Latin)		
▫ Arabic		
▫ Modern german		
▫ Colors		
▫ Numerals		
– Basic word structure	2	
▫ Roots		
▫ Suffix		
▫ Prefix		
– Elements of medical terms	8	
▫ Suffix and compound elements		
▫ Diagnostic suffix and compound elements		

- Operative suffix and compound elements
  - □ Symptomatic and compounding elements
  - □ Roots 4
  - □ Prefixes 4
- • Medical abbreviations 4
  - Anatomy and physiology 24
    - □ Body systems
      - ■ Human body
      - ■ Musculoskeletal system
      - ■ Cardiovascular system
      - ■ Blood and lymphatic system
      - ■ Nervous system
      - ■ Digestive system
      - ■ Endocrine system
      - ■ Respiratory system
      - ■ Senses organs
      - ■ Excretory system
      - ■ Reproductive system
- • Diagnostic procedures and therapeutic interventions 16
  - Description of the diagnostic procedures 6
- • Blood and lymphatic system 1
- • Musculoskeletal system and skin 1
- • Endocrine system 1
- • Cardiovascular and respiratory system 1
- • Digestive system and urinary system 1
- • Female and male reproductive system 1
- • Selective diagnosis with required investigations 3
- • Normal values for laboratory investigations 3
- • Blood test investigations 1
- • Urine investigations 1
- • Semen analysis and cerebrospinal fluid' 1
- • Variations of normal values and resulting diagnosis 4

6. Healthcare information regulations, laws and standards 32 Quality analyst NABA
   - • Licensure, certification and accreditation 4
     - Facility licensure
     - Certification
     - Accreditation
   - • ISO standards 2
     - What is standard?
     - What are the benefits of ISO international standards
     - ISO 9001 healthcare management
     - ISO 9001 health service accreditation
     - ISO 13485 medical device standards
   - • JCAHO standards 4
     - JCAHO information management standards
       - □ JACHO standards for the content and maintenance of patient records
   - • National committee for quality assurance (NCQA)
     - The accreditation of managed care organizations

  - The development and implementation of the health plan employer data
    - Information set (HEDIS)
  - Quality compass
- Health insurance portability accountability act (HIPAA) standards 4
  - HIPAA security standards: Final rule
    - Introduction and background information
    - Administrative simplification
    - Privacy standards—April 14, 2003
    - Transaction and code set standards—Oct 16, 2003
    - Security standards—April 20, 2005
    - Identifier standard–not yet finalized
  - Comparison of the HIPAA final security standards to ISO/IEC
  - Administrative safeguards
    - Security management
    - Assigned security responsibility (required)
    - Workforce security
    - Information access management
    - Security incidence procedures
    - Contingency plan
    - Evaluation report
  - Physical safeguards
    - Facility access controls
    - Workstation (required)
    - Workstation security (required)
      Device and media controls
  - Technical safeguards
    - Access control
    - Audit control
    - Integrity
    - Person or entity authentication (required)
    - Transmission security
- Analysis of comparison between HIPAA standard
  - Implementation and ISO/IEC 17799
- Evidence-based medicine (EBM) 2
  - Introduction
  - Background and definition
  - Evidence-based health services
  - Evidence-based decision making
    - Process and progress
      1. Translation of uncertainty to an answerable question and includes critical questioning, study design and levels of evidence
      2. Systematic retrieval of best evidence available
      3. Critical appraisal of evidence for internal validity that can be broken down into aspects regarding:
         - Systematic errors as a result of selection bias, information bias and confounding
         - Quantitative aspects of diagnosis and treatment
         - The effect size and aspects regarding its precision
         - Clinical importance of results
         - External validity or generalized

4. Application of results in practice
5. Evaluation of performance

- Ranking the quality of service
- Grade work group
- Categories of recommendation
- Statistical measures
- Number needed to treat/harm
- Quality of clinical trails
- Limitations and criticism
- Assessing the teaching of EBM

• Health record as a legal document — 4 MRO/HIM Hosp

- Introduction
- Health record as a legal document
  - Patient-identifiable source data
  - Administrative data
  - Derived data
- Ownership of health information
  - Ownership of masked and aggregate data
  - Multi-provider systems integration arrangements
  - Information systems vendors and clearinghouses
- Electronic health records
  - Introduction
  - Federal laws
  - Retention of health records (manual and electronic) — 3 MRO/HIM
    - Purpose of retention of records
    - Federal/state statutory for retention of records

• Retention schedule

- Patient records
  - Outpatient
  - Inpatient
  - Accident and emergency
  - Medicolegal cases
- X-rays including US, CT scan, MRI, etc.
  - Outpatient
  - Inpatient
  - Accident and emergency
- Registers;
  - Birth
  - Death
  - Patient registration
  - Admission and discharge
  - Medicolegal
  - Narcotic
  - Radiology
  - Laboratory
- Reports
  - Ward census reports
  - Statistical daily, monthly, yearly

- Preservation destruction of health records 1
- Destruction of records process
- Documentation of destruction
- Security, privacy and confidentiality 4
  - Introduction
  - Difference between privacy, confidentiality and security
  - Growth and impact of information technology
  - The impact for health information decurity
  - Model legislative language (AHIMA drafted)
  - Security threat to healthcare information
  - Ensuring healthcare information security
    - □ Development of security organization
    - □ Administrative controls
      - ■ Risk analysis and management
      - ■ Chief security officer
      - ■ System security evaluation
    - □ Physical controls/safeguards
      - ■ Assigned security responsibility
      - ■ Media control
      - ■ Physical access controls
      - ■ Workstation security
    - □ Technical controls/safeguards
      - ■ Access control
      - ■ Entity authentication
      - ■ Audit trails
      - ■ Data encryption
      - ■ Firewall protection
      - ■ Virus checking
- Release of health information 4 MRO/HIM Hosp
  - Release information policies and procedures
    - □ Release of information without authorization
    - □ Release of information with authorization
  - Release of information form

7. Healthcare informatics and management system 32 MRO/HIM Hosp
- Introduction to the healthcare information 3
    - □ Types of healthcare information 1
    - □ Internal data and information: Patient specific clinical 1
      - ■ Purpose of patient records
      - ■ Content of patient records
      - ■ Overview of patient encounter
    - □ Patient-specific data and information—administrative 1
      - ■ Data needed to process reimbursement claims
      - ■ Other uniform data sets
      - ■ Combine clinical and administrative
- History and evolution of healthcare information system 1
  - Definition
  - Types of healthcare information system
  - Evolution of healthcare information system

- Information system
  - Hospital information systems 6
    - Introduction
    - Administration functions
      - Patient registration
      - Patient scheduling
      - Patient admission, discharge and transfers
      - Billing and reimbursement
    - Organizational structure
    - Systems administration
      - Database administrator
      - Application specialist and trainer
      - Hardware/net work engineer
    - Standardization
    - Benefits of HIS
    - Medical record system
      - Purpose
      - Content
        - ID Data
        - Patient care information
      - Administrative issues
        - Legal document
        - Retention of records/information
        - Destruction of records/information
        - Security and privacy of records/information
- Clinic information systems (CIS) 6
  - Introduction
    - What is CIS?
    - How does using the CIS will improve care?
- Laboratory information systems (LIS) 2 Lab Tech. Hosp
  - Introduction
  - Test order
  - Repeated order
  - Quick lab results
  - Pending lab result
  - Visit history
  - Result history
  - Blood request
  - Ultrasound
  - Release/recall details
  - Laboratory components
  - Print investigations
  - Filter investigations
  - Laboratory profile
- Basic features:
  - Patient check in
  - Order entry
  - Specimen processing
  - Result (s) entry
  - Reporting

  - Patient demographics
  - Physician demographics
- Additional features
  - Web-based order entry
  - Web-based results inquiry
  - Faxing and emailing of lab reports
  - Custom report creation
  - HL7 interfaces with reference labs and EMRs
  - Preliminary reporting
  - Final reporting
  - Med tech work sheets
  - Workload balancing
  - Billing
  - Public health reporting
  - Rule engines
  - Report check by reputed pathologist and senior technologist
- Types of laboratory disciplines
  - Hematology
- Chemistry
- Immunology
- Blood bank donor center
- Blood bank transfusion
- Clinical pathology
- Cytology (cytopathology)
- Microbiology
- Flow cytometry
- TB
- Radiology information systems (RIS) 2 Rad. Tech. Hosp.
  - Introduction
  - Radiology procedure
  - Radiology history—visitwise
  - Radiology history—orderwise
  - Referred radiology
    - Printing the referral
    - Printing the report for the patient
- Registration
- Scheduling
- Patient tracking
- Film library management
- Reporting of results
- Department management
- Basic features
  - Patient registration and scheduling
  - Patient list management
  - Interface with modality via worklist
  - Radiology department workflow management
  - Request and documenting scanning
  - Result (s) entry
  - Reporting and printing

  - Result (s) delivery including faxing and e-mailing reports
  - Patient tracking
  - Interactive documents
  - Technical files creation
  - Modality and material management
- Additional features
  - Appointment books
  - PACS workflow
  - Custom report creation
  - HL7 interfaces with a PACS. HL7 also enables communication
  - Between HIS and RIS in addition to RIS and PACS
  - Billing
  - Rule engines
- Pharmacy information systems 2 Pharmacist hosp
  - Medication management system
    - □ Outpatient
    - □ Inpatient
    - □ Emergency patient
    - □ Preoperative patient
    - □ Postoperative patient
  - Delete medicine in the prescribed windows
  - Discontinue prescribed medicine
  - Download medicine prescribed from previous visit
  - Viewing the medical history
  - Activities:
    - □ Clinical screening
    - □ Prescription management
    - □ Inventory
    - □ Patient drug profile
    - □ Report generation
    - □ Interactivity with other systems
- Computerized provider order entry (CPOE) 4 Doctor IT
  - Introduction 1
    - □ Definition and primary function of CPOE system
    - □ Current use of CPOE
    - □ Value of CPOE
  - Benefits of advanced ambulatory CPOE system 1
    - □ Improved patient care
    - □ Cost savings
    - □ Provider revenue enhancement
  - Perspective CPOE implementation 1
    - □ Physician change management
    - □ Workflow change management
    - □ CPOE and decision support
  - Medication administration systems 1
    - □ Barcode-enabled point of care (BPOC)
- Clinical decision support system (CDSS) 6 Doctor IT
  - Introduction
  - Types of CDSS 2

- □ Knowledge based decision support systems
  - ■ Knowledge base
  - ■ Interface engine or reasoning mechanism
- □ Non-knowledge based CDSS
  - ■ Artificial neural networks
  - ■ Genetic algorithms
- □ Effectiveness of CDSS
  - ■ Implementation challenges
- □ Guidelines for selecting and implementing CDSS 2
  - ■ User understand the limitations
  - ■ The knowledge is from reputable source
  - ■ The system is appropriate for the local site
  - ■ The users are properly trained
  - ■ Monitor proper utilization of the installed CDSS
  - ■ The knowledge base is monitored and maintained
- □ Nursing information system (NIS) 2
  - ■ Features
    - Nursing self scheduling
    - Documenting care plans
    - Nursing work distribution
  - ■ Benefits
    - Saving time
    - Review patient care plan from anywhere
    - Make more efficient
    - Reduce stress

8. Scope and sites of electronic health records (EHR) 32 Doctor/HIM Hosp

- • History of electronic health records (EHR) 32
  - The evolution of EHR early work
  - More recent development
- • Scope and site of electronic health records
  - Computer-based patient record (CPR)
  - Electronic medical record (EMR)
- • Setting computer-based patient medical records 16 Network Eng. IT
  - Ambulatory care
  - Integrated delivery system
  - Emergency/urgent care
  - Long-term care
  - Home care
  - Behavioral health
- • Scope of electronic health records
  - Computer architecture
  - Human interface
  - Operating system
  - Data management system
  - Application software
  - Networks
- • Strategic EHR planning 4 Doctor/HIM
  - Strategic planning
    - □ Formulation
    - □ Implementation

- Formulation
- Implementation
  - Gartner generation
  - Collector generation
  - Documenter generation
  - Helper generation
  - Partner generation
  - Mentor generation
- The EHR pathway
  - Conducting strategic planning
  - The components of strategic planning
    - Preparation
    - Strategic analysis
    - Strategic direction
    - Process

• Challenge of EHR adoption	4	Doctor/HIM Hosp.

- Challenges and strategies to EHRR adoption
  - Lack of national information standards and code sets
  - Lack of available funding
  - Concern about physician usage
  - Lack of interoperability
- Strategies
  - Standard and interoperability
  - Expectations for government
  - Hospital strategies
  - Funding and incentives
    - Expectations for government
    - Hospital strategies
  - Physician acceptance
    - Expectations for government
    - Hospital strategies

• HER limitations	2	Doctor/HIM Hosp.

- Difficulty in adding older records to an EHRR system
- Long-term preservation and storage of records
- Synchronization of records
- Privacy
- Hardware limitations
- Cost advantages and disadvantages
- Starting up costs and software maintenance cost
- Inertia
- Legal barriers
- Customization

• HER functional requirements	6	Doctor/HIM Hosp.

- Administration requirements
- Clinical decision requirements

- – Data export requirements
- – Clinical decision support
- – Prescribing requirements
- – Order management requirements
- – Privacy protection and security requirements
- • Functional requirement technolog
  - – Information models for messages
  - – Conformance to international standards
  - – Record server and persistence interfaces and services
  - – Performance and current use
  - – Version control
  - – Exception and errors

9. Implementation of EMR and other systems — 64 — MRO/HIM Hosp
   - • EMR implementation process — 32
     - – The paper-based medical record — 20
       - □ Historical background — 2
         - ■ Introduction
         - ■ Primitive medical records
         - ■ Modern medicine
         - ■ Medical records in western countries
         - ■ Medical records in developing countries
   - • Role of medical records in healthcare delivery — 2
   - • Healthcare delivery system
   - • Purposes of medical records
   - • Importance of medical records
     - – To the patient
     - – To the physician
     - – To the healthcare intuition
     - – To the research team
     - – To the teaching program
     - – To the national health agencies
     - – To the international organizations
   - • Format of medical records — 2
     - – Source-oriented medical records
     - – Integrated-medical record
     - – Problem-oriented medical record (POMR)
   - • Responsibility for medical records — 2
     - – Hospital administration
     - – Healthcare providers
     - – Medical records manager
   - • Standards for medical record services — 2
   - • Hospital must maintain adequate patient records
   - • Outpatient records
     - – Emergency records
     - – Inpatient records
   - • Medical record must be secured confidentially assured
   - • Written policies and procedures for MR maintenance

- MR department must be adequately equipped
- Medical record policies
- Introduction
- General rules and regulations for maintaining MR 4
  - Legal-aspect of medical records 2
    - □ Medico legal cases (MLC) registration
    - □ Patient consent
    - □ Security and privacy
    - □ Release of information
- Quality assurance 2
  - Quality control
  - Quantitative analysis
  - Qualitative analysis
  - Medical audit
  - Formation of medical record committee
- Medical record organization, functions and interdepartmental relationship 6
  - Organization
  - Goal
  - Objectives
  - Organization and function
    - □ Outpatient service
    - □ Accident and emergency
    - □ Inpatient
    - □ Medical record library
    - □ Personal requirement and job description
    - □ Operational policy
    - □ Medical record procedures
      - ■ Central registration
      - ■ Outpatient clinic
      - ■ Accident and emergency
      - ■ Admitting office
      - ■ Nursing wards or unit
      - ■ Processing of OP records
      - ■ Processing of IP records
      - ■ Hospital statistics
      - ■ Filing and retrieving of records and X-rays
      - ■ Medical record library
- Hybrid medical record 2
  - Introduction
  - Definition of hybrid
  - Transformation from paper (manual) to paperless (electronic)
  - Hybrid health record policy
- EMR implementation process 10
  - What is an electronic medical record
    - □ Common healthcare computer systems
    - □ EMR concept
    - □ EMR and CPR

- An introduction to EMR systems 4
  - Software-vendor or tailor-made
  - Hardware and enabling technologies
  - Choosing a successful EMR system
    - Technical features
      - Usage of CPOE and CDSS
      - Role in electronic research work
    - Event monitoring
    - Quality care and costs
  - Implementing EMR system 4
  - Technical standards
    - HL7
    - ANSI × 12 (ED)
    - CEN–CONTSYS (EN 13940)
    - CEN–EHRcom (EN 13606)
    - CEN–HISA (EN 12967)
    - DICOM
  - Regulatory compliance
    - HIPAA
    - HL7
    - DICOM
    - Title 21 CFR part 11
  - Legal issues 1
    - Introduction
    - Ownership of health information
    - Electronic medical records
      - Federal laws
      - State laws
  - Privacy, confidentiality and security

- Checklist for readiness to implement HER 1
- Other systems implementation 32 Doctor Hosp
  - Personal health record (PHR) 4
  - Definition of PHR
  - Purpose of PHR
  - Implementation of PHR
  - PHR components
    - Patient ID format
    - Health summary
    - Immunization
    - Self care
    - Medication
    - Investigations
    - Obstetrics and gynecology
    - Therapy
    - Chronic disease record
    - Dental
  - Telemedicine and tele-health 4 Doctor hosp
  - Telemedicine 2
    - Introduction
    - Definition of telemedicine

Topic	Hours	Faculty
□ Types of technology		
□ Telemedicine concept		
□ Telemedicine program support		
□ Telemedicine challenges		
• Tele-health	2	
– Introduction		
□ Clinical uses of technologies		
– Tele-health modes		
□ Store-and-forward tele-health		
□ Real time tele-health		
❑ Tele-cardiology		
❑ Tele-trauma		
❑ Tele-pharmacy		
❑ Tele-dentistry		
❑ Tele-radiology		
❑ Tele-pathology		
❑ Tele-nursing		
□ Remote patient monitoring		
❑ Home based-nocturnal dialysis		
❑ Cardiac and remote ICUs		
❑ Disease management		
• Mobile technology in healthcare	4	Software Eng. IT
• Smart cards, wireless, RFID	4	
– Smart cards	2	
□ Introduction		
□ History		
□ Integrated circuits		
□ Types of smart cards		
❑ Contact smart cards		
❑ Contact less smart cards		
❑ Combination smart cards		
□ Standards		
❑ ISO 7816		
❑ ISO/IEC 14443		
❑ ETSI		
❑ EMV		
❑ JAVA card		
❑ WHQL		
□ Applications of smart cards		
❑ Identification		
❑ Network access		
❑ Electronic purses		
❑ Telecommunications		
❑ Special applications		
□ Security with smart cards		
❑ Standard security guards		
▪ Authentication		
▪ Confidentiality		

        - Integrity
        - Non-repudiation
    - Wireless — 1
        - Introduction
        - Wireless services
        - Wireless net works
        - Modes
            - Radio
            - Microwave
            - Infrared
    - Applications of wireless technology
        - Mobile telephone
        - Wireless data communications
            - Wi-Fi
            - Cellular data service
            - Mobile satellite communication
    - Categories of wireless implementations
        - Devices standards
        - Radio
        - Broadcasting
        - Armature radio
        - Land mobile radio
        - Cordless telephone
        - Cellular networks
- Radio-frequency identification (RFID) — 1
    - Introduction
    - History
    - Design
    - Miniaturization
- Uses
    - Commerce
    - Transportation
    - Infrastructure
    - Passport
    - Sports
    - Telemetry
- RFID mandates
- Regulations and standardizations
- Health information technology (HIT) — 4 Doctor hosp
    - Introduction
    - Concept and definition
    - Implementation of HIT
    - Types of technology
        - HER
        - Clinical point of care technology—CPOE
- Financial: Revenue and expenditure — 4
- Insurance and billing — 4
- Health informatics professional's role — 2 MRO/HIM
    - Role

– Functions		
– Key responsibilities		
10. Introduction to international classification of diseases (ICD) and surgical procedures	64	MRO/HIM
• Introduction to ICD	12	
– Introduction to ICD and history	1	
– Design and structure of ICD-10	2	
– Difference between ICD-9 and ICD-10	2	
– How to use ICD	2	
– Definition of diagnosis	1	
▫ Other classification systems	1	
▫ Principles and rules of coding	3	
• ICD procedures in medicine	8	
• Introduction and tabular list	7	
– Procedure for medical diagnosis	1	
– Laboratory procedures	1	
– Preventive procedures	1	
– Surgical procedures	1	
– Other therapeutic procedures and ancillary procedures	1	
– Radiology and certain other applications	1	
– Drugs, medicaments and biological agents	1	
• Alphabetical indexing	1	
• Diagnostic coding and indexing procedures	32	
– Inpatient	24	
– Outpatient	8	
• ICD-9CM	8	
• Introduction to ICD-9-CM	1	
• ICD-10-CM and ICD-10-PCS	1	
• HIPAA electronic transactions and coding	1	
• Standards rule		
• Characteristics of ICD-9-CM	1	
• Procedures	3	
• Current procedure terminology (CPT) coding system	4	
– Introduction to CPT		
• Types of categories	2	
• Categories I (six main sections)		
– Codes for evaluation and management		
– Codes for anesthesia		
– Codes for surgery		
– Codes for radiology		
– Codes for pathology		
– Codes for medicine		
• Categories II	1	
– Performance measurements (optional) codes		
• Categories III	1	
– Emerging technology codes		
11. Standards for healthcare informatics	32	
• Digital imaging and communications in medicine (DICOM) and PACS 4 Rad. Doct.		

- Introduction
  - DICOM
  - PACS
  - History
  - Types of images
  - Uses
    - Hardcopy replacement
    - Remote access
    - Electronic image integration
    - Radiology workflow management architecture
  - Querying (C-Find) and image retrieval (C-Move)
  - Image archival and back
  - Integration
  - Regulatory concern
- Health insurance portability and accountability act (HIPAA) 4 HIPAA expert
  - HIPAA security standards: Final rule
    - Introduction and background information
    - Administrative simplification
    - Privacy standards–April 14, 2003
    - Transaction and code set standards—Oct 16, 2003
    - Security standards—April 20, 2005
    - Identifier standard–not yet finalized
  - Comparison of the HIPAA final security standards to ISO/IEC
  - Administrative safeguards
    - Security management
    - Assigned security responsibility (required)
    - Workforce security
    - Information access management
    - Security incidence procedures
    - Contingency plan
    - Evaluation report
  - Physical safeguards
    - Facility access controls
    - Workstation (required)
    - Workstation security (required)
    - Device and media controls
  - Technical safeguards
    - Access control
    - Audit control
    - Integrity
    - Person or entity authentication (required)
    - Transmission security
  - Analysis of comparison between HIPAA standard
    - Implementation and ISO/IEC 17799
- Health level seven (HL-7) 2 HL7 expert
  - Introduction
    - Organization
    - Origin
    - Collaboration

- HL7 standards
  - Membership
  - Sharing information
  - Conceptual standards
- HL7 versions
- Clinical document architecture
  - ISO/HL7 27932
- Methods applied by HL7
  - Services aware interoperability framework
- Arden syntax
- MLLP (minimal lower level protocol)
- CCOW (clinical context object group)

• International organization for standardization (ISO) — 2 — ISO expert NABA NAB

- Introduction
  - History
  - Financing
  - IS and other publications
- Standardization process
  - Stages in the development process of an ISO standard
- ISO document copyright
- Members
- Criticism
- ISO standards — 2
  - What is standard?
  - What are the benefits of ISO international standards
  - ISO 9001 healthcare management
  - ISO 9001 health service accreditation
  - ISO 13485 medical device standards

• American National Standard Institute (ANSI) — 2 — ANSI expert JCI

- Introduction
  - History
  - Membership
- Objectives
  - Consumer empowerment
    - Registration summary
    - Medication history
  - Electronic health record
    - Laboratory result reporting
  - Bio-surveillance
    - Visit
    - Utilization
    - Clinical data
    - Lab and radiology
  - Consumer access to clinical information
    - Access to clinical data
    - Provider permission
    - Personal health record transfer

- ▫ Medication management
  - ▫ Medication reconciliation
  - ▫ Ambulatory prescription
  - ▫ Contraindications
- ▫ Quality
  - ▫ Hospital measurement and reporting
  - ▫ Clinical measurement and reporting
  - ▫ Feedback to clinicians

Topic		
• Standard nomenclature of medicine—clinical terms (SNOMED CT) – Introduction – SNOMED CT in the UMLS – What is SNOMED CT? – Who owns the SNOMED CT? – What impact did the 2007 change in SNOMED CT – Ownership has an existing UMLS licenses? – What SNOMED CT content in the UMLS meta thesaurus? • SNOMED CT Documentation – User guide notes – Technical implication guide – Editorial guide • SNOMED CT in the UMLS meta thesaurus – Insertion of SNOMED CT into the UMLS – Meta thesaurus – Inversion source transparency – Release source transference	2	SNOMED expert
• Logical observation identifier names and codes (LOINC) – Introduction ▫ Functions ▫ Format ▫ Uses ▫ Improved communication ▫ With HL7 ▫ With SNOMED CT • Structure and purpose of LOINC codes • Scope of the current LOINC database • RELMA (registries LOINC mapping assistant) • Distribution and copyright communications and meetings • Conclusion	4	LOINC expert
• CEN prEN 13606 HER com – Introduction – Technical approach – Application standards – Purpose – HER related standards – Scope-CEN/tc 251 enB606-1 – HL7 v2 v3 messages – Archetype paradigm	2	Standard expert Hosp

- HL7 clinical document architecture [HL7 CDA] 2 HL7 expert
  - Introduction
    - What is CDA
      - Define CDA
      - Characteristics of CDA
        - Persistence
        - Stewardship
        - Potential for authentication
        - Context
        - Wholeness
        - Human readability
      - Benefits of CDA
      - Implementation experience
      - Gentle on-ramp to information exchange
      - Improved patient care
      - Lower cost
  - Key aspects of CDA
  - CDA guiding principles
  - Major components of a CDA document
  - CDA is based on
    - Principles of incremental operability
    - CDA2
    - CDA templates
      - Section level templates
      - Entry level templates
- Web access to DICOM persistent objects [WADO] 2 DICOM expert
  - Introduction
    - What is WADO?
  - Scope
  - Conformance
  - Normative references
    - HL7 CDA
    - IETR RFC2616
    - IETF RFC 2396
    - IETP RFC 2616
    - IETP RFC 3240
    - ISO/IEC 10918
  - Terms and definition
    - DICOM persistent object
    - Web client system
    - Web enabled DIOCOM server
    - Web access to DIOCOM persistent object
  - Data communication requirements
    - Interaction
    - HTTP request
      - Parameters of HTTP request
      - List of media types supported in the response
      - List of character sets supported in the response

- HTTP response
  - Body of single DIOCOM MIME sub-type part response
  - Body of non-DIOCOM MIME type response
- Persistent object types
  - Single-frame image objects
  - Multiple-frame image objects
  - Text objects
  - Other objects
- Parameters
  - Parameters available for all DIOCOM persistent objects
  - Parameters for DICOM image persistent objects

- IHE retrieve information for display [RID] 2 MI IT
  - Introduction
    - Summary
    - Benefits
    - Details
    - Systems affected
- RID abstract/scope
  - Access to patient information
  - Access to documents—CDA PDF, JPEG
  - Access to key patient centric information such as allergies
  - current medication
    - Summary of reports
  - Link with other IHE profiles
- RID key technical properties
  - Standards used
    - Web services (WSDL for HTTP get
    - General purpose IT presentation formats XTML, PDF
    - JPEG CDA (HL7)
    - Client in healthcare application display with access to patient ID
  - Two services
    - Retrieve specific information
      - Patient specific information
      - Type of request
      - Date, time and most recent
    - Retrieve a document
      - Object unique instant identifier (OID)
      - Type of request
      - Content type expected
  - Retrieve information for display
    - Display information source
    - Retrieve specific information for display
  - Types of requests
    - Summary of laboratory
    - Summary of radiology
    - Summary of cardiology—retrieve test of ECG XML format
    - Summary of surgery
    - Summary of emergency
    - Summary of ICU
    - Summary of medication

  - Summary of allergies
  - Persistent document—return ECG as PDF or SVG
  - ECG XML list
    - ECG XML List allows advocated display apps to process list
    - XML schema based on HL7 v3 reference information model
  - ECG document
    - ECG information source required to support PDF so its compatible with existing RID clients
    - ECG information source required using vector graphics for waveforms in PDF
  - Option for SVG
- IHE cross-enterprise DICOM/PACS expert
  - Introduction
    - Summary
    - Benefits
    - Details
    - System affected
    - Specifications
- Summary
  - Imaging documents
    - Imaging studies
    - Diagnostic reports for imaging studies
    - Key image selection
- Benefits
  - Imaging component of EHR
  - Effective means to contribute and access imaging documents
  - Scalable sharing of imaging documents
  - Easy access to imaging documents
  - System affected
  - RIS implementation of imaging document source
  - PACS workstations, RIS and non-radiology workstation
- Specifications
  - Profile statistics: Trial implementation
- Document
  - IHE radiology technical framework
    - Supplement for trial implementation revi1-2
- Underlying standards
  - DICOM
  - ebXML (ebRS v30, ehRM v3.o)
  - HL7 CDA release 2.0
  - PDF/A ISO 19005-1
  - MTOM
  - XOP
- Document sharing [XDS] 2
- Introduction
  - Summary
    - A document repository
    - A document registry

- Documents are provided by one or more document sources
- Access by one or more document consumer
- Benefits
  - Facilitate the registration distribution and access
  - Focused on providing a standard-based specification for
  - managing and sharing documents
- Details
  - The cross-enterprise document sharing (XDS) integration profile
- Systems affected
  - Enterprise wide information system that manage patient EHR, e.g. HIS
- Specifications
  - Profile status final text
  - Documents: I HE IT infrastructure technical frame work version 2 or later
  - Vol 1—Secrion 10, appendix, E, J, K
  - Vol 2—Sections 3.18
  - Vol 2b—Sections 3.41, 3.42, 3.43
  - Vol 2x—Appendix A, B, K, L, M, N, V, W
  - Vol 3—Section 4.1, 4.2, 4.3
- Underlying standards:
  - ebMS OASIS/ebXML messaging services specifications v3.0
  - ebRIM OASIS/ebXML registry information model v3.0
  - ebRS OASIS/ebXML registry services specifications v3.0
  - HTTP hyper text transfer protocol HTTP/1.1 (IETF RFC2616)
  - ISO/IEC 9075 database language SQL
- Medical markup language [MML] 2 MML expert
  - Introduction
  - Outline of version 2.3 background to the version
    - Revision of the access right definition
    - Access right
    - Establishment of group ID
    - Revision of the health insurance module
    - Referral module
    - Report information module
    - Test history information module
- Modularization of documents
  - Patient information
  - Health insurance information
  - Diagnosis information
  - Lifestyle information
  - Basic medical information
  - Particular information at the time of first visit
  - Progress course information
  - Surgery information
  - Clinical summary information
  - Test result information
  - Report information
  - Referral information
- Version 3.0 background to the revision
  - Goal for the development of MML version 3.0
  - MML version 3.0 development policy

- Intellectual property
- Referral document
- Overview
  - Clinical document architecture

12.	Preparations and assessment (44)	44
13.	English language (spoken and communication skills) (20)	20
14.	Practical or field work	64
TOTAL:		**576**

COURSE DESCRIPTION

A study of the healthcare delivery services including medical, biomedical and public health and use of health information through healthcare processes by generation of documentation of encounters, application of required technology and regulations for obtaining quality information, and subsequent storage and access for the use of healthcare delivery.

With the emerging information technology, use of electronic medical record documents incorporating CPOE, CDSS in healthcare information systems and application of international medical informatics standards such as DICOM, HL-7, ISO, SNOMED CT, LOINC, and HIPAA in relation to healthcare, privacy, confidentiality, information security for effective, swift, safe and quality care.

A study of basic human anatomy, physiology and medical terminology to help in Classification of diagnosis and surgical procedures by applying international prescribed numerical/alpha medical codes from ICD and CPT manual.

A study of the database knowledge management used in healthcare particularly in patient care, types of database management techniques, file and access techniques, query and update languages, data integrity, use of health record systems, and applications of databases to support the healthcare system for effective maintaining healthcare recording systems for generating quality information for efficient healthcare delivery to the customers.

OBJECTIVES OF THE COURSE

Upon successful completion of the course, the students will be able to:

- Explain the major types of healthcare services and information related to medical and public health
- Differentiate between data and information and explain good quality data
- Describe information flow through the healthcare process in the healthcare system
- Explain how technology that used for competitive advantage for the healthcare system
- Describe the security, privacy and confidentiality issues associated with healthcare
- State the healthcare regulations, laws and standards
- Explain how technology impacts implementation of EMR and its importance
- Understand the impact of technology on the healthcare system
- State the rules for building medical terms combing forms, prefixes, and suffixes
- Describe the purpose of codified and classification of health records
- Differentiate ICD-9-CM, ICD-10, CPT codes the use for each code
- Explain the advantages of computerized databases over manual record processing in healthcare system
- Describe effective management of healthcare information using a database
- Understand the use of technology standards in hospital information system.

Chapter 17

Syllabus for Four-Week Nursing Medical Information Technology

INTRODUCTION

The nursing profession due to implementation of electronic system in healthcare environment encounters the use of technology daily. Clinical information systems have replaced manual paper charting and duplicate documentations are eliminated. The use of physician order entry systems allows orders to be entered at the point of care (POC) and provides alerts to possible contradictions or patient alerts eliminating errors. Standards of care are also tracked through computerized programs. Blood pressure, temperature, and other vital signs are now taken electronically, recorded and tracked for trends. Nurses are alerted to any abnormal results based on previously established parameters programmed into the systems. This has become integral link to staff development and continue education. Nursing administrators have begun to utilize informatics applications to assist with staffing, managing, budgeting and disseminating information. Precisely, the technology, helping in preventing medication errors, data capturing and reporting tools which meet quality care, risk management and other quality assurance programs. Handheld units are utilized to transmit patient information directly to electronic medical records (EMR) providing more efficient documentation with increased accuracy and consistency.

1. Introduction to nursing 1

   Nursing definition

   Nursing profession

   Nursing objectives

   - To provide professional care for patients' recovery and physical and mental health.
   - To provide non-professional care for patients' comfort and safety such as bed making.
   - To perform administrative duties such as safe-custody of drugs and maintenance of equipment and materials in satisfactory condition.
   - To maintain comprehensive patient records for the services rendered.
   - To provide continuing education for professional nurses and nursing assistants.

- To undertake understanding, or assist with, research for improved nursing care.
- To provide, where necessary, clinical experience for student nurses.

2. Nursing standards, policies and procedures 2

Nursing standards

Nursing standardis a practice that enjoys general recognition and conformity among professionals or an authoritative statement by which the quality of practice, service or education can be judged. Standard is an established rule or basis of comparison in measuring or judging capacity, quantity and quality, value of other products in the same category.

Nursing policies

- To restore patients to the highest level of health individually possible.
- To get patients' families to participate where appropriate, in tasks such as patients' feeding, washing, and dressing.
- To group patients in large wards by degree of illness with groups needing most care located nearest the nurses' station.
- To change locations in ward periodically for long stay patients' psychological benefit.

Nursing procedures

- Receiving admitted patients
- Administration of medication.
- Assisting physicians.
- Performing simple diagnostic procedures.
- Collecting and sending specimens to laboratory.
- Recording and maintaining medical records
- Recording of vital signs
- Performing gastric lavage and giving enema
- Preoperative preparations
- Delivering bed-side nursing
- Coordinating patient care with other team members
- Maintaining clean and safe environment
- Bed making and providing privacy to patients

3. Nursing functional organization 8

a. Nursing professional practice 1

- Assessment, planning, intervention and evaluation of human responses to health and illness.
- Provision of nursing care to individuals to restore optimum health.
- Procurement, coordination and management of essential patient resources.
- Provision of health counseling and education.
- Establishment of standards of practice for nursing care.
- Development of policies, procedures and protocols.
- Supervision of those assist in the practice of nursing.
- Administration of medications and treatment as prescribed by qualified medical professionals.

b. Nursing ward management 1

- Admission, transfer and discharge management
- Supervising, directing and controlling staff
- Diet ordering
- Maintaining poisonous and narcotic drug controls and registers
- Communicating
- Maintaining records pertaining to patient care, investigation reports, inventory, medico-legal cases, etc.
- Nursing education
- Safe custody of patients' valuables
- Visitors control
- Follow-up scheduling
- Discharge and bill settlement

c. Nursing operation theatre management 1

- Aseptic environment maintenance
- Autoclaving
- Receiving patients from wards
- Coordinating trolley traffic
- Assisting surgeon and anesthetist
- Indenting and procuring surgical instruments and surgical sundries
- Maintaining records and reports
- Safe maintenance of theatre equipment and apparatus

d. Labor room management 1

- Preparation of expectant mother for aseptic safe delivery.
- Conducting normal deliveries
- Assisting doctors in obstetrical emergencies
- Assisting difficult and abnormal deliveries.
- Taking care of newborn and premature babies
- Indenting and procuring drugs, linen, etc.
- Maintaining records and reports pertaining to labor room

e. Postoperative/ICU/burns unit management 1

- Indenting and procuring drugs, equipment and oxygen cylinders.
- Operating ECG, EEG, cardiac resuscitation
- Assisting physicians in operating other high-tech equipment and apparatus
- Observing and documenting the progress of the patient monitor

f. Public health nursing: Functions 1

- To promote maternal and child health (MCH) program
- To promote health and nutrition education activities
- To coordinate the activities of health visitors in MCH, family planning and health and nutrition education.
- To coordinate and conduct immunization program.
- To help in school health program in the district.
- To ensure regular supply of equipment, records, registers, drugs, vaccines and other sundries for MCH program.

- To ensure the maintenance of prescribed records and submission of periodical progress of MCH/family planning/nutrition program
- To help the statistical officer in compiling periodical progress reports of program
- To review the progress of public health program.
- To supervise and give technical guidance and support to ANMs and health visitors.
- To investigate complaints against public health workers.
- To provide continuing education for public health workers.
- To work with other functionaries of social welfare, rural development and voluntary organizations

g. Documentation of records 1

- Direct patient care related documents
- Temperature, pulse, respiration form
- Nursing progress record form
- Operation/special procedures consent form
- Fluid balance sheet
- Medication sheet
- Laboratory mount sheet
- Preoperative check list
- Intake qutput record
- Nursing information sheet
- Nursing care plan
- 24 hours bed turning
- 24 hours ward returns
- Diet orders
- Report form—absconded patient
- Incident report form

Indirect patient care related documents/registers and records

- Day and night report book
- Treatment book/injection book
- Instructions book—the head nurse carries with her when she accompanies the medical officer during ward rounds
- Dangerous drugs register
- Dispatch book
- Inventory book
- Breakages account book
- Standing orders for patients
- Telephone message book (specially maintained for receiving laboratory results of serious patients when required urgently)
- Demand/indent book
- Maintenance/repairs request book

h. Staff development and educational 1

- Induction to new staff and students
- In-service education and training
- Continuing education

- Assisting in research programs
- Utilization of nursing services
- Professional issues
- Negligence
- Do it absolutely right and safe
- Right patient
- Right documentation
- Right medication
- Right dose
- Right route
- Right authentication
- Right date and time

4. Nursing staff and operational organization 2

   a. Staff organization: 1
   - Nursing director
   - Assistant director
   - Nursing supervisor
   - Night supervisor
   - Nursing sister
   - Senior staff nurse or head nurse
   - Staff nurse

   b. Nursing operational fields: 1
   - Accident and emergency
   - Outpatient clinics
   - Wards including special care units
   - Delivery suites
   - CSSD
   - Operating rooms
   - Radiology
   - Public health
   - Nursing education

5. Introduction of basic computers 8

   i. Introduction to computers 1
      a. Functionality of computer
      b. Benefits of using a computer over manual

   ii. Data and information 2
      a. Inputting data into the database
      b. Retrieval of data
      c. Accessing information from a database

   iii. Introduction to software 4
      a. System software
      b. Application software
         i. Types of application software used in a hospital
         ii. Functionality of the software used in the hospitals

iii. Entering data and retrieval of data from the application software
iv. Data and reports 1

6. Healthcare information regulations, laws and standards 2
   - ISO standards
   - JACHO standard
   - HIPAA standards
   - Evidence based medicine (EBM)
   - Health record as a legal document
   - Security, privacy and confidentiality
7. Healthcare information management system 5
   - Introduction to healthcare information 2
     - Hospital information system
     - Nursing information system
   - Clinical information system 3
     - Laboratory
     - Radiology
     - Pharmacy
     - Computerized physician order entry (CPOE)
     - Computerized decision support system (CDSS)
8. Implementation of EHRR and other system 4
   - Paper based medical records 1
   - Hybrid of medical records 1
   - HER implementation process 1
   - Other system implementation 1
     - PHR
     - Telemedicine and tele-health
     - Mobile technology
     - Introduction to ICD
9. Preparations and assessment 8
10. Practical or fieldwork 20

COURSE DESCRIPTION

This certificate in nursing medical informatics program developed to suit the nursing personnel who have no background of information technology that is used in healthcare environment. Nursing informatics can be defined as the integration of nursing, computer and information sciences to manage and distribute information, data and knowledge in the practice of nursing. This integration helps to better serve patients while assisting nurses and other healthcare providers in making effective, timely decisions regarding patient care.

The main objective of this program is to train students to become technologically competent nurses who assist those who are responsible for maintaining of health, the improvement of health status, the prevention of illness, and the alleviation of suffering.

Theoretical lectures will cover the computer and human interface components, the ethics involved in nursing informatics, ergonomics, and confidentiality and privacy. Students will learn which technologies to use under various situations and how to apply best technologies to manage and communicate various types of information and data. Students will also learn to apply data principles and to document information appropriately within various computer applications designed specifically for nursing and healthcare administration.

The practical and field work "hands-on-the job" will enlighten how to operate and implement the competency that will facilitate in daily carryings out the responsibilities. The practical experience and skills with theoretical knowledge will help the nursing staff meeting the day to day work and in achieving swift, safe, improved quality care.

OBJECTIVES OF THE COURSE

Upon successful completion of the course, the students with IT knowledge will be able to:

- Provide professional care for patients' recovery and physical and mental health.
- To perform administrative duties, such as safe-custody of drugs and maintenance of equipment and materials in satisfactory condition.
- Maintaining comprehensive patient records for the services rendered.
- Provide continuing education to professional nurses and nursing assistants.
- Communicate with investigation departments to send and receive orders investigations
- Coordinate with the allied departments for the services required for effective patient care.
- To assist in the medical education and research programs.
- Teach the use of technology used to new staff and students.
- Work within the environment where the technology has become part of the healthcare delivery system.
- Utilize for routine jobs such as admissions, discharges, transfers, sending orders and receiving reports.
- Understand the care team orders and requests to carry out the responsibility.
- Get acquainted with the physician order entry (CPOE) and able to be entered at the point of care (POC).
- Understand the different standards used for providing alert to possible contradictions to eliminate errors.
- Track the status of patient care through computerized programs.
- To take electronically; blood pressure, temperature, and other vital signs.
- Utilize the technology for staff development and continuing education.
- Utilize informatics applications to assist with staffing, managing, budgeting and disseminating information.
- Acquainted with the handheld, PDA units, mobile communication technology and other wireless local networks used in the facility.

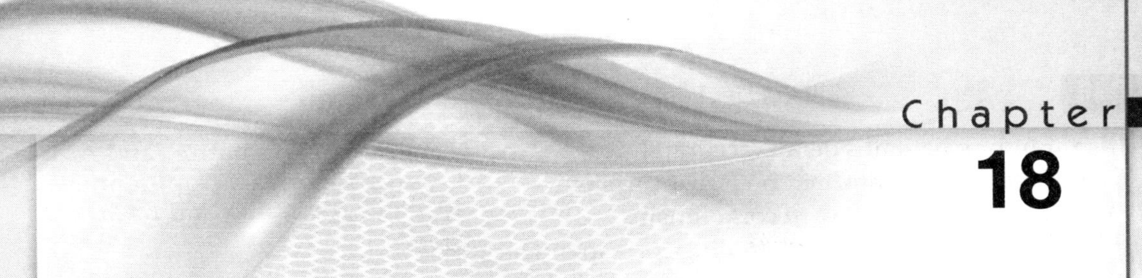

Chapter 18

Syllabus for Four-Week Information Technology (IT) for Front Office

INTRODUCTION

A "Front Office" is suitably located at the main entrance of the hospital or a department to facilitate easy accessible to patient or public and equipped with patient and physician related information, works as a liaison between the hospital staff and the patient/relatives/ and public. People encounter the front office when they visit hospital clinic first time for information. A medical front office is a busy intersection where healthcare workers and patients and public interact. Depending on the size of the practice or hospital, there may be multiple people working at a time in the front desk or just one covering 24 × 7.

1. Introduction to front office 1

   Objective
   - Meeting and greeting patients and visitors
   - Registration and appointment scheduling and other functions
   - Attending and responding to enquiries personally and telephonically

   Location
   - Main entrance, easily accessible to patients and visitors

   Amenities
   - Pleasant appearance of the front office
   - Keeping hospital information related to patient and physician
   - Waiting hall for patients, relatives and visitors
   - Front office equipped with working devices
2. Duties and responsibilities of front office 2

   General administrative duties 1
   - Greet patients and visitors
   - Answering phones, registering, scheduling appointments
   - Track patient flow, and incoming faxes
   - Collect co-pays from patients and verify insurance
   - Scan documents into the EMR

- Enquire patient's details accurately
- Enter correct information into the system
- To attend the call with compliments
- Taking messages and handling correspondence
- Efficientl transactions and paper work in a time-bound manner

Medical specific duties and documentation 1

- Updating and filing patient medical records
- General understanding of a medical terminology
- Help patients, arrange for laboratory services or hospital admittance.
- Collecting patient information and making appointments
- Billing tasks and coding payment posting
- Serve as a liaison between patient and medical staff
- Patient appointment scheduling, insurance authorizations

Document maintaining

Documentation

- OP register
- IP register
- MLC register
- Biomedical register
- Deposit register
- Breakdown register
- Inventory register

3. Organization of front office 2

Organization by staff of front office 1

Characteristics of personnel

- Strong customer service skills
- Positive Attitude, excellent phone skills, with strong work ethics
- Self-motivated, reliable, able to prioritize the task
- Ability to deal with multitask issues with patient or staff efficiently
- Experience with different types of health insurance benefit verification
- Professional bilingual or trilingual languages to deal with customers
- Computer skills, windows, and microsoft outlook and experience with EMR practice management
- Experience and training as a front office assistant, officer, executive
- Skill in greeting patients and answering busy multi-line telephone in peasant and helpful manner
- Excellent interpersonal skills

Organization by function 1

Functions of front office

- Welcoming and greeting the customers who encounter
- Operating telephone switchboard
- Responding authorized calls
- Maintaining records
- Updating the front office required information
- Handling financial transaction

- Maintaining diary for management
- Registration of new and repeat patients
- Making appointment schedule for patients
- Handling complains and issue about

4. Organization of hospitals and clinics 4
   Introduction to hospital organization 1
   - Outpatient services
   - Emergency services
   - Inpatient services

   Introduction to clinics 1
   Introduction to insurance and billing 1
   Communication skills 1
5. Work environment and enquiries 1
   Work environment
   - Front office staff work indoors in an office environment
   - Interact with people regularly
   - Spend a significant amount of time on phone and computer
   - Diplomatic, courteous and helpful
   - Maintain confidentiality of patient information

   Enquiries
   Patient related enquiries
   - Bed allotment
   - Admission details
   - Demographic details
   - Payment details
   - Discharge details
   - Patient hospitalization details

   Doctor related enquiries
   - Bed allotment
   - OP clinic details
   - Appointment schedules
   - Operation schedules
   - Charge details
   - Patient condition details
   - Patient related documentation details
6. Medical terminology course 5
   - Basic medical terminology origin 1
   - Prefix 1
   - Suffix 1
   - Medical abbreviations 1
   - Hospital terms 1
7. Introduction of basic computers 8
   i. Introduction to computers 1
      a. Functionality of computer
      b. Benefits of using a computer over manual

ii. Data and information 2
   a. Inputting data into the database
   b. Retrieval of data
   c. Accessing information from a database
iii. Introduction to software 4
   a. System software
   b. Application software
      i. Types of application software used in a hospital
      ii. Functionality of the software used in the hospitals
      iii. Entering data and retrieval of data from the application software
      iv. Data and reports 1
8. Implementation front office management modules 9
   Registration and appointment management
   - Inpatient admission, discharge and transfer (ADT) management
   - Electronic medical record management
   - Pharmacy management
   - Laboratory management
   - Radiology management (PACS)
   - Service rendered processing and billing
   - Ambulance service management
   - Bed allocation of patient management
9. Preparations and assessment 8
10. Practical or fieldwork 20

COURSE DESCRIPTION

A study of brief hospital organization including general information on outpatient, emergency and inpatient services and also information on independent government of private clinics and physician's clinics. This study includes front office organization, its objectives, location, amenities and organization by staff and function, characteristics of staff, duties and responsibilities. A study of basic medical terminology including prefixes, origin and suffixes with medical abbreviations and hospital terms will enlighten the front desk staff to deal effectively with patients, visitors and public in triaging and assisting with required information promptly.

The course specially designed to teach basic computers for personnel working in front office which includes functionality of computer, advantages of using computer over manual. The information technology includes inputting and retrieval of information from database, introduction of software that encompasses; types of applications used, functionality of the software used in the hospital and data reporting particularly for front office. Designing and implementation aspect of front office management including, registration, appointment scheduling, admission and discharge information and other patient care related information is captured for front office to assist the visitors with required information.

OBJECTIVES OF THE COURSE

Upon successful completion of the course, the students will be able to:

- Greet patients and visitors in a courteous way
- Answer phone calls, register and make appointments

- Use computers for entering and retrieving data efficiently
- Track patient flow information and incoming faxes
- Collect co-pays from patient and verify insurance information
- Enquire patient's detail and enter correct information in the system
- Attend the call with compliments and respond promptly
- Scan the documents into the EMR
- Take messages and handling correspondence
- Transact paper work in time-bound manner
- Update and file patient medical records
- Serve as a liaison between patient and medical and administrative staff
- Guide the patients, relatives and visitors promptly with right information
- Prepare bills and forward to the required destiny
- Maintain registers, e.g. OP, IP, MLC, and other registers
- Work under pressure
- Work with utmost kindness and consideration
- Handle multi-functions effectively
- Understand of patient's or customers issue properly
- Update and assist the patients, physicians and administrators
- Deal with persons diplomatically, courteously and helpfully
- Maintain confidentiality of patient and others information
- Distinguish between elective and emergency patients
- Communicate with the staff and customers clearly.

Chapter

19

Syllabus for Four-Week Information Technology (IT) for Operation Theatre Staff

INTRODUCTION

The operation theatre (OT) being a critical area of the hospital with the application of technology functions effectively. By developing and installing different computer modules in the system with features like generic dynamic template for capturing various types of data, generic consent forms, alert facility, vital monitoring and graph plotting facility, use of touch pane, etc. Design aspects related to check list facility, patient monitoring utility, video streaming, and decision support system, etc. computer modules handles both major and minor operations performed referred from IPD, emergency and OPD. The operation theatre management system (OTMS) streamlines the flow of operations performed in the hospitals and encompasses information about the availability of all the theatres, and equipment/tools, scheduling of operations, etc. operating surgeons names, and specific transactions for preanesthesia checks (PAC), request made, PAC result entry, updating operation list, updating patient records with the type and dose of anesthesia and the surgical procedures carried out along with any transfusion of blood or any other fluid given is accounted scrupulously.

1. Introduction to OT management	4
Services	1
Surgical services	
• Anesthesia services	
• Respiratory care department RT	
Classification of surgeries	1
• General surgery	
• Obstetrics and gynecology	
• Pediatric surgery	
• Ortho-surgery	
• Otorhinolaryngology (ENT)	
• Ophthalmology	
• Plastic surgery	

- Urology
- Neurosurgery
- Cardiac thoracic surgery
- Dentistry

Anesthesiology specialties 1

- Neuroanesthesiology
- Obstetrics anesthesiology
- Pediatric anesthesiology
- Cardiac and thoracic anesthesiology
- ENT anesthesiology

Anesthesiology outside OT 1

- Situations
- Cath lab
- Radiology
- ECT
- Day care anesthesia
- Geriatric anesthesia
- Anesthesia for trauma shock

2. OT objectives: 1
   - To perform surgical procedures for inpatients, emergency and outpatients
   - To use best sterilized, aseptic techniques and infection free equipment and instruments during the surgery
   - To operate only those who are fit for operation with accepting informed consent
   - To maintain patient stability in pre, during and postoperative procedures
   - To follow up for postoperative care in recovery room
   - To assist in teaching and continued education program for interns, residents and other students
   - To undertake medical research for medical science advancement
   - To maintain comprehensive patient operation record
   - To collect and send the tissue and specimen for histopathological test for diagnosis
3. OT organization 6
   a. Organization chart by staff 1
      - Head of OT
      - Head or chief anesthesiologist
        - Anesthetist
        - Anesthesia nurse
        - Surgical theatre head nurse
          - Scrub nurse
          - Circulating nurse
          - Operation recovery room nurse
          - Surgical theatre assistant
          - Medical secretary
      - Respiratory therapist

   b. OT organization by function 1

      Aseptic environment maintenance
      - Autoclaving

- Receiving patients from wards
- Coordinating trolley traffic
- Assisting surgeon and anesthetist
- Indenting and procuring surgical instruments and surgical sundries
- Maintaining records and reports
- Safe maintenance of theatre equipment and apparatus
  - Sterilization process
  - Sterile storage area
  - Non-sterile storage area
  - Work area

c. Postoperative/ICU/burns unit management: 1
- Indenting and procuring drugs, equipment and oxygen cylinders.
- Operating ECG, EEG, cardiac resuscitation
- Assisting physicians in operating other high-tech equipment and apparatus
- Observing and documenting the progress of the patient monitor

d. OT management 1
- OT booking
- OT scheduling
- Patient tracking
- OT reports

f. OT maintenance 1
- Building maintenance
- Maintenance of equipment and instruments
- Manufacture of dressings and drapes, eye pads, swabs
- Sterilization and disinfection procedures
  - Autoclave
  - Autoclave times
- Dry heat oven
- Boiling
- Chemical solutions
  - Stock keeping, storage and security
  - Managing with limited recourses
  - Infection control

g. Interdepartmental relationship with OT 1
- Inpatient
- Accident and emergency
- Outpatient clinics
- Daycare
- ICU, CCU, NICU
- Delivery suites
- CSSD
- Operating rooms
- Laboratory
- Radiology
- Pharmacy
- Biomedical engineering

4. Key duties and responsibilities of clinical team	2
• Chief surgeon	1
• Anesthetist	1
5. Key duties and responsibilities of theatre nurse	3
• Scrub nurse	1
• Circulation nurse	1
• Recovery room nurse	1
6. Introduction of basic computers	8
i. Introduction to computers	1
a. Functionality of computer	
b. Benefits of using a computer over manual	
ii. Data and information	2
a. Inputting data into the database	
b. Retrieval of data	
c. Accessing information from a database	
iii. Introduction to software	4
a. System software	
b. Application software	
i. Types of application software used in a hospital	
ii. Functionality of the software used in the hospitals	
iii. Entering data and retrieval of data from the application software	
iv. Data and reports	1
7. Design and implementation OT management modules	8
• Introduction to OT management	1
• Workflow of OT module	1
• Dynamic template utility	1
• Check list facility	1
Patient monitoring utility	3
i. Vital monitoring	
ii. Intake monitoring	
iii. Outtake monitoring	
Video screening	1
8. Preparations and sssessment	8
9. Practical or fieldwork	20

COURSE DESCRIPTION

The study will project on overall management of operation theatre (OT) including maintenance of building, equipment and instruments, sterilization and disinfection procedures, stock keeping and storage and security. The OT team comprises surgeons, anesthetists, OT nursing staff and their duties and responsibilities related to preoperative, during and postoperative stages of patient operation. The different modules provide information on supplies, stock availability before, during and after operation. The administrative management such as booking and scheduling the patient for OT, tracking of status of patient, and receiving satirized packs, blood for transfusion, drugs and other requirements. The computer dynamic templates with various controls like, text boxes, labels, text areas, control boxes, etc. will help in patient monitoring throughout before, during and after operation.

The course specially designed to teach basic computers for personnel working in OT, which includes functionality of computer, advantages of using computer over manual. The information technology includes inputting and retrieval of information from database, introduction of software that encompasses; types of applications used, functionality of the software used in the hospital and data reporting particularly for OT. Designing and implementation aspect of OT management module that includes workflow, dynamic templates for various functions, template utility, check list facility, patient monitoring utility including vital monitoring, intake and outtake monitoring, video screening.

The course contains introduction to operation theatre (OT) management including surgical, anesthesia and respiratory services and categorization of different specialty of surgeries, OT objectives and organization by function and staff. The equipment and instrument used in OT, and nursing management include aseptic environment, safe maintenance of theatre equipment and apparatus, autoclaving, receiving patient from wards, coordinating with allied departments such as wards, emergency, recovery room, ICU, CCU, CSSD, laboratory, radiology, blood bank, pharmacy, indenting and procuring surgical instruments and surgical sundries, assisting surgeon and anesthetist and maintaining records and reports. Other OT management includes OT booking, scheduling, accounting OT consumable and instrument used during operation.

OBJECTIVES OF THE COURSE

Upon successful completion of the course, the students with IT knowledge will be able to:

- Explain the staff involved in OT and their major functions
- Differentiate elective and emergency operations and process involved
- State the different types of anesthesia given to patient and the role of anesthetist
- Understand different types of preoperative checklist used in OT prior to surgery
- Explain the relationship with OP, ward, emergency, ICU, CCU, recovery room, etc.
- Link OT with CSSD, blood bank, laboratory, radiology, biomedical engineering, etc.
- Explain the measures adopted during surgical procedure in the OT
- Distinguish different sterilized packs for different surgical procedures.
- Understand the equipment and instruments used in the OT and their upkeep
- Understands the responsibilities of OT nursing staff
- Explain the measures used for controlling infection in OT
- Carryout OT booking, scheduling and prepare OT reports using IT
- Explain the procedures used in OT preoperative, during and postoperative
- State the OT organization by staff and functions
- Use the computers in OT and it functionalities and knows the benefits over manual system
- Enter data and able to retrieve required data from database
- Understand and operate different modules used in the OT
- Describe types of application software used in OT
- State different functionality of the software used in the hospital
- Describe the various types of reports generated from OT computer.

Chapter

20

Syllabus for Four-Week Information Technology (IT) for Wards

INTRODUCTION

Ward is the most vital section where all inpatients are hospitalized and treated and headed by a senior nursing staff. From the time a patient is admitted till he/she is discharged, the major responsibility rests with the in-charge nurse and her ward team as they are custodian of patient till he/she is discharged. During the hospitalization of patients, there are innumerable functions of general and critical nature that have to be carried out by nursing staffs under the treating physician's guidance without interruption (24 × 7) to ensure the admitted patient is getting utmost care as planned by the healthcare team. Any delay or deviation could be detrimental to the patient care process and results. With the implementation of information technology in the hospital including ward setting enhances the efficiency of the nursing staffs dealing with innumerable work/service formats, personnel, communictions, interactions, etc. while working in the ward. The treating physician and his medical team are responsible for treatment of patient, in reality the care and treatment is practically executed by the nursing service.

1. Introduction of ward management 2
   - Objectives 1
     - Quality care
     - Economic operation
     - Patient satisfaction and comfort
     - Efficient ward services
     - Ethical practice of care
     - Privacy of patient
   - Ward functions 1
2. Responsibilities care providers 1
   - Medical staff
   - Nursing staff
   - Paramedical staff
   - Administrators

3. Components 5
   - Patient care 1
   - Ward round by physician
     - Unit head with team
     - Physician on call
     - Documentation
     - Patient care plan on admission
     - Patient discharge process
   - Personnel management 1
   - Supply and equipment 1
   - Environment cleanliness 1
   - Policies and procedures 1
     - Policies
     - Procedures
4. Ward organizational 5
   - Organization by staff 2
     - Treating physician (consultant)
       - Physician/surgeon/obstetrician/pediatrician
       - Assistant medical staff
       - Medical consultations
     - Head nurse
     - Asstistant head nurse
       - Nurse
         - Auxiliary nurse
         - Nursing aide
         - Ward clerk
   - Organizational by/functions 3
     - Nursing administration 1
     - Patient care related
       - Admission of patient
       - Vital signs
       - Medication
       - Diet
       - Rounds with physician
       - Laboratory
       - Radiology/radiation
       - Blood bank
       - Pharmacy
       - Follow-up appointments
       - Medical record
       - Medical billing
       - Administration
   - Support services 1
     - CSSD
     - Laundry
     - Housekeeping

- Biomedical
- Maintenance
- Patient valuables
- Transportation

• Reports 1
- Daily admission and discharge report
- Daily ward census report
- Medico-legal report
- Absconded patient report
- Incident/occurrence report
- VIP admissions
- Seriously Ill patient report
- Nurses on-duty and on leave
- Waiting list of patient admissions

5. Classification of hospitals and beds 2
• Hospital classification by size and care 1
- Classification by size
    - Small
    - Medium
    - Large
    - Extra large
- Classification by care
    - Primary care hospital
    - Secondary care hospital
    - Tertiary care hospital
- Ward service and bed classification
    - Ward services 1
        - Medical
        - Surgical
        - Obstetrics and gynecology
        - Pediatrics
        - Psychiatric
        - Geriatrics
        - Oncology
        - Isolation
- Beds classification
    - General beds
    - Private (special)
    - Semi-private

6. Introduction of basic computers 8
i. Introduction to computers 1
a. Functionality of computer
b. Benefits of using a computer over manual
ii. Data and information 2
a. Inputting data into the database

b. Retrieval of data
c. Accessing information from a database
iii. Introduction to software 4
a. System software
b. Application software
i. Types of application software used in a hospital
ii. Functionality of the software used in the hospitals
iii. Entering data and retrieval of data from the application software
iv. Data and reports 1

7. Design and implementation ward management modules 8
- Nursing ward management
- Registration and appointment management
- Electronic medical record management
- Inpatient admission, discharge and transfer (ADT) management
- Pharmacy management
- Laboratory management
- Radiology management (PACS)
- OT management
- Blood bank management
- Service rendered processing and billing
- Ambulance service management
- Bed census management
- Quality assurance management
- Stores and inventory management

8. Ward nursing station 1
- Nursing amenities
- Nursing documentation
  - Clinical
  - Non-clinical
- Ward maintenance
- Inter service relationship
  - Accident and emergency
  - Outpatient clinics
  - Daycare
  - ICU, CCU, NICU
  - Delivery suites
  - CSSD
  - Operating rooms
  - Laboratory
  - Radiology
  - Pharmacy
  - Blood bank
  - Biomedical engineering

9. Preparations and assessment 8
10. Practical or fieldwork 20

COURSE DESCRIPTION

The study will project on overall management of ward including maintenance of ward equipment and instruments, sterilization and disinfection procedures, stock keeping and storage and security. The ward team comprises medical staff ranging from consultant to junior staff and ward nursing staff from head (In charge) nurse to junior nurses, nursing orderlies and their duties and responsibilities related to hospitalization of patient from admission till discharge stages of patient. The different IT modules provide information on supplies, stock availability before, during and after discharge. The administrative management such as booking and scheduling the patient for admission, tracking of status of patient, and ordering and receiving investigation reports, blood for transfusion, drugs and other requirements. The computer dynamic templates with various controls like, text boxes, labels, text areas, control boxes, etc. will help in patient monitoring throughout before, during and after hospitalization of patient.

The course specially designed to teach basic computers for personnel working in ward, which includes functionality of computer, advantages of using computer over manual. The information technology includes inputting and retrieval of information from database, introduction of software that encompasses; types of applications used, functionality of the software used in the hospital and data reporting particularly for ward. Designing and implementation aspect of ward management Module that includes workflow, dynamic templates for various functions, template utility, check list facility, patient monitoring utility including vital monitoring, intake and outtake monitoring, video screening.

The course contains introduction to ward management including admission, discharge, transfers, bed allocation and utilization, and other consultancy, investigations, pharmacy, blood bank, and other support services, such as ward objectives and organization by function and staff. The amenities and instruments used in ward, and nursing management include patient care related taking vital information, medication, diet, sending and receiving patient from OT, and coordinating with allied departments such as wards, emergency, recovery room, ICU, CCU, CSSD, laboratory, radiology, blood bank, pharmacy, indenting and procuring linen, CSSD sterilized instruments, assisting physician rounds and other medical consultants and maintaining records and reports. Other ward management includes follow-up booking, waiting admissions, accounting ward consumable and instrument used during hospitalized of patients.

OBJECTIVES OF THE COURSE

Upon successful completion of the course, the students with IT knowledge will be able to:

- Explain the staff involved in ward and their major functions
- Differentiate between medical and surgical patients.
- State the different types of wards and beds
- Understand different types of patients referred to investigations departments
- Explain the relationship with OP, OT, emergency, ICU, CCU, recovery room, etc.
- Link ward with CSSD, blood bank, laboratory, radiology, biomedical engineering, etc.
- Explain the measures adopted during patient sent to OT or other departments
- Distinguish the responsibilities of medical staff and nursing staff during hospitalized patient
- Understand the patient care procedure from admission till discharge of patient
- Understands the responsibilities of ward nursing staff
- Explain the measures used for well-being and privacy of patient during hospitalization

- Carryout follow-up booking OT booking, ward census, other legal and administrative financial report
- Explain the procedures observed during consultant/physician round in the ward
- State the ward organization by staff and functions
- Use the computers in ward and its functionalities and know the benefits over manual system
- Enter data and able to retrieve required data from database
- Understand and operate different modules used in the ward
- Describe types of application software used in ward management
- State different functionality of the software used in the hospital
- Describe the various types of reports generated from ward computer
- Use of touch pane in the ward.

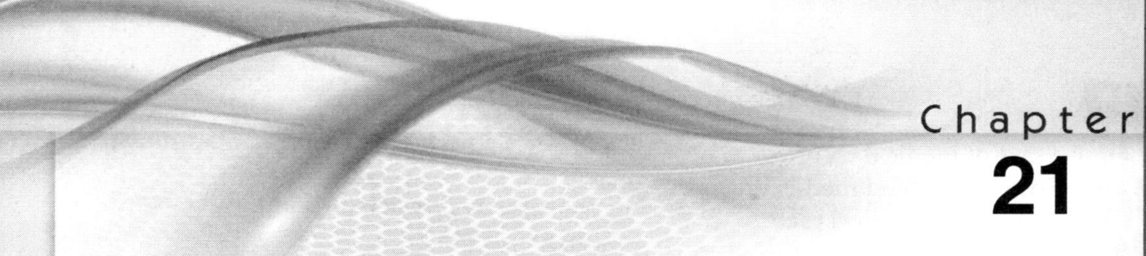

Chapter

21

Syllabus for Twelve-Week EMR for Medical Records and Medical Coding

PART I: MEDICAL RECORDS (MR)

INTRODUCTION

The medical records are vital documents contain accurate, timely written, and complete health information, such as patient history, physical examination, progress notes, physician's orders, investigations carried out, diagnosis, treatment rendered—medical or surgical by healthcare providers to the patient during his/her admission to outpatient, emergency, ICU or CCU and inpatient. The medical records are classified as per the international classifications of diseases and surgical procedures for morbidity and mortality information, and considered confidential and legal document that are to be preserved and retained as per the national schedule for the use of patient care, medical education and research and to meet the needs of insurance and legal requirements.

1. The introduction to medical records 2
   - Historical background
     - Primitive medical records
     - Modern medicine
     - Medical records in developed countries
     - Medical records in developing countries
2. Role of medical records 2
   - Purposes of medical records
   - Importance of medical records
     - To the patient
     - To the physician
     - To the healthcare intuition
     - To the research team
     - To the teaching program
     - To the national health agencies
     - To the international organizations

3. Format of medical records 2
    - Source-oriented medical records
    - Integrated medical record
    - Problem-oriented medical record (POMR)
4. Responsibility for medical records 2
    - Hospital administration
    - Healthcare providers
    - Medical records manager
5. Responsibility for contents of MR 2
    - Medical record staff
    - Medical staff
    - Nursing staff
    - Paramedical staff
6. Functions of medical record department (MRD) 4
    - Definition of MRD
    - Registration and appointment schedule
    - Admission, discharge and transfers
    - Maintaining hospital functional registers
    - Investigation reports
        - Laboratory
        - Radiology
        - Other
    - Control and movement of records
        - Emergency records
        - Outpatient records
        - Inpatient records
            - Ward census
    - Patient medical files sent to other hospitals
    - Patient medical files received from other hospitals
    - Registration of births and deaths
    - Registration of oncology (cancer) patients
    - Classification of diseases and operations
    - Hospital statistics
        - Outpatient
        - Emergency
        - Inpatient
        - Administrative
    - Orientation and training of staff
7. Terms and definitions 2
8. Standards for medical record services 2
    - Outpatient records
    - Emergency records
    - Inpatient records
        - Medical record must be secured confidentially assured
        - Written policies and procedures for MR maintenance
        - MR Department must be adequately equipped

9. Hospital's general rules and regulations 2
   - Legal aspects of medical records
     - Personal document
     - Impersonal document
     - Medical legal registration
     - Patient consent
     - Authorized staff
     - Release of information
       - With patient permission
       - Without patient permission
   - Retention and preservation of records
     - Retention of records
       - Retention schedule
     - Perseveration of records
   - Medical record procedures 2
     - Central registration
     - Outpatient clinic
     - Accident and emergency
     - Admitting office
     - Nursing wards or unit
     - Processing of OP records
     - Processing of IP records
     - Hospital statistics
     - Filing and retrieving of records and X-rays
     - Medical record library
10. Organization, functions and interdepartmental relationship 4
    - Organization
      - Goal
      - Objectives
      - Organization and functions
        - Outpatient service
        - Accident and emergency
        - Inpatient
        - Medical record library
11. Needs of medical record department (MRD) 2
    - Introduction
    - Location and space
    - Equipment
    - HR and job descriptions
    - Standards, policies and procedures
12. Introduction to healthcare delivery 1
    - Primary healthcare
    - Secondary healthcare
    - Tertiary healthcare

13. Quality assurance 2
    - Quality control
    - Quantitative analysis
    - Qualitative analysis
    - Medical audit
    - Patient care evaluation
    - Formation of medical record committee
      – Medical record forms
    - Role of MRD in quality assurance program
    - Evaluation of medical record services
14. Rights and responsibilities of a patient 1
    - Rights of patent
    - Responsibilities of a patient

COURSE DESCRIPTION

This course encompasses the introduction to medical records, historical background; primitive medical records and medical practice. The role of medical record includes the purpose, and the importance to patient, physician, hospital, medical education and research, national and international health organizations.

The syllabus describes the format and the responsibilities for content and maintaining medical records. The study contain the functions of medical record department including registration, appointment schedule, maintenance of outpatient, emergency and inpatient medical records, preparation of statistics and performance of quality assurance, medical audit and patient care evaluation programs.

The course includes the needs for organizing the department such as location, space, personnel, job descriptions, orientation and training of staff. Development of standards, policies and procedures, maintain legal aspects of medical records, retention and preservation of medical records, of quality assurance programs.

OBJECTIVES OF THE COURSE

Upon successful completion of the course, the students will be able to:

- Describe the historical background including primitive medical records and medical practice
- Explain the role of medical records including its purpose and importance
- Elucidate the format including source, integrated and problem oriented medical records
- Recognize the responsibilities for content and management of medical records
- Elaborate the functions of medical records department
- Explain the required standards, policies and procedures for maintaining medical records
- Know the legal aspects, retention, preservation of medical records and release of information
- Portray the needs of medical record department including training of the new staff
- Organize the medical record department to meet the patient care services of the hospital
- Classify the primary, secondary and tertiary care services of healthcare delivery system
- Classify the diseases and operations as per the international classification of diseases/ operations
- Perform quality assurance, patient care evaluation or medical audit programs
- Know the rights and responsibilities of a patient

PART II: ELECTRONIC MEDICAL RECORDS (EMR) 32

1. Introduction to information technology (IT) 1
   - Computer
     - Hardware
     - Software
       - Systems software
       - Applications software
     - Overview of networking
       - Intranets
       - Extranet
       - Internet services
2. Healthcare information regulations, laws and standards 7
   - Licensure, certification and accreditation 1
     - Facility licensure
     - Certification
     - Accreditation
   - ISO standards 1
     - What is standard?
     - What are the benefits of ISO international standards
     - ISO 9001 healthcare management
     - ISO 9001 health service accreditation
     - ISO 13485 medical device standards
   - JCAHO standards 1
     - JCAHO information management standards
       - JACHO standards for the content and maintenance of patient records
   - Health insurance portability accountability act (HIPAA) standards 1
     - Administrative safeguards
       - Security management
       - Assigned security responsibility (required)
       - Workforce security
       - Information access management
       - Security incidence procedures
       - Contingency plan
       - Evaluation report
     - Physical safeguards
       - Facility access controls
       - Workstation (required)
       - Workstation security (required)
       - Device and media controls
     - Technical safeguards
       - Access control
       - Audit control
       - Integrity

- ◻ Person or entity authentication (required)
- ◻ Transmission security

- Analysis of comparison between HIPAA standard
  - Implementation and ISO/IEC 17799
- Evidence based medicine (EBM) 1
  - Introduction
  - Background and definition
  - Evidence-based health services
  - Evidence-based decision making
  - Process and progress
  1. Translation of uncertainty to an answerable question and includes critical questioning, study design and levels of evidence
  2. Systematic retrieval of best evidence available
  3. Critical appraisal of evidence for internal validity that can be broken down into aspects regarding:
     - ◻ Systematic errors as a result of selection bias, information bias and confounding
     - ◻ Quantitative aspects of diagnosis and treatment
     - ◻ The effect size and aspects regarding its precision
     - ◻ Clinical importance of results
     - ◻ External validity or generalized
  4. Application of results in practice
  5. Evaluation of performance
- Ranking the quality of service
- Grade work group
- Categories of recommendation
- Statistical measures
- Number needed to treat/harm
- Quality of clinical trails
- Limitations and criticism
- Assessing the teaching of EBM
- Health record as a legal document 1
  - Introduction
  - Health record as a legal document
    - ◻ Patient-identifiable source data
    - ◻ Administrative data
    - ◻ Derived data
  - Ownership of health information
    - ◻ Ownership of masked and aggregate data
    - ◻ Multi-provider systems integration arrangements
    - ◻ Information systems vendors and clearinghouses
- Electronic health records
  - Introduction
  - Federal laws
  - Retention of health records (manual and electronic)

- – Purpose of retention of records
  - ▫ Federal/state statutory for retention of records
  - ▫ Retention schedule
- • Security, privacy and confidentiality 1
  - – Introduction
  - – Difference between privacy, confidentiality and security
    - ▫ Growth and impact of information technology
    - ▫ The impact for health information security
    - ▫ Model legislative language (AHIMA drafted)
    - ▫ Security threat to healthcare information
    - ▫ Ensuring healthcare information security
      - ❑ Development of security organization
      - ❑ Administrative controls
        - ■ Risk analysis and management
        - ■ Chief security officer
        - ■ System security evaluation
      - ❑ Physical controls/safeguards
        - ■ Assigned security responsibility
        - ■ Media control
        - ■ Physical access controls
        - ■ Workstation security
      - ❑ Technical controls/safeguards
        - ■ Access control
        - ■ Entity authentication
        - ■ Audit trails
        - ■ Data encryption
        - ■ Firewall protection
        - ■ Virus checking

3. Healthcare informatics and management system 10
   - • Information system 2
     - – Hospital information systems 1
       - ▫ Introduction
       - ▫ Administration functions
         - ❑ Patient registration
         - ❑ Patient scheduling
         - ❑ Patient admission, discharge and transfers
         - ❑ Billing and reimbursement
       - ▫ Organizational structure
       - ▫ Systems administration
         - ❑ Database administrator
         - ❑ Application specialist and trainer
         - ❑ Hardware/network engineer
       - ▫ Standardization
       - ▫ Benefits of HIS
       - ▫ Medical record system
         - ❑ Purpose

- Content
  - ID Data
  - Patient care information
- Administrative issues
  - Legal document
  - Retention of records/information
  - Destruction of records/information
  - Security and privacy of records/information

- Clinic information systems (CIS) 1
  - Introduction
    - What is CIS?
    - How does using the CIS will improve care?
- Laboratory information systems (LIS) 1 Lab tech. Hosp
  - Introduction
  - Test order
  - Repeated order
  - Quick lab results
  - Pending lab result
  - Visit history
  - Result history
  - Blood request
  - Ultrasound
  - Release/recall details
  - Laboratory components
  - Print investigations
  - Filter investigations
  - Lab profile
- Basic features
  - Patient check in
  - Order entry
  - Specimen processing
  - Result (s) entry
  - Reporting
  - Patient demographics
  - Physician demographics
- Additional features
  - Web-based order entry
  - Web-based results inquiry
  - Faxing and emailing of lab reports
  - Custom report creation
  - HL7 interfaces with reference labs and EMRs
  - Preliminary reporting
  - Final reporting
  - Med tech work sheets
  - Workload balancing

  - Billing
  - Public health reporting
  - Rule engines
  - Report check by reputed pathologist and senior technologist
- Types of laboratory disciplines
  - Hematology
- Chemistry
- Immunology
- Blood bank donor center
- Blood bank transfusion
- Clinical pathology
- Cytology (cytopathology)
- Microbiology
- Flow cytometry
- TB
- Radiology information systems (RIS) 1 Rad. Tech. Hosp.
  - Introduction
  - Radiology procedure
- Radiology history—visitwise
- Radiology history—orderwise
- Referred radiology
  - Printing the referral
  - Printing the report for the patient
- Registration
- Scheduling
- Patient tracking
- Film library management
- Reporting of results
- Department management
- Basic features
  - Patient registration and scheduling
  - Patient list management
  - Interface with modality via work list
  - Radiology department workflow management
  - Request and documenting scanning
  - Result (s) entry
  - Reporting and printing
  - Result (s) delivery including faxing and e-mailing reports
  - Patient tracking
  - Interactive documents
  - Technical files creation
  - Modality and material management
- Additional features
  - Appointment books
  - PACS workflow

- Custom report creation
- HL7 interfaces with a PACS. HL7 also enables ommunication
- Between HIS and RIS in addition to RIS and PACS
- Billing
- Rule engines

• Pharmacy information systems	1	Pharmacist Hosp
– Medication management system		
– Outpatient		
– Inpatient		
– Emergency patient		
– Preoperative patient		
– Postoperative patient		
• Delete medicine in the prescribed windows		
• Discontinue prescribed medicine		
• Download medicine prescribed from previous visit		
• Viewing the medical history		
• Activities:		
– Clinical screening		
– Prescription management		
– Inventory		
– Patient drug profile		
– Report generation		
– Interactivity with other systems		
• Computerized provider order entry (CPOE)	1	Doctor IT
– Introduction		
– Definition and primary function of CPOE system		
– Current use of CPOE		
– Value of CPOE		
• Benefits of advanced ambulatory CPOE system		
– Improved patient care		
– Cost savings		
– Provider revenue enhancement		
• Perspective CPOE implementation		
– Physician change management		
– Workflow change management		
– CPOE and decision support		
• Medication administration systems		
– Barcode-enabled point of care (BPOC)		
• Clinical decision support system (CDSS)	1	Doctor IT
– Introduction		
– Types of CDSS		
▫ Knowledge based decision support systems		
▫ Knowledge base		
▫ Interface engine or reasoning mechanism		

- Non-knowledge based CDSS
  - Artificial neural networks
  - Genetic algorithms
- Effectiveness of CDSS
- Implementation challenges

* Nursing information system (NIS) 1
  - Features
    - Nursing self scheduling
    - Documenting care plans
    - Nursing work distribution
  - Benefits
    - Saving time
    - Review patient care plan from anywhere
    - Make more efficient
    - Reduce stress
* Financial: Revenue and expenditure 1
* Insurance and billing 1

4. Hybrid medical record 2
   - Introduction
     - Definition of hybrid
       - Transformation from paper (manual) to paperless (electronic)
       - Hybrid health record policy
5. EMR implementation process 7
   - What is an electronic medical record 1
     - Common healthcare computer systems
     - EMR concept
     - EMR and CPR
   - An introduction to EMR systems 2
     - Software vendor or tailor-made
       - Hardware and enabling technologies
       - Choosing a successful EMR system
         - Technical features
           - Usage of CPOE and CDSS
           - Role in electronic research work
         - Event monitoring
         - Quality care and costs
       - Implementing EMR system
       - Technical standards 1
         - HL7
         - ANSI × 12 (ED)
         - CEN—CONTSYS (EN 13940)
         - CEN—EHRcom (EN 13606)
         - CEN—HISA (EN 12967)
         - DICOM
       - Regulatory compliance 1
         - HIPAA

- HL7
- DICOM
- Title 21 CFR part II
- Legal issues 1
  - Introduction
  - Ownership of health information
  - Electronic medical records
    - Federal laws
    - State laws
  - Privacy, confidentiality and security
- Checklist for readiness to implement HER 1

6. Other systems implementation 5
   - Personal health record (PHR) 1
     - Definition of PHR
     - Purpose of PHR
     - Implementation of PHR
     - PHR Components
       - Patient ID format
       - Health summary
       - Immunization
       - Self care
       - Medication
       - Investigations
       - Obstetrics and gynecology
       - Therapy
       - Chronic disease record
       - Dental
   - Telemedicine and tele-health 1
   - Telemedicine
     - Introduction
     - Definition of telemedicine
     - Types of technology
     - Telemedicine concepts
     - Telemedicine program support
     - Telemedicine challenges
   - Tele-health
     - Introduction
       - Clinical uses of technologies
     - Tele-health modes
       - Store-and-forward tele-health
       - Real time tele-health
         - Tele-cardiology
         - Tele-trauma
         - Tele-pharmacy
         - Tele-dentistry

        - Tele-radiology
        - Tele-pathology
        - Tele-nursing
    - Remote patient monitoring
        - Home based nocturnal dialysis
        - Cardiac and remote ICUs
        - Disease management
- Mobile technology in healthcare 1
- Smart cards, wireless, RFID 1
    - Smart cards
    - History
    - Integrated circuits
    - Types of smart cards
        - Contact smart cards
        - Contact less smart cards
        - Combination smart cards
- Standards
    - ISO 7816
    - ISO/IEC 14443
    - ETSI
    - EMV
    - JAVA card
    - WHQL
- Applications of smart cards
    - Identification
    - Net work access
    - Electronic purses
    - Telecommunications
    - Special applications
- Security with smart cards
    - Standard security guards
        - Authentication
        - Confidentiality
        - Integrity
        - Non-repudiation
- Wireless
    - Introduction
    - Wireless services
    - Wireless net works
    - Modes
        - Radio
        - Microwave
        - Infrared
- Applications of wireless technology
    - Mobile telephone

- Wireless data communications
  - Wi-Fi
  - Cellular data service
  - Mobile satellite communication
- Categories of wireless implementations
  - Devices standards
  - Radio
  - Broadcasting
  - Armature radio
  - Land mobile radio
  - Cordless telephone
  - Cellular networks
- Radio-frequency identification (RFID)
  - Introduction
  - History
  - Design
    - Miniaturization
  - Uses
    - Commerce
    - Transportation
    - Infrastructure
    - Passport
    - Sports
    - Telemetry
  - RFID mandates
  - Regulations and standardizations
- Health informatics professional's role 1
  - Role
  - Functions
  - Key responsibilities

COURSE DESCRIPTION

The course outline includes computer hardware, systems and application software, overview of network consisting intra-, extra- and internet services. The study encompasses healthcare information regulations, laws and standards, e.g. ISO, JCAHO, HIPAA, evidence based medicine (EBM), health record legal document. The procedure for EMR retention period, security, privacy and confidentiality.

The course incorporates hospital information system including administrative, functions organizational structure, administrative system and clinical information system including; laboratory, radiology, pharmacy, computer physician order entry (CPOE), computer decision support system (CDSS), nursing information system and others. EMR implementation process include hybrid medical records, technical standards, e.g. HL7, ANSI, CEN, DIOCOM and other system implementation. The other system includes personal health records (PHR), telemedicine and telehealth, mobile technology, smart cards, wireless and RFID. The course incorporates the role of health information professional in the implementation and maintaining the electronic medical records.

OBJECTIVES OF THE COURSE

Upon successful completion of the course, the students will be able to:

- Understand basics of computer hardware, software and overview of intra-, extra- and internet
- Describe healthcare information regulations, laws and standards, e.g. ISO, JCAHO, HIPAA, etc.
- Recognize the procedure for security, privacy and confidentiality
- Elaborate healthcare information and management system including hospital and clinical system
- Describe lab, radiology, pharmacy, CPOE, CDSS, financial and insurance information systems
- Understand the technical standards such as HL7, ANSI, CEN, DICOM and others
- Illustrate hybrid medical record system in implementation of electronic medical records
- Expound EMR realization process; technical standards, regulatory compliance and legal issues.
- Explain other systems execution, e.g. PHR, telemedicine, telehealth, mobile and smart cards
- Reveal the health information professional's role in development of electronic medical records

PART III: MEDICAL CODING (MC) 32

Introduction

- Description of the ICD and related health problems 4
  - Introduction to ICD-10
  - Purpose and applicability
  - The concept of a "family" of disease and health related classifications
  - General principles of disease classification
  - The basic structure and principles of classification of the IC
  - How to use ICD-10 2
- How to use the ICD volume 1
  - Introduction
  - Use of the tabular list of inclusions and four characters
  - Sub-categories
  - Two codes for certain conditions
  - Conventions used in the tabular list
  - Categories with common characteristics
- How to use volume 3 2
  - Arrangement of the alphabetical index
  - Structure
  - Code numbers
  - Conventions
- Rules and guidelines for mortality and morbidity coding
- Notes for interpretation of entries of causes of death
- Perinatal mortality: Guidelines for certification and rules for coding

- Morbidity
- Statistical presentation 2
  - Introduction
  - Source of data
  - Level of detail of cause in tabulations
  - The recommended special tabulation lists for mortality
  - The special tabulation list for morbidity
- Recommendations in relation to statistical tables for 1
  - International comparison
- Standards and reporting requirements related to fetal, perinatal, neonatal and infant mortality 1
- Standards and reporting requirements related to maternal mortality 1
- Proportion of deaths classified to ill-defined causes 1
- Morbidity
- History of the development of ICD 1
  - Early history
  - Adoption of the international list of causes of death
  - The fifth decennial revision conference
  - The sixth revision of the international lists
  - The seventh and eighth revision
  - The ninth revision
  - Preparations for the tenth revision
- Difference between ICD-9 and ICD-10 1
  - Definition of diagnosis
  - Other classification systems
  - Principles and rules of coding
  - Alphabetic indexing
- ICD procedures in medicine 2
  - Introduction and tabular list
    - Procedure for medical diagnosis
    - Laboratory procedures
    - Preventive procedures
    - Surgical procedures
    - Other therapeutic procedures and ancillary procedures
    - Radiology and certain other applications
    - Drugs, medicaments and biological agents
    - Alphabetical indexing
- Diagnostic coding and indexing procedures 2
  - Inpatient
    - Outpatient
- ICD-9CM 2
  - Introduction to ICD-9-CM
  - HIPAA electronic transactions and coding
  - Standards rule
  - Characteristics of ICD-9-CM
  - Procedures

- – Current procedure terminology (CPT) coding system 2
  - □ Introduction to CPT
- Types of categories
  - – Categories I (six main sections)
    - □ Codes for evaluation and management
    - □ Codes for anesthesia
    - □ Codes for surgery
    - □ Codes for radiology
    - □ Codes for pathology
    - □ Codes for medicine
  - – Categories II
    - □ Performance measurements (optional) codes
  - – Categories III
    - □ Emerging technology codes
- ICD-10-CM guidelines for coding and reporting 8
  - – Introduction 1
  - – Conventions, general coding guidelines 1
    - □ The alphabetical index and tabular list
    - □ Format and structure
    - □ Use of codes for reporting purposes
  - – General coding guidelines 1
    - □ Locating a code in the ICD-CM
    - □ Level of detail in coding
    - □ Signs and symptoms
    - □ Multiple coding for a single condition
  - – Chapter—specific coding guidelines (Chapters 1 to 21) 1s
    - □ Selection of principal diagnosis 1
    - □ Reporting additional diagnosis 1
    - □ Diagnostic coding and reporting 1
    - □ Guidelines for outpatient services 1
    - □ ICD-10-CM and ICD-10-PCS

COURSE DESCRIPTION

This course encompasses the introduction to international classification of disease and related health problems, its historical background, revisions from fifth to tenth. The syllabus includes ICD general, ICD-9 CM, ICD-10, procedures in medicine and CPT coding system and also brief introduction to ICD-10 CM PCS.

The course describes the use of three volumes of ICD-10; in detail the volume 1 including list of three-character categories, and tabular list of inclusions and four-character subcategories. While volume 2 contains guidelines for recording and coding, together with outlines of historical background to the classification. And detailed instructions on the use of alphabetical index are contained in the introduction to volume 3.

The syllabus explains the ICD-9 CM its characteristics procedures and provides guidelines for ICD-10 CM coding and reporting and brief introduction to ICD-10 CM –PCS (procedure coding system). And also the course covers introduction to current terminology procedure (CPT) coding system and its main categories.

The course includes the statistical presentation, source of data, recommended special tabular lists for Mortality and morbidity. The course includes the distinction between the ICD-9 and ICD-10. And also covers the use of ICD procedures in medicine including tabular list of different specialties.

OBJECTIVES OF THE COURSE

Upon successful completion of the course, the students will be able to:

- Describe international classification of diseases (ICD) and related health problems
- Explain how to use ICD-10—volume 1 including tabular list
- Elucidate the use of volume 3 with arrangement of alphabetical index, structure, code numbers and conventions
- Enumerate the guidelines for mortality and morbidity coding
- Explicate statistical source of data, collection, compilation and presentation
- Recognize the special tabular list for mortality and morbidity
- Narrate history of the development of ICD including adoption of international list of cause of death, and revision of fifth to ninth and preparation of tenth revision
- Differentiate between ICD-9 and ICD-10 coding system
- Recognize the ICD procedures in medicine including tabular list of different specialties
- Describe the ICD-9 CM and its characteristics and procedures
- Code diagnostic and surgical procedures for OP and IP for ICD- 9 CM and ICD-10
- Recognize the current procedure terminology (CPT) coding system and its main categories
- Provide guidelines for ICD-10 CM coding and reporting
- Enlighten ICD-10 PCS (procedure coding system).

Chapter 22

Health Information Management Center for Excellence

I. VISION

To establish health information management center (HIMC) to meet the needs of 21st century in the field of healthcare management. The future vision is to earn as one of the renowned centers for health information management of the world and to be a model to other nations.

II. MISSION

Is to contribute significantly to the national healthcare delivery system in general and health information management program in particular to provide the best possible health to all the citizens and residents of India at par with international standards.

III. GOALS

The HIM center main goal is to develop an international standard center specialized in health information management center to contribute greatly in providing services that require in achieving the national goal of providing best possible swift, safe healthcare with reasonable cost to the people India.

IV. OBJECTIVES

The main objective of this centre is to focus on: Research, education, quality, innovation, association, sustain, cost, conferences, accreditation and advice to accomplish unification and standardization of systems throughout the nation.

1. **Research:** Conduct research to find problems and provide solutions.
2. **Education:** Educate in right direction to generate able and competent Professionals who can deliver the efficient service in 21st century
3. **Quality:** To ensure that high quality of services are rendered.
4. **Innovation:** To search continuously the modern and novelty methods.
5. **Association:** Public participation to serve better the community.
6. **Sustain:** Keep going or carry on to uphold the set goals and objectives

7. **Cost:** To study the price/charge trends in order to develop the cost standards to contain cost
8. **Conferences:** Conduct conferences, symposia, seminars and workshops to exchange ideas, knowledge and skills.
9. **Accreditation:** To develop accreditation standards and provide official approvals and certification to the needy institutions.
10. **Advice:** Offer opinion, counsel and information.

V. STRUCTURE OF THE HIMC

This center besides health information management department will have units such as information technology, epidemiology and biostatistics, quality improvement and management.

The health information management and technology center (HIMC) will be equipped with best possible infrastructure that would facilitate involving fully with the nations needs in the field of healthcare and successfully delivering best possible healthcare to the people. In order to participate actively in this process, the HIMC would carry out the following:

1. Develop best medical record (health information) management systems and procedures, standards, policies and procedures to maintain excellent health information that would inspire other institutions take as a model, that would help in providing best possible healthcare, swiftly, safely and with reasonable cost.
2. The center will establish a modern information technology (IT) department within the centre to develop e-Health information system that could help in maintaining electronic health records and hospital information system so that the patient records are on-line and can be easily accessible to authorized from any part of the world.
3. The center will have an of epidemiology and biostatistical department that will carry out in depth research and maintain demographic and health data/information that would meet the current and future needs of the nation in particular and international in general. This center will maintain demographic database for all the health institutions of the country. Research is the main focus through which many surveys would be conducted and results are found. The morbidity and mortality information, disease pattern, underlying causes for mortality and case mix studies would be main task of this department.
4. **Quality improvement (QI):** This unit will be equipped with the continuous quality improvement programs, explore new methods and techniques in carrying out QI and performance improvement studies. Develop strategies that will meet the set goals and objectives.
5. **Management:** This unit will be responsible for developing the best practicable organizational and managerial structures related to health field that would facilitate in effective organization and efficiently managed systems. This unit also includes human resource management, finance, and support services.

All the five wings (units/departments) will work as one body and all will focus their energy and efforts towards common goal and objectives set by the center.

VI. REQUIREMENTS FOR ESTABLISHING A HIM CENTER

The following are some of main needs:

1. **Location:** Appropriate location with required space to be allocated to be adequate enough to accommodate the convention (conference) hall, 5 seminar rooms, library, medical records and information technology laboratories, administration wing, units such as research, management, quality, statistics, MR and IT. And also to accommodate

car parking areas for guests and staff, landscape, gift shop, book shop, cafeteria and security, etc.

2. **Building:** A suitable modern building to be designed by renowned architect to meet the current requirement and scope for future expansion for next five to ten years.
3. **Personnel:** Obviously this is a very sensitive issue needs to be tackled very carefully. Number and type of personnel required have to be worked out in consultation with HRD and each of the department stipulated above.
4. **Infrastructure:** Selection of appropriate equipment and furniture needs to be worked out with the concerned units, administration, and finance and purchase department to have right equipment for the departments.
5. **Technology:** Software and hardware and related accessories form a major component of the center, involves exorbitant cost. This needs to be worked out critically taking into present and future requirements.
6. **Books and periodicals and also online facilities:** Books and Periodicals and online information facilities play a very vital role in the management of HIMC. Hence, the selecting and purchase of books of different topics and contributing to various related periodicals is also quite cumbersome and expensive issue need to be tackled.
7. **Budget:** Once we have hypothetical project in hand, the need to work out budgetary requirements for the present and future requirements. Initial one time budget that is non-recurrent and recurrent budget which is essential has to be calculated and presented every year.
8. Hierarchical organizational set up to be drawn and job descriptions have to be prepared and duties and responsibilities have to be clearly laid down.
9. **Policies and procedures:** The rules and regulations for the functioning of the center and all allied departments have to be prepared to avoid any ambiguous situations.
10. **Continuing education:** There should be clear strategic plans for conducting continuous educational program for HIM personnel. There should be half yearly or yearly program schedule prepared in advance wherever and whenever possible and implemented accordingly.
11. **Training of trainers:** This is another area needs special attention to impart trainers training, orientations on very specially selected subjects that emerged as new to be conducted.
12. **Manpower development:** The major responsibility of this center would be providing leadership direction for development of professional manpower. It is essential to take the national, regional and local, government and private needs for the current and future, with addition of 15 to 20% to the total manpower to be calculated and ways to generate the same to be worked out.
13. **Collaboration within and outside organizations:** The objective of this center is to become renowned in the international arena, needs to collaborate within and outside organizations engaged in similar fields to cooperate in exchange of technology. This entails inviting renowned international experts from different parts of the world and also center staff to visit other places, all these needs have to be considered.
14. **Innovation:** The modernization issues have to be continuously carried out by varied ways including research, studies, surveys, interviews and observations and so on.

VII. SCOPE: MAJOR SCOPE

- **Education:** To find new methods of learning and teaching
- Quality and performance improvement
- Manpower development and utilization

- Cost containment; effective allocation and utilization
- **Systems and method development:** For providing efficient tools and techniques to carry out set work.
- Conducting improved managerial programs for high executives, policy makers such as ministers, director generals, hospital CEOs, and other directors/mangers.

Moderate Scope

- Develop work culture
- Develop job descriptions
- Develop work systems and methods
- Develop appropriate standards, policies and procedures
- Education and training for all health related personnel in all the stipulated fields:
  - Health information (medical records) management
  - Information technology (IT)
  - Quality and performance improvement management (QM/PI)
- Develop E library (electronic library online media)
- Establish virtual E education center for HIM program
- Develop accreditation center for HIM program
- Develop required HIM manpower for the country
- Collaborate with overseas countries in the areas of education and, research.

Accreditation and Affiliation

- Develop regional centers for easy access of information and transforming/transporting the outcomes of the center.
- Develop Licensing Authority to accredit the professional qualifications by registering the HIM related professionals.
- Continuing education on latest (modern trends) on HIM fields to be conducted within and outside the center.
- Collaborate with HIM Association of India for professional development.

VIII. HOW TO ACCOMPLISH HIM CENTER FOR EXCELLENCE

The following are some of the suggestions for action.

- Invite International expert/s to participate and give their insight and input in the development and managing the center successfully.
- Collaborate with centers of similar nature to exchange expertise, knowledge, skills through well established coordination and cooperation
- To prepare a good comprehensive scheme with full justification, how the center would play a role in solving innumerable unsolved national issues related to education, professional manpower development, and incredible contribution in healthcare delivery and benefits derived by the community as a whole though the center.
- Conduct regular conferences, symposia, workshops to build up our research project work and to raise funds. And also use the center as platform for surveying and evaluating the current situations in different fields that would benefit tremendously in carrying out successful research.
- Maintain list of resource persons in different fields within, and outside the center to utilize their expertise, guidance, consultation services wherever and whenever needed.
- To fulfill the centers goals and objectives, requires adequate budget (for short and long term) to develop infrastructure. The proposal with full justification; how this center is

going to benefit to the nation in general and the university in particular to be submitted to the higher authority for their approval, not only for establishing but also to maintain the center.

IX. PROPOSED BUILDING PLAN

Selection of location is very vital, once this is done, the need for proper building with other environmental requirements for drawing an appropriate architecture plans for constructing the building and other areas such as landscape, parking for staff, outside guests, security, and other requirements have to be covered in the building plan.

Some of the major departments of the center for HIM for excellence are furnished: The center can be housed in two story building with an area of 400 to 500 Sq. meters. The entire area can be divided mainly into 3 parts:

PART I

1. Main front gate with security room
2. **Front location of the building:** Open area for landscape, guest parking

PART II

1. Administrative wing
2. Conference/convention hall
3. Seminar/classrooms
4. Central library
5. Medical record and IT laboratories
6. Accreditation unit
7. Medical record (health information) deptartment
8. Information technology (IT) unit
9. Epidemiology and biostatistical unit
10. Quality improvement init
11. Research unit
12. Multimedia unit
13. Management unit (MU) for HR; finance and others
14. Other units/services:
    - Reception
    - Public relations
    - Gift shop
    - Book shop
    - Cafeteria
    - Internet conference
    - Telephone/fax services
    - Waiting halls
    - Meeting rooms
    - Examination rooms
    - First aid unit
    - HIM Association of Office or representative or Honorary HIM Adviser

- Community center for public participation and opinion
- Rest rooms for men and women
- Security
- Disaster plan equipped room.

PART III

- Rear emergency gate with security if needed
- Rear location of the building: Open area for landscape, staff parking, etc.

X. BUILDING PLAN (A MODEL BUILDING PLAN): ANNEXURE I

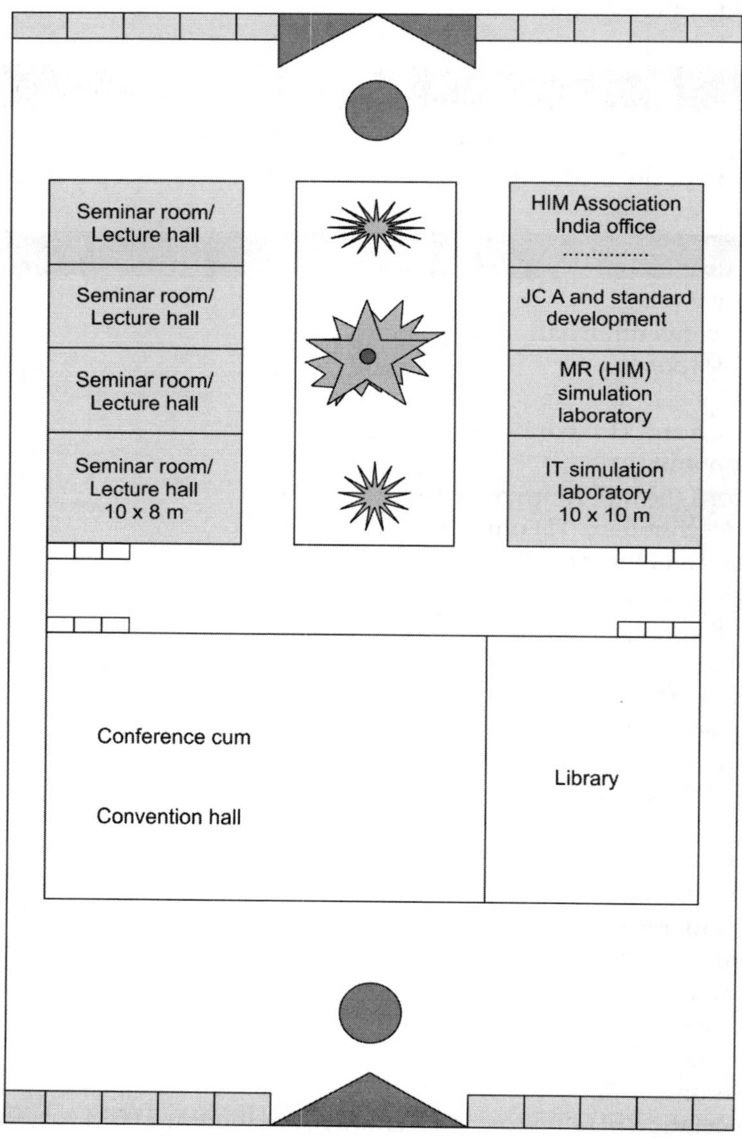

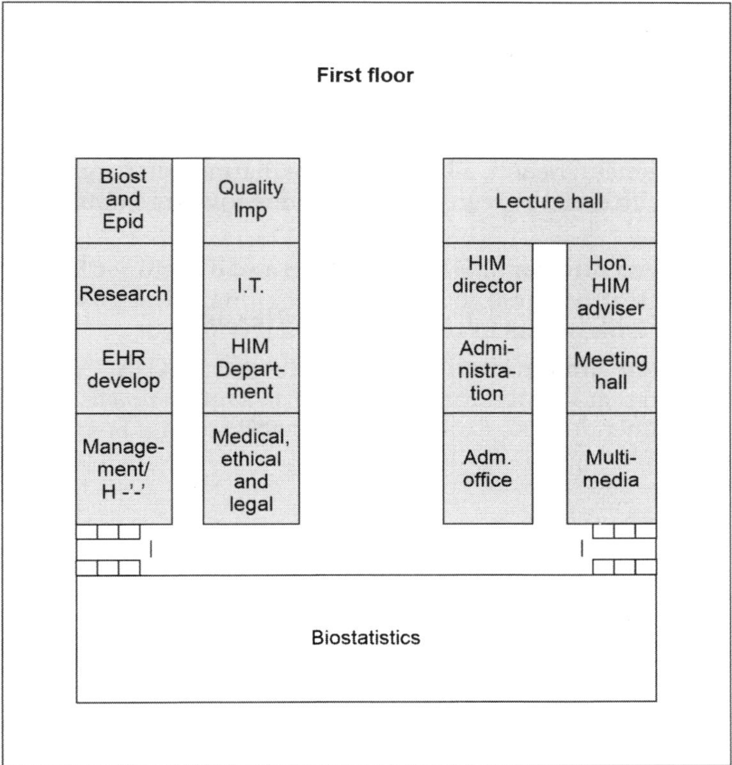

NATIONAL INSTITUTE OF ALLIED HEALTH SCIENCES (NIAHS), MINISTRY OF HEALTH AND FAMILY WELFARE, GOVERNMENT OF INDIA

INTRODUCTION

On similar lines as suggested for Health Information Management Center (HIMC) for excellence, the National Institute of Allied Health Sciences (NIAHS) building could be planned which includes all the core allied health sciences, such as physiotherapy, optometry, health information management and sanitary inspector, etc.

Each department will have similar facilities or some of them can be shared by combining such as conventional center, library including online library, seminar rooms and lecture halls, or board meeting room, etc.

Mechanism of allocation: Each allied health science field will be as part of NIAHS, and be located in separate wing, e.g. HIMC will be in "Wing-A", "Physiotherapy in Wing-B", Optometry in "Wing-C" and Sanitary Inspector in "Wing-D"., and so on.

Management: The national institute of allied health sciences will be managed by the ministry of health and family welfare under the supervision and guidance of an additional director general of health services. Each allied health science department will have a director to oversee the department; he/she is supported by administrative and technical staff. Each director will have a retired honorary senior advisor in the field to advice.

National Institute of Regional Allied Health Sciences (NIRAHS): Under the NIAHS there are eight Regional Institutes of Allied Health Ssciences (RIAHS). Each region will have a deputy director general of health services to oversee the RIAHS. Each specialty department will be headed by a director, e.g. physiotherapy, optometry, health information management and sanitary inspector department and supported by a retired honorary senior adviser in the field to advice.

Coordination between NIAHS and RIAHS: Under the supervision and guidance of additional director general health, all the RIAHS will function. Any policy discussions will be held at the head office, all the regional deputy directors of general health services will be invited.

Coordination between director of HIM at NIAHS and director of HIM at RIAHS: During any policy meetings at national level, all the regional directors of region along with honorary retired senior advisors too will be invited if required.

Continuing education and monitoring by NIAHS and RIAHS: Continuing education in all the specialties and regular monitoring has to be on a regular basis to ensure all are within the standards recommended and expected quality and target is being maintained.

Chapter 23

Medical Records Diploma Education Program in Kuwait

INTRODUCTION

Kuwait is the gateway to the Arabian peninsula, it is bounded in the east by the Arabian Gulf, in the south-west by the Kingdom of Saudi Arabia and in the north and west by the Republic of Iraq, Modem Kuwait is identified with oil, and has a total population of 3,695, 316; out of this nationals 1,403, 962, (33%) and immigrants accounting 67% (2013) a total area of 17, 818 Sq. km., with Kuwait Gross Domestic Product (GDP); 175.8 billion USD (2013).

The Public Authority for Applied Education and Training (PAAET) is an academic institute in Kuwait; it is considered one of the largest institutes in the Middle East in terms of the number of enrolled students, the PAAET offers a wide variety of programs across its different colleges and training institutes. It was established on December 28, 1982, by law number (63) with the objective of developing and upgrading manpower to meet the challenge of shortfall in technical manpower created by industrial development and economic development of the country.

The foundation of applied education and training was laid along with the initiation of oil exploration, production and export in Kuwait. In the 1950s, the state began to establish training centers and organized programs to prepare the manpower needed for the oil industry. After building the fundamental structure of the education system, the Ministry of Education established a number of specialized institutions to meet the increasing demand for skilled manpower. The other ministries established their own training centres and institutes as well. The state found it essential to establish a central body to supervise and coordinate the activities of these numerous institutes with the main objective is to develop the national technical manpower to meet the human resource needs of the country through its two sectors; education and training. The college of health sciences is the part of the public authority for applied education and training.

Medical Records Program

The College of Health Sciences previously (The Kuwait Institute of Health Sciences), was started the medical record program 1985, the two-year diploma program was developed by Dr Mogli and other committee members and was started by Dr GD Mogli, who was working as Medical Records Advisor to the Ministry of Health. The public authority had requested his services from the ministry of health to teach the two years diploma program in medical records. The same program is being run till now. The program consists of 68 credits which can be shown as follows:

The Medical Records Technician Program Courses

1st Course

Code and course No.	*Subject*	*Credit*	*No. of hours weekly*
EL III	English for medical technician	5	10
MED 120	Medical terminology	3	3
MED 156	Anatomy and physiology	3	3
MR 103	Introduction to medical record field	2	2
MR 104	Health care delivery system	2	2
LiB 104	Research and library	1	2
		16	**22**

2nd Course

Code and course No.	*Subject*	*Credit*	*No. of hours weekly*
EL 161	English for medical technician	2	4
MED 160	Clinical medicine	4	4
Pharm 156	Pharmacology	1	1
MR 105	Filing systems	5	12
Typ 155	English typing	2	4
	Elective course*	2	2
		16	**27**

*Elective courses (select any one)
114—Introduction to psychology
123—Human relations
Kuwait history

3rd Course

Code and course No.	*Subject*	*Credit*	*No. of hours weekly*
EL 211	English for medical record technician	2	4
MED 204	Content and analysis of medical record	4	8
MED 205	Coding and indexing	4	9
MR 107	Introduction to statistic	4	6
Comp. 108	Introduction to computer	3	4
		17	**31**

4th Course

Code and Course No.	Subject	Credit	No. of hours weekly
R 206	Managing medical record	5	12
MR 207	Health information system	4	8
MR 208	Computer application for medical record	3	4
IE 101	Islamic education	2	2
TYP 155	Arabic typing	2	4
		16	**30**

Summer Practicum

Code and course No	Credit	No. of hours weekly
MR 209	3	30

The period of study of this program is two years (4 semester courses) and summer practical (6 weeks). The above courses consist of theoretical lectures and laboratory and clinical practice at hospital setting in the ministry of health.

All courses taught in English languages except elective courses taught in Arabic. The program starts from September to January and second from February to June and summer practicum starts from June to August.

Admission to the program

- Passed general secondary education with minimum 55%
- Passed an interview.

The number of admission to the program is 30 candidates per course admitted both girls and boys. Graduate student will receive Diploma in health science (medical records). Student after finishing program will work at the ministry of health hospitals as medical records technician.

Conclusion

The syllabus curriculum, content and the teaching program developed since 1985 has been used for many years (till now), due to advent of technology and also the transformation of medical records into health information management. I had personally consulted Dr GD Mogli and other professionals in order to develop the medical record program to be consistent with recent development and with special emphasis on technology as most of the health institutions are converting the manual paper record into electronic records. It became necessary to teach such subjects which will help medical records students for the career build-up.

Now, the two years diploma program of medical records at the college of health sciences is being reviewed for development under the direct supervision of qualified professionals with a mission that new developed program should provide instructions and clinical experience to assist students in developing the technical skills necessary to maintain components of health information system consistent with the medical administrative, ethical, legal accreditation and regulatory requirement of health care delivery system of the ministry of health and consistent with recent developed program and with other university around the world.

Chapter

24

Recommendations on Electronic Medical Records Standards in India

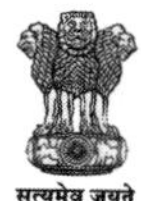

Government of India

Ministry of Health and Family Welfare
Department of Health and Family Welfare
Nirman Bhawan, New Delhi-110108

APRIL 2013

Recommendations of EMR standards committee constituted by an order of Ministry of Health and Family Welfare, Government of India and coordinated by FICCI on its behalf.

EXECUTIVE SUMMARY

Healthcare systems are highly complex, fragmented and use multiple information technology systems. With vendors incorporating different standards for similar or same systems, it is little wonder that all-round inefficiency, waste and errors in healthcare information and delivery management are all too common place an occurrence. Consequently, a patient's medical information often gets trapped in silos of legacy systems, unable to be shared with members of the healthcare community. These are some of the several motivations driving an effort to encourage standardization, integration and electronic information exchange amongst the various healthcare providers.

Developmental origins of health and diseases (DOHAD) have successfully proven the importance of developmental records of individuals in predicting and/or explaining the diseases that a person is suffering from. In the current largely paper-based medical records world, invaluable data is more often than not unavailable at the right time in the hands of the clinical care providers to permit better care. This is largely due to the inefficiencies inherent in the paper-based system. In an electronic world, it is very much possible, provided certain important steps are taken beforehand, to ensure the availability of the right information at the right time.

In order to be meaningful, the health record of an individual needs to be from conception (better) or birth (at the very least). As one progresses through one's life, every record of every clinical encounter represents an event in one's life. Each of these records may be insignificant or significant depending on the current problems that the person suffers from. Thus, it becomes imperative that these records be arranged chronologically to provide a summary of the various clinical events in the lifetime of a person.

Electronic health records are a summary of the various electronic medical records that get generated during any clinical encounter. Without standards, a lifelong summary is not possible as different records from different sources spread across ~80+ years will potentially need to be brought into one summary. To achieve this, a set of pre-defined standards for information exchange that includes images, clinical codes and a minimum data set is imperative.

This report provides a structured overview of the key EMR standards with respect to Indian conditions. A detailed discussion on the interoperability and standards that include a discussion on the goals, categories of adoption of standards, clinical standards, EMR/EHR, ownership, privacy and security aspects, healthcare informatics standards, and the various coding systems are carried out followed by the detailing of the minimum data set that any Indian EMR must have. A background on EMR and EHR and its use is provided, followed by a list of the various stakeholders. A short study of the efforts world-wide including country-wise analysis of similar efforts and their current state is also outlined.

While any vendor may choose to have any additionally relevant information captured and presented, all must conform to the MDS. A short reference section and a detailed section of acronyms, definitions and glossary are added for everyone's benefit.

In conclusion, it must be added that these standards cannot be considered either in isolation or as "etched in stone for all eternity". These will need to undergo periodic (at a maximum of 24 month interval) review and update as necessary. This document must be a "living document".

1. BACKGROUND

Healthcare sector in India has witnessed significant growth during the last few years, both in quality and capacity. The relatively lower cost of healthcare, as compared to developed countries, coupled with international quality, has positioned India as a major destination for healthcare services. The private sector has also initiated massive investments in various facets of healthcare. This is expected to position healthcare as one of the largest service sectors and a significant contributor to the GDP. As the health sector is poised for major growth in next decade, the sheer size of healthcare sector in the country will necessitate extensive use of information and communication technology (ICT) infrastructure, services and databases for policy planning and implementation. Such a framework would require services based on inter-operable and sharable technology, standards utilization, connecting various institutions and service providers. The use of international experience, best practices and open technologies may be necessary in some scenarios.

Technology is a critical tool in achieving the benefits of health information exchange (HIE). However, technology alone is not sufficient. Healthcare industry stakeholders that base their HIE solutions solely on technology do so at the expense of underlying health information management principles. An abundance of disparate HIE principles, models, definitions, products, and standards camouflages some crucial policy and process decisions an HIE initiative must make in the early stages of its development. Transmitting patient data electronically without attending to the business processes surrounding data capture, translation, and transmission has the potential to increase patient risks and healthcare costs. Data accessibility, reliability, and accuracy are therefore critical success factors in obtaining the trust of stakeholders, including consumers, and in sustaining long-term data exchange on a large scale.

Electronic health records (EHRs) can improve care by enabling functions that paper medical records cannot deliver:

- EHRs can make a patient's health information available when and where it is needed—too often care has to wait because the chart is in one place and needed in another. EHRs enable clinicians secure access to information needed to support high quality and efficient care.
- EHRs can bring a patient's total health information together to support better healthcare decisions, and more coordinated care.
- EHRs can support better follow-up information for patients, for example, after a clinical visit or hospital stay, instructions and information for the patient can be effortlessly provided and reminders for other follow-up care can be sent easily or even automatically to the patient.
- EHRs can improve patient and provider convenience—patients can have their prescriptions ordered and ready even before they leave the provider's office, and insurance claims can be filed immediately from the provider's office.

It is important to note that a number of initiatives proposing standardization and health information exchange (HIE) including telemedicine had been undertaken by the Government of India from time to time. In 2003, MCIT had prepared and published a recommended framework for IT infrastructure for healthcare including recommendations on guidelines, standards and practices for telemedicine in India. The taskforce set up by MoHFW in 2005 for telemedicine also looked at the issues and standards related to EMR.

The current recommendations are a result of the deliberations of the EMR Standards Committee set up by MoHFW, GoI in September 2010. FICCI is the nodal agency for coordination of the exercise nominated by the ministry.

2. MAJOR STAKEHOLDERS

This list includes the following:

- Citizens
- Healthcare providers
- Payers, i.e. insurance companies including TPA
- Education, research institutions and investigators
- Government departments and institutions including law enforcement and courts of law
- Public health agencies and NGOs
- Pharmaceutical industry and medical device makers
- Telemedicine institutions
- Software and hardware vendors

It must be noted that while there are a number of stakeholders who have a vested interest in the data collected in an electronic health record system, the only two of these stakeholders have an active interest are the citizens and healthcare providers.

Therefore, the standards, guidelines and regulations mentioned in this document will apply to the following[1]*:*

- Healthcare providers
- Healthcare institutions

- Patients
- Independent software vendors including EHR/EMR system designers, manufacturers, suppliers, and re-sellers

3. ELECTRONIC HEALTH RECORDS (EHR) ELECTRONIC MEDICAL RECORDS (EMRs)

According to the "Integrated Care EHR", as defined in ISO/DTR 20514, an "*EMR is a repository of information regarding the health of a subject of care in computer-processable form that is able to be stored and transmitted securely, and is accessible by multiple authorized users*".

It has a commonly agreed logical information model which is independent of EHR systems and its chief purpose is the support of continuing, efficient and quality integrated healthcare and it contains information which is retrospective, concurrent and prospective.

Broadly speaking, an EMR is a specific recording/episode of encounter and is case or purpose specific—telemedicine/care, while an EHR is an aggregation of EMRs and is usually life-long.

The benefits that an EMR is expected to bring in are:

- Paperless medical history
- Reduced healthcare costs
- Empowering the stakeholders to be able to deliver right treatment at the right time
- Promote the practice of evidence-based medicine
- Accelerate research and building effective medical practices
- Usher in ease in maintaining health information of patients
- With proper backup policies increase lifespan of health records of individuals that is from conception to cremation
- Safety with access, audit and authorization control mechanisms
- Faster search and updates

Study and Analysis of National EHR/EMR Programs around the World*

Table 24.1: Review of healthcare IT programs world-wide

Country	*National healthcare IT program*
Australia	Health connect
Austria	ELGA
Canada	EHRS blueprint
Denmark	Medcom
England	Spine
Hong Kong	eHR infrastructure
Netherlands	AORTA
Singapore	EMRX
Sweden	National patient summary (NPO)
Taiwan	Health information network (HIN)

*Conducted by Medical Informatics Group, C-DAC, Pune as part of project for building distributed National EHR funded by DIT, MCIT, Govt. of India 10

Table 24.2: Country-wise HCIT standards usage

	Australia	*Austria*	*Canada*	*Denmark*	*England*	*Hong Kong*	*Netherlands*	*Sweden*	*Singapore*	*Taiwan*
HL7v2.5	N	N	N	N	N	Y	N	N	N	N
HL7v only	N	Y	Y	N	Y	Y	Y	Y	N	N
CDA	Y	Y	Y	N	Y	Y	N	N	N	Y
ASTM CCR	N	N	N	N	Y	N	N	N	N	N
CCD	N	N	N	N	Y	N	N	N	N	N
Open EHR	Y	N	N	Y	N	N	N	Y	N	N
IHE	N	Y	Y	N	N	N	N	N	N	N
DICOM	N	Y	Y	N	N	N	N	N	N	N
EDIFACT	N	N	N	Y	N	N	N	N	N	N
EHR Com	N	N	N	N	N	N	N	Y	N	N

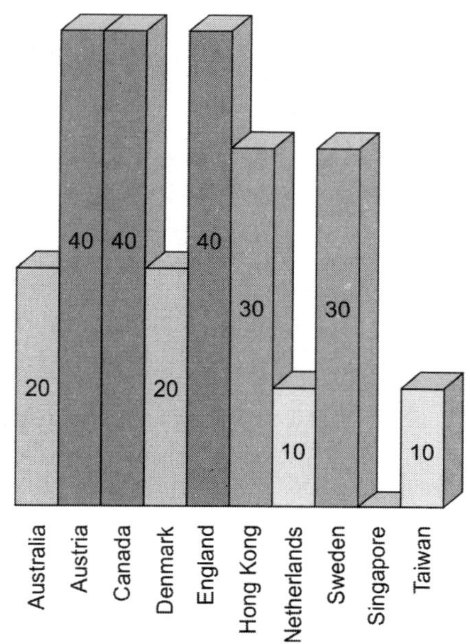

Fig. 24.1: Country-wise data exchange standards usage

4. INTEROPERABILITY AND STANDARDS

The recommendations outlined in this section are an incremental approach to adopting standards, implementation specifications, and criteria to enhance the interoperability, functionality, utility, and security of health information technology and to support its widespread adoption. It is to be kept in mind that these standards should be flexible and modifiable to adapt to the demographic and resource variance observed in a large and developing country like India.

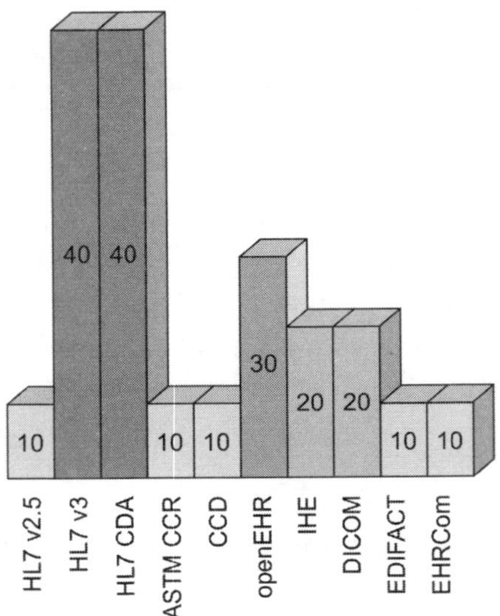

Fig. 24.2: Country-wise standards adoption statistics

It is important to recognize that interoperability and standardization can occur at many different levels. To achieve interoperability, information models would need to be harmonized into a consistent representation.[8]

In other cases, organizations may use the same information model, but use different vocabularies or code sets (for example, systematized nomenclature of medicine clinical Terms (SNOMED CT®) or ICD10-CM within those information models. To achieve interoperability at this level, standardizing vocabularies, or mapping between different vocabularies (using tools like Unified Medical Language System (UMLS)) may be necessary. For some levels (such as the network transport protocol), an industry standard that is widely used (e.g. transmission control protocol TCP) and the Internet Protocol [(IP) (TCP/IP)] will likely be the most appropriate. Ultimately, to achieve semantic interoperability, it is anticipated that multiple layers—network transportation protocols, data and services descriptions, information models, and vocabularies and code sets—will need to be standardized and/or harmonized to produce an inclusive, consistent representation of the interoperability requirements.

It is further anticipated that using a harmonization process will integrate different representations of healthcare information into a consistent representation and maintain and update that consistent representation over time. For an information model, this process could include merging related concepts, adding new concepts, and mapping concepts from one representation of healthcare information to another. Similar processes to support standardization of data and services descriptions and vocabularies and codes sets may also be needed.

It is also recognized that a sustainable and incremental approach to the adoption of standards will require processes for harmonizing both current and future standards. This will allow the incremental updating of the initial set of standards, implementation specifications, and certification criteria and provide a framework to maintain them. The decision to adopt such updates will be informed and guided by recommendations from an appropriate authority akin to a National Health Information Authority.

Goals

- Promote interoperability and where necessary be specific about certain content exchange and vocabulary standards to establish a path forward toward semantic interoperability
- Support the evolution and timely maintenance of adopted standards
- Promote technical innovation using adopted standards
- Encourage participation and adoption by all vendors and stakeholders
- Keep implementation costs as low as reasonably possible
- Consider best practices, experiences, policies and frameworks
- To the extent possible, adopt standards that are modular and not interdependent.

Categories for Adoption of Standards

Vocabulary Standards

Standardized nomenclatures and code sets used to describe clinical problems and procedures, medications, and allergies.

This is to be achieved through the extensive use of Controlled Medical Vocabularies (CMV) that is detailed as follows:

a. **Logical observation identifiers names and codes (LOINC®):** The purpose of LOINC® is to facilitate the exchange and pooling of clinical results for clinical care, outcomes management, and research by providing a set of universal codes and names to identify laboratory and other clinical observations. The Regenstrief Institute Inc., an internationally renowned healthcare and informatics research organization, maintains the LOINC database and supporting documentation, and the RELMA mapping program.

b. **International classification of diseases (ICD-10):** The ICD is the international standard diagnostic classification for all general epidemiological, many health management purposes and clinical use.

c. **Systematized nomenclature of medicine: Clinical terms (SNOMED: CT):** Is a comprehensive clinical terminology, originally created by the College of American Pathologists (CAP) and owned, maintained, and distributed by the International Health Terminology Standards Development Organization (IHTSDO), a non-for-profit association in Denmark.

d. **Current Procedural Terminology, 4th edition (CPT-4):** The CPT-4 is a uniform coding system consisting of descriptive terms and identifying codes that are used primarily to identify medical services and procedures furnished by physicians and other healthcare professionals.

e. **RxNorm:** RxNorm, produced by the national library of medicine (NLM) provides normalized names for clinical drugs and links its names to many of the drug vocabularies commonly used in pharmacy management and drug interaction software, including those of first databank, micromedex, medi span, gold standard alchemy, and Multum. By providing links between these vocabularies, RxNorm can mediate messages between systems not using the same software and vocabulary.

f. **ATC—anatomic therapeutic chemical classification of drugs:** It is used for the classification of drugs. It is controlled by the WHO collaborating centre for drug statistics methodology (WHOCC), and was first published in 1976. This pharmaceutical coding system divides drugs into different groups according to the organ or system on which they act and/or their therapeutic and chemical characteristics. Each bottom-level ATC code stands for a pharmaceutically used substance in a single indication (or use). This means that one drug can have more than one code: acetylsalicylic acid (aspirin), for example, has A01AD05 as a drug for local oral treatment, B01AC06 as a platelet inhibitor, and N02BA01 as an analgesic and antipyretic. On the other hand, several different brands share the same code if they have the same active substance and indications.

Content Exchange Standards

Standards used to share clinical information such as clinical summaries, prescriptions, and structured electronic documents.

a. **Health level seven (HL7) clinical document architecture:** Is an XML-based mark-up standard intended to specify the encoding, structure and semantics of clinical documents for exchange. CDA is being used also in electronic health records projects to provide a standard format for entry, retrieval and storage of health information.

b. **HL7 2.5.1:** Defines a series of electronic messages to support administrative, logistical, financial as well as clinical processes and mostly uses a textual, non-XML encoding syntax based on delimiters. HL7 v2.x has allowed for the interoperability between electronic patient administration systems (PAS), electronic practice management (EPM) systems, laboratory information systems (LIS), dietary, pharmacy and billing systems as well as electronic medical record (EMR) or electronic health record (EHR) systems.

c. **Continuity of care record (CCR)** is a health record standard specification developed jointly by ASTM international, the Massachusetts Medical Society (MMS), the Healthcare Information and Management Systems Society (HIMSS), the American Academy of Family Physicians (AAFP), the American Academy of Pediatrics (AAP), and other health informatics vendors. It is a core data set of the most relevant administrative, demographic, and clinical information facts about a patient's healthcare, covering one or more healthcare encounters. It provides a means for one healthcare practitioner, system, or setting to aggregate all of the pertinent data about a patient and forward it to another practitioner, system, or setting to support the continuity of care. The primary use case for the CCR is to provide a snapshot in time containing the pertinent clinical, demographic, and administrative data for a specific patient. To ensure interchange ability of electronic CCRs, this specification specifies XML coding that is required when the CCR is created in a structured electronic format. Conditions of security and privacy for a CCR instance must be established in a way that allows only properly authenticated and authorized access to the CCR document instance or its elements. The CCR consists of three core components: the CCR header, the CCR body, and the CCR Footer.

d. **Digital imaging and communications in medicine (DICOM):** The DICOM standards committee exists to create and maintain international standards for communication of biomedical diagnostic and therapeutic information in disciplines that use digital images and associated data. The goals of DICOM are to achieve compatibility and to improve workflow efficiency between imaging systems and other information systems in healthcare environments worldwide. DICOM currently defines an upper layer protocol (ULP) that is used over TCP/IP (independent of the physical network), messages, services, information objects and an association negotiation mechanism. These definitions ensure that any two implementations of a compatible set of services and information objects can effectively communicate.

Clinical Standards

Clinical standards are health information standards to capture a patient's health information in a more coherent manner. This health information can include all or part thereof as relevant of the following:

- The illness a patient is suffering from
- The physician's observation of the patient's illness
- The diagnostic tests that need to be carried out to ascertain the patient's illness and to give the patient better treatment
- The results of the diagnostic tests
- The kind of treatment to be given to the patient
- The way the treatment should be given to the patient.

Table 24.3: HCIT standards (relevant to India—Initial set)

	Recommended healthcare IT standards (for India)	
Name	*Class*	*Comments*
Phase 1		
UHID	Unique health identifier—to act as patient identifier	UID as a unique (primary or secondary) patient identifier. The UID should be used to identify a particular patient across all organizations (and their EMR systems); Aadhar number is recommended for use in EMR as either the primary or secondary, where the primary is an internal unique health identifier used by the healthcare provider organisation
XML (eXtensible markup language)	for data capture, integration department documents (the CDA CCD)	To access via SOAP—simple object and presentation layer access protocol CCD (HL7/ASTM) clinical data for inter likely to be used for exchanging the clinical documentation between two EHR solutions both within an organisation and outside
RxNorm/ATC pharmacologic-therapeutic classification/NDC—national drug classification, FDB—first databank (USA) Indian drugs—MIMS/CIMS from CMPMedica	Medicines	Needs to be researched as there is no universal drug reference database. The WHO drug dictionary ATC (anatomic therapeutic classification) may be a good choice to begin with
Dictionary of medicine and devices, UK	Medicines and medical devices	UK standard used in NHS includes devices and drugs

Contd...

Table 24.3: HCIT standards (relevant to India—Initial set) *(Contd…)*

	Recommended healthcare IT standards (for India)	
Name	*Class*	*Comments*
LOINC	Clinica laboratory observations	Published and maintained by the Regenstrief Institute, USA, this is a universally accepted code for laboratory observations
HL7 V2.x	Messaging	Propose V2.3
HL7 V3.0 RIM	Reference information model	As this version is being superceded by FHIR from HL7, it would be preferable to adopt FHIR instead of V3.0 RIM
DICOM 3.0–2004	Medical images	The latest version
CPT 4 or 5, US	Procedure and therapy classification	As this will involve paying a licensing fee, this is optional
OPCS4, UK	Procedure and therapy classification	
SNOMED-CT	Clinical terminology	Provide comprehensive clinical granularity, used to capture problem list, allergies, diagnosis, procedures, etc.—will immensely aid in clinical analytics, clinical decision support systems, automated clinical care pathway management systems, support evidence based practice, etc.
WHO ICD 10	Disease classification	WHO is actively working with IHTSDO to converge SNOMED-CT with ICD
WHO—PCS	Procedure coding system	
WHO—ICF	International classification of functioning, disability and health	
Phase 2		
DSM	Psychiatric conditions	Diagnostic and statistical manual of mental disorders
NIC/NOC/NANDA	Nursing interventions classification	
CDT 2, US	Dental procedures	
Unknown	AYUSH clinical terminology, treatment planning including medication details	Ayurveda, Yoga, Unani, Siddha, Homoeopathy systems of medicine as distinct from the allopathic (Western) system of medicine

Table 24.4: Health informatics standards

Relevant healthcare informatics standards (as adopted internationally)	
Organization	*Standards*
National recommendations for health information infrastructure in India	• Information technology infrastructure for health (ITIH) framework • Recommendations on guidelines, standards and practices for telemedicine in India • Indian health information network development (iHIND) recommendations from the national knowledge
International organization for standardization (ISO)	Requirements for electronic health record architecture (ISO/TS 18308)
European committee for standardization (CEN)	CEN/TC 251 EN 13606
Code of federal regulations (CFR)	Health information technology standards, implementation specifications, and certification criteria and certification programs for health information technology (title 45, part 170)
American Society for Testing and Materials (ASTM)	Continuity of care record (CCR)
Health level 7 (HL7)	HL7 v2.x HL7 v3 CDA-2 FHIR (fast health interoperable resources)—the newest version; easy upgrade from v2.x to FHIR EHR—system functional model
HL7 and ASTM collaboration	Continuity of care document (CCD)
National electrical Manufacturer's (NEMA)	Digital imaging and communications in medicine (DICOM PS Association 3.0 2004 onwards)
Office of national coordinator for health information Technology (ONCHIT)—USA	EHR meaningful use

Issues

- Unique identification
- Interoperability/sharing
- Integrated systems require consistent use of standards in, e.g. medical terminologies and high quality data to support information sharing across wide networks
- Ethical, legal and technical issues linked to the accuracy, security confidentiality and access rights.
- Common record architectures, structures
- Clinical information standards and communications protocols

Trends

- National UID and healthcare
- Distributed EHR concept

Table 24.5: EMR MDS

Data item	*Data type*	*Data length*	*Format/values*	*Status*	*Additional observations*
UHID	Numeric	12	As per Aadhar specifications	Mandatory if no other concomitant ID is used inthe system, else optional	Only the public key will be used and that too only for identification, aid in patient search, patient merge and demerge functionalities
Alternate UHID	Any	Any	As per institution/ vendor's specifications	Mandatory if no other concomitant ID is used in the system, else optional	Wherever Adhaar number is unavailable and the healthcare provider wishes to use their own ID system, this field should be used; this ID may be used in addition to the UHID above
Patient name	Alphanumeric	Sufficiently large	To be split into first name, middle name and last (family) name	Mandatory	MDDS (http://egovstandards.gov.in/standards and Framework/metadata-and-data-standards/MDDS-Demographic%20Ver%201.1.pdf/at_download/file) may be referred to for patient demographics data; only the person identification part of the meta data and data standards are applicable
Patient date of birth	Date	Fixed	dd.mm.yyyy	Optional	
Patient age	Numeric	Fixed	999,99,999 no preceding zero [years, months, days]	Mandatory	Age is to be automatically calculated if date of birth is entered/available; once the patient's age is available, all client systems must automatically "age" the patient. For this, unless the patient's date of birth is available, the age will be approximated with the assumption that the patient was born on the 1st day

Contd.

Table 24.5: EMR MDS *(Contd.)*

Data item	*Data type*	*Data length*	*Format/values*	*Status*	*Additional observations*
					of January of the year that the entered age appears to point to. The record display will need to clearly show that this age is an approximated one and that the patient may actually be older by 1 additional year maximally
Patient Gender	Alphanumeric	1	To be shortened to one byte as M, F, U or T for male, female, unknown and transgender. Systems should translate and show the full form on user screens	Mandatory	
Patient Occupation	Alphanumeric	Sufficiently large		Mandatory	
Patient address Type	Alphanumeric	9	Current/ permanent/ previous	Mandatory	
Patient address Line 1	Alphanumeric	Sufficiently large		Mandatory	It is recommended that MDDS be followed; details are given above
Patient address Line 2	Alphanumeric	Sufficiently large		Optional	It is recommended that MDDS be followed; details are given above
Patient city/town/ village/police station	Alphanumeric village	Sufficiently large		Mandatory	It is recommended that MDDS be followed; details are given above
Patient district	Alphanumeric	Sufficiently large		Optional	It is recommended that MDDS be followed; details are given above

(Contd.)

Table 24.5: EMR MDS *(Contd.)*

Data item	*Data type*	*Data length*	*Format/values*	*Status*	*Additional observations*
Patient state	Alphanumeric	Sufficiently large		Optional	It is recommended that MDDS be followed; details are given above
Patient pin code	Alphanumeric	Sufficiently large		Optional	It is recommended that MDDS be followed; details are given above
Patient country code	Alphanumeric	Sufficiently large	As per ISO Country codes	Optional	
Patient phone type	Alphanumeric	20	Landline/mobile/ PP- Landline/neigh bour landline/relation landline/ neighbour mobile/relation mobile	Optional	
Patient phone number	Alphanumeric	16	(099)9999999999	Optional	
Patient email ID	Alphanumeric	255	Must contain '@' and "." at Appr. position	Optional	
Emergency/contact person name	Alphanumeric	Sufficiently large		Optional	It is recommended that MDDS be followed; details are given above
Emergency contact person relationship	Alphanumeric	9	Spouse/parent/C hild/partner/cous in/friend/neigh bour/other	Mandatory, if used, else optional	
Emergency contact person address type	Alphanumeric	9	Current/permanent/previous	Mandatory, if used, else optional	
Emergency Contact person Address line 1	Alphanumeric	Sufficiently large		Mandatory, if used, else Optional	It is recommended that MDDS be followed; details are given above

(Contd.)

Table 24.5: EMR MDS *(Contd.)*

Data item	*Data type*	*Data length*	*Format/values*	*Status*	*Additional observations*
Emergency contact person address line 1	Alphanumeric	Sufficiently large		Mandatory, if used, else Optional	It is recommended that MDDS be followed; details are given above
Emergency contact person Address line 2	Alphanumeric	Sufficiently large		Optional	It is recommended that MDDS be followed; details are given above
Emergency contact person City/town/village/police stat.	Alphanumeric	Sufficiently large		Mandatory, if used, else optional	It is recommended that MDDS be followed; details are given above
Emergency	Alphanumeric	Sufficiently		Optional, if used	It is recommended that MDDS be
Care provider address type	Alphanumeric	9	Current/ permanent/ previous	Mandatory, if used, else optional	
Care provider address line 1	Alphanumeric	Sufficiently large		Mandatory, if used, else Optional	It is recommended that MDDS be followed; details are given above
Care provider address line 2	Alphanumeric	Sufficiently large		Optional	It is recommended that MDDS be followed; details are given above
Care provider	Alphanumeric city/town/ villa ge/police station	Sufficiently large		Mandatory, if used, else Optional	It is recommended that MDDS be followed; details are given above
Care provider district	Alphanumeric	Sufficiently large		Optional, if used	It is recommended that MDDS be followed; details are given above
Care provider state	Alphanumeric	Sufficiently large		Optional, if used	It is recommended that MDDS be followed; details are given above
Care provider pin code	Alphanumeric	Sufficiently large		Optional, if used	It is recommended that MDDS be followed; details are given above
Care provider country code	Alphanumeric	Sufficiently large	As per ISO country codes	Optional, if used	

(Contd.)

Table 24.5: EMR MDS *(Contd.)*

Data item	*Data type*	*Data length*	*Format/values*	*Status*	*Additional observations*
Care provider phone type	Alphanumeric	20	Landline/mobile/ PP-landline/ neighbour landline/relation landline/ neighbour mobile/relation mobile	Optional	
Care provider phone number	Alphanumeric	16	(099)9999999999	Optional	
Encounter number	Numeric	4	9999 format – no prefixed 0	Mandatory	It must be ensured that the no encounter number is arbitrarily assigned. The system will need to ensure this. When linking records from diverse systems, episode and encounter reconciliation through appropriate merging and demerging will need to take place. However, this is a design and development issue, and out of scope for the work of MDS proposal
Encounter date and Time	Datetime	Fixed	Complete date plus hours, minutes and seconds/complete date plus hours, minutes, seconds and a decimal fraction of a second	Mandatory; should be auto-inserted by the system from system time that is synchronised with Indian standard time	
Reason for visit	Alphanumeric	4096		Mandatory	More than one reason for visit may be entered

(Contd.)

Table 24.5: EMR MDS *(Contd.)*

Data item	*Data type*	*Data length*	*Format/values*	*Status*	*Additional observations*
Present history	Alphanumeric	4096		Optional	Both structured and unstructured data can be used wherever the data type is alphanumeric and data length is 4096 and if necessary, it can be made longer-this is true for all fields in the MDS wherever they occur
Past history	Alphanumeric	4096		Optional	
Personal history	Alphanumeric	4096		Optional	
Family history	Alphanumeric	4096		Optional	
Menstrual and obstetric history	Alphanumeric	4096	LMP, cycle duration, gravida, parity to be captured as structured data where LMP: date type; cycle duration, gravida, parity: numeric type;	Optional	Menstrual and obstetric history to be available only if the chosen gender is female
Socio-economic status	Alphanumeric	Sufficiently large		Optional	
Immunization history	Alphanumeric	4096		Optional	It is preferable that the details are captured in as granular a manner as is practical; multiple entries should be possible, with a list of values for each vaccine type and dates administered with current status (administered/not-administered)

(Contd.)

Table 24.5: EMR MDS *(Contd.)*

Data item	*Data type*	*Data length*	*Format/values*	*Status*	*Additional observations*
Allergy status	Alphanumeric	8	Active/Inactive		Optional
Allergy history	Alphanumeric	4096		Optional	Allergies will be a list of values (drug generics, etc.) that would, in future, allow allergy alerts to be activated
Clinical exam vitals systolic BP	Numeric	3	999–no preceding 0	Optional	Unit of measurement is mmHg
Clinical exam vitals diastolic BP	Numeric	3	999–no preceding 0	Optional	Unit of measurement is mmHg
Clinical exam pulse rate	Numeric	3	999–no preceding 0	Optional	Unit of measurement is per minute
Clinical exam temperature (°C)	Floating	2 digits, 2 decimals	99.99	Optional	Unit of measurement is degrees centigrade; if degrees Fahrenheit is to be used, then this may be converted at run time for display or data manipulation purposes by the system
Clinical exam temperature source	Alphanumeric	6	Oral/Armpit/Groin/Rectal		Mandatory, if Temperature is captured
Clinical exam respiration rate	Numeric	3	999–no preceding 0	Optional	Unit of measurement is per minute
Clinical exam height (cm)	Floating	3 digits, 2 decimals	999.99	Optional	Unit of measurement is centimetres; if any other unit of measurement, like feet, is to be used, then this may be converted at run time for display or data manipulation purposes by the system

(Contd.)

Table 24.5: EMR MDS *(Contd.)*

Data item	*Data type*	*Data length*	*Format/values*	*Status*	*Additional observations*
Clinical exam weight (kg)	Floating	3 digits, 2 decimals	999.99	Optional	Unit of measurement is kilograms; if any other unit of measurement, like pounds, is to be used, then this may be converted at run time for display or data manipulation purposes by the system
Blood group	Alphanumeric	3	A+/A-/B+/B-/AB+/AB-/O+/O-	Optional	
Clinical exam observation	Alphanumeric	4096		Optional	It is recommended that SNOMED-CT be used for all clinical terms/observations
Investigation results	Alphanumeric	4096		Optional	It is recommended that LOINC be used for all laboratory observations
Clinical summary	Alphanumeric	4096		Mandatory	It is recommended that SNOMED-CT be used for all clinical terms/observations
Diagnosis type	Alphanumeric	11	Provisional/final/admission/interim/working/discharge	Mandatory	
Diagnosis code name	Alphanumeric	Sufficiently large	ICD/SNOMED-CT/Free	Mandatory	
Diagnosis code	Alphanumeric	Sufficiently large	Coding system dependent	Mandatory	Diagnosis code should allow multiple entries per encounter record
Diagnosis (description)	Alphanumeric	4096		Mandatory	
Treatment plan Investigations	Alphanumeric	4096		Optional	The user may or may not enter any value
Treatment plan Medication	Alphanumeric	4096		Optional	It is preferable that the details are captured in as granular a manner as is practical; for the allopathic system of medicine, it is suggested that something similar to the contents of the table below be followed—this requirement is not mandatory

(Contd.)

Table 24.5: EMR MDS *(Contd.)*

Data item	*Data type*	*Data length*	*Format/values*	*Status*	*Additional observations*
Treatment plan procedure	Alphanumeric	4096		Optional	
Treatment plan referral	Alphanumeric	4096		Optional	For use in referral cases only
Other treatment plan	Alphanumeric	10	Diet/life-style/ others	Optional	
Type other	Alphanumeric	4096		Mandatory if other	
Treatment plan details				Treatment type is selected	
Current clinical status	Alphanumeric	255	[Free text]	Mandatory	Captures the current clinical status; synonymous with clinical outcome or condition at discharge; it is preferable that terms such as "Fair", "Relieved", "Better", "Same", "Worse",

Table 24.6: Medication details (for allopathic system of medicine only)

Data item	*Data type*	*Data length*	*Format/values*	*Status*	*Additional observations*
Medication name	Alphanumeric	Sufficiently large	As per the drug database	Mandatory	Should preferably be generic
Drug code	Alphanumeric	Sufficiently large	As per the drug database	Mandatory	Auto populated by the system
Strength	Alphanumeric	Sufficiently large	As per the drug database	Mandatory	Should be presented as a LOV
Dose	Alphanumeric	Sufficiently large		Mandatory	To be entered by the care provider
Route	Alphanumeric	Sufficiently large		Mandatory	To be entered by the care provider
Frequency	Alphanumeric	Sufficiently large		Mandatory	To be entered by the care provider

5. EHR MINIMUM DATA SET (MDS)

The following MDS is recommended for an EMR to be used in India. Vendors are free and indeed encouraged to opt for additional data to satisfy additional and the unmet needs of the various stakeholders, principally the patients and the clinical care providers.

6. GUIDELINES

Hardware

- The IT hardware used should meet (and preferably be better than) the optimal requirement given by the software (to be) used.
- The medical and IT hardware used must meet the relevant applicable specifications from BIS, NEMA, ISO, CE, RoHS, EnergyStar, apart from medical and IT standards for the equipment.
- A backup or data preservation mechanism should be considered. Data capacity should be planned to meet the storage requirement as per the mandated rule/law.
- System redundancy at various levels (disk, power, network, etc.) should be planned to meet the organizational system availability requirement.
- Network and data security should be planned, implemented, and periodically audited. Please see section on security and privacy for requirements and functions to be supported and implemented.
- Hardware should be checked periodically for correctness and completeness of operation expected from them. An appropriate maintenance cycle should be planned and followed.
- Planned and expected capacity and quality requirement of the organization should be met by the hardware used. Periodic updates and upgrades should be carried out to meet the requirements.

Networking and Connectivity

- Should be able to harness any telecommunications-related connectivity like the Internet, LAN, WAN, WAP, CDMA, GSM or even cloud computing that will permit the various EMRs of an individual to be integrated into a single lifelong electronic health record
- As far as practical and affordable, the connectivity medium chosen should be reliable and fast enough to sustain a secure data exchange for the period expected for transaction of records and data. The speed of the connectivity medium should be chosen from among available options so as to provide an acceptable user experience and not cause software/system fault due to delays/noise/failure.
- Should be able to ensure that data exchange is performed in a secure manner to ensure data validity and non-repudiability
- The data exchange must further ensure that data integrity is maintained at all times.

Software Standards

The software Should

- Conform to the specified standards
- Satisfy specified requirements
- Be interoperable should be able to ensure role based access control at all times
- Should be able to support privacy, secrecy and audit trail
- Possess advanced search, merge, and demerge functionality to ensure that duplicates are robustly resolved
- Should be able to support conception-to-current medical records of a person

- Should be able to support digital archiving and retrieval of medical records after the death of a person for the total duration as specified by Government of India from time to time
- Should be able to construct a medical/clinical summary based on available records from the very first visit to current
- Should be able to support for rapid data capture-storage-retrieval-display of data
- Should be able to ensure user authentication and authorisation.

Proposed Mobile Health Record

As patients move around the healthcare system there is a need to carry essential information to ensure quality healthcare which will give their treating clinician basic information, viz. medical condition, drug/allergy information, etc. CCR standard XML file format, with demographics, insurance info, problem list/diagnoses, medications, allergy and alerts, vital signs, and lab results, consultation reports, hospital discharge and operative reports and investigative and diagnostic results (e.g. ECG reports, tread mill test results, biochemistry results, histopathological findings, ultrasound findings, etc.) kept current and accurate by a person's healthcare team (nurses, doctors and pharmacists) which includes the patient. Conformance to m-governance guidelines of DEITY is imperative (http://www.deity. gov.in/content/framework-mobile-governance).

7. DATA OWNERSHIP OF EMR

The ethical, legal, social issues (ELSI) guidelines for Electronic Medical Record (EMR) are recommended as follows.

For the purposes of these recommendations, the term "privacy" shall mean that only those person or person(s) including organisations duly authorized by the patient may view the recorded data or part thereof. The term "security" shall mean that all recorded personally identifiable data will at all times be protected from any unauthorized access, particularly during transport (e.g. from healthcare provider to provider, healthcare provider to patient). The term "trust" shall mean that person, persons or organisations (doctors, hospitals, patients) are those who they claim they are.

The following approaches are to be adopted wherever applicable

- Privacy would refer to authorization by the owner of the data (the patient)
- Security would have as components both public and private key encryption; the encryptions used in transit and at rest need to be through a different methodology.
- Trust would be accepted whenever a trusted third party confirms identify.

Protected health information (PHI) would refer to any individually identifiable information whether oral or recorded in any form or medium that (1) is created, or received by a stakeholder; and (2) relates to past, present, or future physical or mental health conditions of an individual; the provision of healthcare to the individual; or past, present, or future payments for healthcare to an individual.

Electronic protected health information (ePHI) would refer to any protected health information (PHI) that is created, stored, transmitted, or received electronically. Electronic protected health information includes any medium used to store, transmit, or receive PHI electronically.

The following and any future technologies used for accessing, transmitting, or receiving PHI electronically are covered:

- Media containing data at rest (data storage)
  - Personal computers with internal hard drives used at work, home, or traveling

  - External portable hard drives, including iPods and similar devices
  - Magnetic tape
  - Removable storage devices, such as USB memory sticks, CDs, DVDs, and floppy disks
  - PDAs and smartphones
- Data in transit, via wireless, ethernet, modem, DSL, or cable network connections
  - Email
  - File transfer

For data ownership, a distinction is to be made between

a. The physical or electronic records, which are owned by the healthcare provider. These are held in trust on behalf of the patient, and
b. The contained data which are the sensitive personal data of the patient is owned by the patient itself.
c. The healthcare provider will have the privilege to change/append/modify any record in relation to the medical care of the patient as necessary with a complete documented trail of such change. No alteration of the previously saved data will be permitted. No update or update like command shall be utilised by the system to store a record or part thereof. A new record will be created with the unaltered parts of the existing record. The changed/appended/modified data will replace the relevant parts of that record. This record shall then be stored and marked as active while rendering the previous version or versions of the same record marked inactive. A strict audit trail shall be maintained of all activities at all times that may be suitably reviewed by an appropriate authority like auditor, legal representatives of the patient, the patient, healthcare provider, privacy officer, court appointed/authorised person, etc.
d. The medium of storage or transmission of such electronic medical record will be owned by the healthcare provider.
e. The "sensitive personal information (SPI) and personal information (PI)" of the patient is owned by the patient themselves. Refer to IT Act 2000 for the definition of SPI and PI.
f. Sensitive data—as per the Information Technology Act 2000, Data Privacy Rules,refer to 'sensitive personal data or information' (sensitive data) as the subject of protection, but also refer, with respect to certain obligations, to 'personal information'. Sensitive Data is defined as a subset of 'personal information'. Sensitive data is defined as personal information that relates to:
   i. Passwords,
   ii. Financial information such as bank account or credit card or debit card or other payment instrument details,
   iii. Physical, psychological and mental health condition,
   iv. Sexual orientation,
   v. Medical records and history,
   vi. Biometric information,
   vii. Any detail relating to (points i–vi) above received by the body corporate for provision of services, or
   viii. Any information relating to (points i–vii) that is received, stored or processed by the body corporate under a lawful contract or otherwise.

Data access and confidentiality would refer to:

a. Regulations are to be enforced to ensure confidentiality of the recorded patient/medical data and the patient should have a control over this.

b. Patients will have the sufficient privileges to inspect and view their medical records without any time limit. Patient's privileges to amend data shall be limited to correction of errors in the recorded patient/medical details. This shall need to be performed through a recorded request made to the healthcare provider within a period of 30 days from the date of discharge in all inpatient care settings or 30 days from the date of clinical encounter in outpatient care settings. An audit of all such changes shall be strictly maintained. Both the request and audit trail records shall be maintained within the system. Patients will have the privileges to restrict access to and disclosure of individually identifiable health information.

c. All recorded data will be available to care providers on 'as required on demand' basis.

d. Minimum data standards.

Disclosure of information would be applicable as follows:

a. For use for treatment, payments and other healthcare operations—in all such cases, a general consent must be taken from the patient or next of kin, etc. as defined by applicable laws by MCI.

b. Fair use for non-routine and most non-healthcare purposes—a specific consent must be taken from the patient; format as defined by MCI.

c. Certain national priority activities, including notifiable/communicable diseases, will be specified for which health information may be disclosed to appropriate authority as mandated by law without the patient's prior authorization

Responsibilities of any healthcare provider would include:

a. Protect and secure the stored health information, as per the guidelines specified in this document (*see* Data Privacy and Security).

b. While providing patient information, revove patient identifying information, if it is not neecesary to be provided.

c. Will ensure that there are appropriate means of informing the patient of policies relating to his/her rights to health record privacy

d. Document all its privacy policies and ensure that they are implemented and followed. This will include:

   i. Develop internal privacy policies

   ii. Designate a privacy officer (preferably external, may be internal) who will be responsible for implementing privacy policies, audit and quality assurance

   iii. Provide privacy training to all its staff.

Patient will have the privilege to appoint a personal representative to carry out the activities detailed below.

a. Patients will have the privilege to ask for a copy of its medical records held by a healthcare organization.

b. Patients will have the privilege to request a healthcare organization which holds its medical records, to withhold specific information that he/she does not want disclosed to other organizations or individuals.

c. Patient can demand information from a healthcare provider on the details of disclosures performed on the patients medical records.

Instances where denial of information will apply are as follows:

Healthcare provider will be able to deny information to a patient or representative or third party, in contravention of normal regulations, if in the opinion of a licensed healthcare professional the release of information would endanger the life or safety of the patients and others. This will include but not be limited to as follows:

a. Information obtained from an anonymous source under a promise of confidentiality.
b. Psychotherapy notes.
c. Information compiled for civil, criminal or administrative action.

Instances where use and disclosure without individual authorization will be possible are as follows:

Disclosures can be performed without individual authorization in the following situations.

- With identifiers, on production of court order
- However, as far as possible, and where appropriate, the data so provided should be anonymised to remove information that will allow identification of the patient. (Removing identifiers as indicated below).

Digital signatures are to be used to prevent non-repudiation (establishing authenticity of author of the document) and trust by the recipient.

Follow e-Pramaan National e-Authentication service offered by DeitY, Govt. of India

http://epramaan.gov.in/

Reference Framework for e-authentication – ePramaan

http://egovstandards.gov.in/policy/framework-document-for-e-authentication-epramaan

Reference Guidelines for Digital Signatures, available at http://egovstandards.gov.in/guidelines/Guidelines%20for%20Digital-signature/view

Additional Reference Guidelines for Information Security, available at http://egovstandards.gov.in/guidelines/guidelines-for-information-security/view

Patient Identifying Information

Data are "individually identifiable" if they include any of the under mentioned identifiers for an individual or for the individual's employer or family member, or if the provider or researcher is aware that the information could be used, either alone or in combination with other information, to identify an individual. These identifiers are as follows:

1. Name
2. Address (all geographic subdivisions smaller than street address, and PIN code)
3. All elements (except years) of dates related to an individual (including birth date, date of death)
4. Telephone and/or Fax numbers
5. Email address
6. Medical record number
7. Health plan beneficiary number
8. Bank account and/or credit card number
9. Certificate/license number
10. Any vehicle or other any other device identifier or serial numbers
11. PAN number
12. Passport number
13. ADHAAR card
14. Voter ID card
15. Fingerprints/biometrics
16. Voice recordings that are non-clinical in nature

17. Photographic images and that possibly can individually identify the person
18. Any other unique identifying number, characteristic, or code.

8. DATA PRIVACY AND SECURITY

Security of Electronic Health Information

The privacy standards and the security standards are necessarily linked. Any health record system requires safeguards to ensure the data is available when needed and that information is not used, disclosed, accessed, altered, or deleted inappropriately while being stored or transmitted. The security standards work together with the privacy standards to establish appropriate controls and protections. Health sector entities that are required to comply with the privacy standards also must comply with the security standards.

Organizations must consider several factors when adopting security measures. How a healthcare provider satisfies the security requirements and which technology it decides to use are business decisions left to the individual organization. In deciding what security measures to adopt, an organization must consider its size, complexity, and capabilities; its technical infrastructure, hardware, and software security capabilities; the cost of particular security measures; and the probability and degree of the potential risks to the ePHI it stores and transmits.

The security standards require healthcare providers to implement reasonable and appropriate administrative, physical, and technical safeguards. These safeguards seek to ensure the confidentiality, integrity, and availability of all the ePHI they create, transmit, receive, or maintain; protect against reasonably anticipated threats or hazards to the security or integrity of their ePHI; protect against uses or disclosures of the ePHI that are not required or permitted under the privacy standards; and ensure their workforce will comply with their security policies and procedures.

Standards

Purpose of the Security Standards

The security standards require healthcare providers to implement reasonable and appropriate administrative, physical, and technical safeguards to:

- Ensure the confidentiality, integrity, and availability of all the e-PHI they create, transmit, receive, or maintain.
- Protect against reasonably anticipated threats or hazards to the security or integrity of their e-PHI.
- Protect against uses or disclosures of the e-PHI that are not required or permitted under the privacy standards ensure their workforce will comply with their security policies and procedures.

Technical Standards

To protect the ePHI handles by a healthcare provider, the provider must implement technical safeguards as part of its security plan. Technical safeguards refer to using technology to protect ePHI by controlling access to it. Therefore, they must address the following standards focusing on the following. It is worth noting that they will need to use an EHR/EMR solution that is able to successfully and robustly demonstrate the possession and working of these functionalities.

Access control: The solution must assign a unique name and/or number for identifying andtracking user identity and establish controls that permit only authorized users to access electronic health information. In cases of emergency where access controls need to be suspended in order to save a live, authorized users (who are authorized for emergency situations) must be permitted to have unfettered access electronic health information during the duration of the emergency.

Automatic log-off: An electronic session after a predetermined time of inactivity must beforcibly terminated. To log in back, the user will have to initiate a new log in session. However, for the sake of ergonomics, it is recommended that the unsaved state of the system at the time of automatic log-off be saved and presented back to the user for further action. This should be a user-specific feature.

Audit log

- All actions related to electronic health information in accordance with the standard specified in this document including viewing should be recorded.
- Based on user-defined events must be provided.
- All or a specified set of recorded information upon request or at a set period of time must be electronically displayed and printed.

Integrity

- During data transit the fact that the electronic health information has not been altered intransit in accordance with the standard specified in this document must be verifiable.
- Detection of events—all alterations and deletions of electronic health information and audit logs, in accordance with the standard specified in this document must be detected.

Authentication

- Locally within the system the fact that a person or entity seeking access to electronic health information is the one claimed and is authorized to access such information must be verifiable.
- Across the network, however extensive it might be–that a person or entity seeking access to electronic health information across a network is the one claimed and is authorized to access such information in accordance with the standard specified in this document must be verifiable.

Encryption

- Generally, all electronic health information must be encrypted and decrypted as necessary according to user defined preferences in accordance with the best available encryption key strength.
- During data exchange all electronic health information must be suitably encrypted and decrypted when exchanged in accordance with an encrypted and integrity protected link.
- All actions related to electronic health information must be recorded with the date, time, patient identification, and user identification whenever any electronic health information is created, modified, deleted, or printed; and an indication of which action(s) took place must also be recorded.
- Appropriate verification that electronic health information has not been altered in transit shall be possible at any point in time. A secure hashing algorithm must be used to verify that electronic health information has not been altered in transit and it is recommended that the secure hash algorithm (SHA) used must be SHA-1 or higher.
- A cross-enterprise secure transaction that contains sufficient identity information such that the receiver can make access control decisions and produce detailed and accurate security audit trails must be used within the system.

Administrative Safeguards Standards

The Administrative Safeguards require healthcare providers to develop and implement a security management process that includes policies and procedures that address the full range of their security vulnerabilities. Being administrative in nature, these need to be internally designed and developed as SOP that must be published for all users to see and adhere to. Conformance to adherence may be delegated to the Privacy Officer detailed in the Data Ownership of EMR. To comply with the Administrative Safeguards, a healthcare provider must implement the following standards.

- The security management process standard, to prevent security violations.
- Assigned security responsibility, to identify a security officer.
- Workforce security, to determine ePHI user access privileges.
- Information access management, to authorize access to ePHI.
- Security awareness training, to train staff members in security awareness.
- Security incident procedures, to handle security incidents.
- Contingency plan, to protect ePHI during an unexpected event, and
- Evaluation, to evaluate an organization's security safeguards.

Physical Safeguards Standards

Physical safeguards are security measures to protect a healthcare provider's electronic information systems, related equipment, and the buildings housing the systems from natural and environmental hazards, and unauthorized intrusion. Covered entities must fulfill four standards. However, because most of the implementation specifications in this category are addressable, healthcare providers will have considerable flexibility in how to comply with the requirements as long as these are internally designed and developed as SOP and published for all users to see and adhere to. Conformance to adherence may be delegated to the Privacy Officer detailed in the Data Ownership of EMR.

The required physical standards are

- The facility access control standard, to limit actual physical access to electronic information systems and the facilities where they are located.
- The workstation use standard, to control the physical attributes of a specific workstation or group of workstations, to maximize security.
- The workstation security standard, to implement physical safeguards to deter the unauthorized access of a workstation, and
- The device and media controls standard, to control the movement of any electronic media containing ePHI from or within the facility.

REFERENCES

1. Final Recommendation, Framework for Information Technology Infrastructure for Health in India (ITIHI), Volumes I and II, DIT, MCIT, Govt. of India.
2. Recommendations on Guidelines, Standards and Practices for Telemedicine in India, DIT, MCIT, Govt. of India.
3. HIM Principles in Health Information Exchange (Practice Brief).
4. 2006 HIMSS RHIO Definition Workgroup.
5. http://healthit.hhs.gov/portal/server.pt?open=512&objID=2996&mode=2 (see below)
6. Institute of Medicine (2000). "To Err Is Human: Building a Safer Health System (2000)". The National Academies Press. http://fermat.nap.edu/catalog/9728.html#toc. Retrieved 2006-06-20.
7. Charatan, Fred (2000). "Clinton acts to reduce medical mistakes". BMJ Publishing Group.http://bmj.bmjjournals.com/cgi/content/full/320/7235/597?ijkey=190e9b6d d6e8fec4ca3c2e353f290efb 8237b334&keytype2=tf_ipsecsha. Retrieved 2006-03-17
8. Department of Health and Human Services, USA, USA Billing Code: 4150-45
9. HIPAA Laws: Privacy and Security 45 CFR 142
10. EHR Meaningful Use
11. CCR—http://www.astm.org/Standards/E2369.htm
12. ATC—http://www.whocc.no/atc_ddd_index/

ACRONYMS, DEFINITIONS AND GLOSSARY

[A]

ADSL (asymmetric digital subscriber line): A type of DSL that uses copper telephone lines to transmit data faster than a traditional modem. ADSL only works within short distances because it uses high frequencies with short signals.

Allergy list: This is a list of all the patient's allergies.

Allopathic, allopathy: Defined as relating to or being a system of medicine that aims to combat disease by using remedies (as drugs or surgery) which produce effects that are different from or incompatible with those of the disease being treated.

Ambulatory care: Any medical care delivered on an outpatient basis.

ANM: Auxillary nurse midwife.

ASHA: Accredited social health activist is usually a literate 25–45 years old married/widowed/divorced lady selected from the village itself and accountable to it and trained to work as an interface between the community and the public health system. This is position is one of the key components of the national rural health mission aimed at providing every village in the country with a trained female community health activist.

ATC: Anatomical therapeutic chemical classification system, controlled by the WHO collaborating centre for drug statistics methodology (WHOCC), is used for drug classification.

Authentication: The verification of the identity of a person or process.

Authorization: Any document designating any permission. Authorization or waiver ofauthorization for the use or disclosure of identifiable health information for research (among other activities) is required. The authorization must indicate if the health information used or disclosed is existing information and/or new information that will be created. The authorization form may be combined with the informed consent form, so that a patient need sign only one form. An authorization must include the following specific elements: A description of what information will be used and disclosed and for what purposes; a description of any information that will not be disclosed, if applicable; a list of who will disclose the information and to whom it will be disclosed; an expiration date for the disclosure; a statement that the authorization can be revoked; a statement that disclosed information may be re-disclosed and no longer protected; a statement that if the individual does not provide an authorization, she/he may not be able to receive the intended treatment; the subject's signature and date.

AYUSH: Ayurveda, Yoga, Unani, Siddha and Homeopathy. Falls under the broad category of Indian Systems of Medicines and Homoeopathy (ISM&H) governed by Ministry of Health and Family Welfare, Government of India.

[C]

CCD (continuity of care document): A joint effort of HL7 International and ASTM. CCD fosters interoperability of clinical data by allowing physicians to send electronic medical information to other providers without loss of meaning and enabling improvement of patient care. CCD is an implementation guide for sharing Continuity of Care Record (CCR) patient summary data using the HL7 Version 3. Clinical Document Architecture (CDA), Release 2. It establishes a rich set of templates representing the typical sections of a summary record, and these same templates for vital signs, family history, plan of care, and so on can then be used for establishing interoperability across a wide range of clinical use cases.

CDT: Common dental terminology

Chain of trust agreement: A contract needed to extend the responsibility to protect healthcare data across a series of sub-contractual relationships.

Chief complaint (CC), reason for consultation (RFC), reason for visit (ROV): For recording apatient's disease symptoms.

Client/server architecture: An information-transmission arrangement, in which a client program sends a request to a server. When the server receives the request, it disconnects from the client and processes the request. When the request is processed, the server reconnects to the client program and the information is transferred to the client. This usually implies that the server is located on site as opposed to the ASP (application server provider) architecture.

Clinical care: Synonymous to healthcare.

Clinical care provider: Synonymous to healthcare provider.

Clinical data repository (CDR): A real-time database that consolidates data from a variety of clinical sources to present a unified view of a single patient. It is optimized to allow clinicians to retrieve data for a single patient rather than to identify a population of patients with common characteristics or to facilitate the management of a specific clinical department.

Clinical decision support system (CDSS): A clinical decision support system (CDSS) is software designed to aid clinicians in decision-making by matching individual patient characteristics to computerized knowledge bases for the purpose of generating patient-specific assessments or recommendations.

Clinical establishment: Clinical establishment means (1) a hospital, maternity home, nursing home, dispensary, clinic, sanatorium or an institution by whatever name called that offers services, facilities requiring diagnosis, treatment or care for illness, injury, deformity, abnormality or pregnancy in any recognised system of medicine established and administered or maintained by any person or body of persons, whether incorporated or not; or (2) a place established as an independent entity or part of an establishment referred to above, in connection with the diagnosis or treatment of diseases where pathological, bacteriological, genetic, radiological, chemical, biological investigations or other diagnostic or investigative services with the aid of laboratory or other medical equipment, are usually carried on, established and administered or maintained by any person or body of persons, whether incorporated or not. (Clinical Establishment Act—CEA 2010.)

Clinical guidelines (protocols): Clinical guidelines are recommendations based on the latestavailable evidence for the appropriate treatment and care of a patient's condition.

Clinical messaging: Communication of clinical information within the electronic medical record to other healthcare personnel.

Code set: Any set of codes used to encode data elements, such as tables of terms, medical concepts, medical diagnostic codes, or medical procedure codes. This includes both the codes and their descriptions.

Coded data: Data are separated from personal identifiers through use of a code. As long as alink exists, data are considered indirectly identifiable and not anonymous or anonymized.

Coding: A mechanism for identifying and defining physicians' and hospitals' services. Codingprovides universal definition and recognition of diagnoses, procedures and level of care. Coders usually work in medical records departments and coding is a function of billing. Medicare fraud investigators look closely at the medical record documentation, which supports codes and looks for consistency. Lack of consistency of documentation can earmark a record as "up-coded" which is considered fraud. A national certification exists for coding professionals and many compliance programs are raising standards of quality for their coding procedures.

Computer-based patient record (CPR): A term for the process of replacing the traditional paper-based chart through automated electronic means; generally includes the collection of patient-specific information from various supplemental treatment systems, i.e. a day program and a personal care provider; its display in graphical format; and its storage for individual and aggregate purposes. CPR is also called "digital medical record" or "electronic medical record".

Computerized patient record (CPR): Also known as an EMR or EHR. A patient's past, present, and future clinical data stored in a server.

Computerized physician order entry (CPOE): A system for physicians to electronically order labs, imaging and prescriptions.

CPT (current procedural terminology) code: A recognizable five-digit number used to represent a service provided by a healthcare provider. It is a manual that assigns five digit codes to medical services and procedures to standardize claims processing and data analysis. The coding system for physicians' services developed by the CPT Editorial Panel of the American Medical Association.

[D]

Data content: All the data elements and code sets inherent to a transaction, and not related to the format of the transaction.

Data: This is factual information (as measurements or statistics) used as a basis for reasoning, discussion, or calculation. It additionally points to the information output by a sensing device or organ that includes both useful and irrelevant or redundant information and must be processed to be meaningful.

Database management system (DBMS): The separation of data from the computer application that allows entry or editing of data.

DICOM (digital imaging and communications in medicine): Digital imaging and Communications in medicine (DICOM) is a standard to define the connectivity and communication between medical imaging devices.

Disease management: A type of product or service now being offered by many large pharmaceutical companies to get them into broader healthcare services. Bundles use of prescription drugs with physician and allied professionals, linked to large databases created by the pharmaceutical companies, to treat people with specific diseases. The claim is that this type of service provides higher quality of care at more reasonable price than alternative, presumably more fragmented, care. The development of such products by hugely capitalized companies should be the entire indicator necessary to convince a provider of how the healthcare market is changing. Competition is coming from every direction—other providers of all types, payers, employers who are developing their own in-house service systems, the drug companies.

Document imaging: It is a process of converting paper documents into an electronic format usually through a scanning process.

Document management: The document manager allows the medical institution to store vital patient documents such as X-ray's, paper reports, and lab reports, etc.

Documentation: The process of recording information.

DOHAD: Developmental origins of health and diseases

Drug formulary: Varying lists of prescription drugs approved by a given health plan for distribution to a covered person through specific pharmacies. Health plans often restrict or limit the type and number of medicines allowed for reimbursement by limiting the drug formulary list. The list of prescription drugs for which a particular employer or State Medicaid program will pay. Formularies are either "closed," including only certain drugs or "open," including all drugs. Both types of formularies typically impose a cost scale requiring consumers to pay more for certain brands or types of drugs. *See* also formulary.

Drug formulary database: This EMR feature is used for electronic prescribing, electronicmedical record (EMR), and computerized physician order entry (CPOE) systems to present formulary status to the provider while during the prescribing decision.

DSM: Diagnostic and statistical manual for mental diseases.

[E]

EDI: Acronym for electronic data interchange. Electronic communication between two parties, generally for the filing of electronic claims to payers.

EDI translator: Used in electronic claims and medical record transmissions, this is a software tool for accepting an EDI transmission and converting the data into another format, or for converting a non-EDI data file into an EDI format for transmission. *See* also electronic data interchange.

EHR/EMR system designer, developer, manufacturer, vendor, supplier, retailer, re-seller: Any entity that is involved in the design, development, testing, manufacturing, supplying, selling including re-selling of electronic health records or electronic medical records systems as a whole or part thereof.

Electronic data interchange (EDI): The automated exchange of data and documents in a standardized format. In healthcare, some common uses of this technology include claims submission and payment, eligibility, and referral authorization. This refers to the exchange of routine business transactions from one computer to another in a standard format, using standard communications protocols.

Electronic health records (EHR): It is a distributed personal health record in digital format. The EHR provides secure, real-time, patient-centric information to aid clinical decision-making by providing access to a patient's health information at the point of care. Patient health records including treatment history, medical test reports, and images stored in an electronic format that can be accessed by healthcare providers on a computer network.

Electronic medical records (EMR): A computer-based record containing healthcareinformation. This technology, when EMR fully developed, meets provider needs for real-time data access and evaluation in medical care. Together with clinical workstations and clinical data repository technologies, it provides the mechanism for longitudinal data storage and access. A motivation for healthcare entities to implement this technology derives from the need for medical outcome studies, more efficient care, speedier communication among providers and management of health plans. This record may contain some, but not necessarily all, of the information that is in an individual's paper-based medical record.

Electronic protected health information (ePHI): Electronic protected health information (ePHI)is any protected health information (PHI) that is created, stored, transmitted, or received electronically. Electronic protected health information includes any medium used to store, transmit, or receive PHI electronically. The following and any future technologies used for accessing, transmitting, or receiving PHI electronically are covered. Media containing data at rest (data storage) like personal computers with internal hard drives used at work, home, or traveling, external portable hard drives, including iPods and similar devices, magnetic tape, removable storage devices, such as USB memory sticks, CDs, DVDs, and floppy disks, PDAs and smartphones and data in transit, via wireless, Ethernet, modem, DSL, or cable network connections, email, file transfer (for Protected Health Information—PHI, please *see* below).

Encounter: A clinical encounter is defined by ASTM as "(1) an instance of direct provider/practitioner to patient interaction, regardless of the setting, between a patient and a practitioner vested with primary responsibility for diagnosing, evaluating or treating the patient's condition, or both, or providing social worker services. (2) A contact between a patient and a practitioner who has primary responsibility for assessing and treating the patient at a given contact, exercising independent judgment." Encounter serves as a focal point linking clinical, administrative and financial information. Encounters occur in many different settings—ambulatory care, inpatient care, emergency care, home healthcare, field and virtual (telemedicine). [http://www.ncvhs.hhs.gov/040127p1.htm]

Episode: An episode of care consists of all clinically related services for one patient for adiscrete diagnostic condition from the onset of symptoms until the treatment is complete [http://www.ncmedsoc.org/non_members/pai/PAI-FinalWorkbookforVideo.pdf] Thus, for every new problem or set of problems that a person visits his clinical care provider, it is considered a new episode. Within that episode the patient will have one to many encounters with his clinical care providers till the treatment for that episode is complete. Even before the resolution of an episode, the person may have a new episode that is considered as a distinctly separate event altogether. Thus, there may be none, one or several ongoing active episodes. All resolved episodes are considered inactive. Hence they become part of the patient's past history. A notable point here is that all chronic diseases are considered active and may never get resolved during the life-time of the person, e.g. diabetes mellitus, hypertension, etc.

EPR: Broadly defined, a personal health record is the documentation of any form of patient information–including medical history, medicines, allergies, visit history, or vaccinations–that patients themselves may view, carry, amend, annotate, or maintain. Today, when we refer to PHRs, we typically mean an online personal health record–which may variously be referred to as an ePHR, an Internet PHR, an Internet medical record, or a consumer Internet Medical Record (CIMR). Generally, such records are maintained in a secure and confidential environment, allowing only the individual, or people authorized by the individual, to access the medical information. Not all electronic PHRs are Internet PHRs. PC-based PHRs may be set up to capture medical information offline.

Evidence based medicine: Evidence-based medicine (EBM) is the integration of best researchevidence with clinical expertise to aid in the diagnosis and management of patients.

[F]

Family history: A list of the patient's family medical history including the chronic medicalproblems of parents, siblings, grandparents, etc.

FHIR: Fast health interoperable resources, the newest version from HL7 org for messaging.

Formatting and protocol standards: Data exchange standards which are needed between CPR systems, as well as CPT and other provider systems, to ensure uniformity in methods for data collection, data storage and data presentation. Proactive providers are current in their knowledge of these standards and work to ensure their information systems conform to the standards.

Formulary: An approved list of prescription drugs; a list of selected pharmaceuticals and their appropriate dosages felt to be the most useful and cost effective for patient care. Organizations often develop a formulary under the aegis of a pharmacy and therapeutics committee. In HMOs, physicians are often required to prescribe from the formulary. *See* also drug formulary.

[G]

Growth chart: A feature for a primary care or EMR that can be used for paediatric patients. Age, height, weight, and head measurements can be entered over the patient's lifetime, and the feature creates a line graph.

[H]

Healthcare operations: Institutional activities that is necessary to maintain and monitor the operations of the institution. Examples include but are not limited to: Conducting quality assessment and improvement activities; developing clinical guidelines; case management; reviewing the competence or qualifications of healthcare professionals; education and training of students, trainees and practitioners; fraud and abuse programs; business planning and management; and customer service. Under the HIPAA Privacy Rule, these are allowable uses and disclosures of identifiable information "without specific authorization." Research is not considered part of healthcare operations.

Healthcare, healthcare: Care, services, and supplies related to the health of an individual. Healthcare includes preventive, diagnostic, therapeutic, rehabilitative, maintenance, or palliative care, and counseling, among other services. Healthcare also includes the sale and dispensing of prescription drugs or devices.

Health information: Information in any form (oral, written or otherwise) that relates to the past, present or future physical or mental health of an individual. That information could be created or received by a healthcare provider, a health plan, a public health authority, an employer, a life insurer, a school, a university or a healthcare clearing house. All health information is protected by state and federal confidentiality laws and by HIPAA privacy rules.

Health level seven (HL7): A data interchange protocol for healthcare computer applicationsthat simplifies the ability of different vendor-supplied IS systems to interconnect. Although not a software program in itself, HL7 requires that each healthcare software vendor program HL7 interfaces for its products. The organisation is one of the American National Standards Institute accredited Standard Developing Organization (SDO)—Health Level 7 domain is the standards for electronic interchange of clinical, financial and administrative info among healthcare oriented computer systems. It is a not-for-profit volunteer organization. It develops specifications, most widely used is the messaging standard that enables disparate healthcare applications to exchange key sets of clinical and administrative data. It promotes the use of standards within and among healthcare organizations to increase the effectiveness and efficiency of healthcare delivery. It is an international community of healthcare subject matter experts and information scientists collaborating to create standards for the exchange, management and integration of electronic healthcare information.

Health: The state of complete physical, mental, and social well-being and not merely the absence of disease or infirmity. It is recognized, however, that health has many dimensions (anatomical, physiological, and mental) and is largely culturally defined. The relative importance of various disabilities will differ depending upon the cultural milieu and the role of the affected individual in that culture. Most attempts at measurement have been assessed in terms or morbidity and mortality.

Healthcare provider: A healthcare provider is an individual or an institution that providespreventive, curative, promotional or rehabilitative healthcare services in a systematic way to individuals, families or communities. An individual healthcare provider may be a healthcare professional, an allied health professional, a community health worker, any or other person trained and knowledgeable in medicine, nursing or other allied health professions, or public/community health workers like, ASHA, ANM, midwives, paramedical staff, OT/lab/radio-diagnostic technicians, etc. An institution will include hospitals, clinics, primary care centres and other service delivery points of healthcare individual clinics, polyclinics, diagnostic centres, etc., i.e. any place where a medical record is generated during a patient-care provider encounter (in conformance to CEA 2010—please refer to Clinical Establishment item above)

History of present illness (HPI): The HPI is the history of the patient's chief complaint.

Human subject: Refers to a living subject participating in research about whom directly orindirectly identifiable health information or data are obtained or created.

Hybrid record: Term used for when a provider uses a combination of paper and electronicmedical records during the transition phase to EMR.

[I]

Independent software vendor (ISV): A company specializing in making or selling softwareproducts that runs on one or more computer hardware or operating system platforms.

Immunisation: A complete list of all immunizations that the patient has had.

Informatics: The application of computer technology to the management of information.

Integration: Integration allows for secure communication between enterprise applications.

Interface: A means of communication between two computer systems, two software applications or two modules. Real time interface is a key element in healthcare information systems due to the need to access patient care information and financial information instantaneously and comprehensively. Such real time communication is the key to managing healthcare in a cost effective manner because it provides the necessary decision-making information for clinicians, providers, other stakeholders, etc.

International classification of diseases: This is the universal coding method used to document the incidence of disease, injury, mortality and illness. A diagnosis and procedure classification system designed to facilitate collection of uniform and comparable health information. The ICD-9-CM was issued in 1979. This system is used to group patients into DRGs, prepare hospital and physician billings and prepare cost reports. Classification of disease by diagnosis codified into six-digit numbers. See also coding.

International health terminology standards development organization (IHTSDO): Denmark-based organization that maintains and licenses SNOMED codes worldwide.

Interoperability: The capability to provide successful communication between end-users across a mixed environment of different domains, networks, facilities and equipment.

ISP: Internet service provider

[J]

J-codes: A subset of the HCPCS Level II code set with a high-order value of "J" that has been used to identify certain drugs and other items.

[L]

LAN (local area network): A LAN supplies networking capability to a group of computers inclose proximity to each other such as in an office building, a school, or a home.

Legacy system integration: The integration of data between a legacy system and some other software program most commonly using HL-7 standards.

Legacy systems: Computer applications, both hardware and software, which have been inherited through previous acquisition and installation. Most often, these systems run business applications that are not integrated with each other. Newer systems which stress open design and distributed processing capacity are gradually replacing such systems.

Length of stay (LOS): The duration of an episode of care for a covered person. The number of days an individual stays in a hospital or inpatient facility. May also be reviewed as Average Length of Stay (ALOS).

LEPR (longitudinal patient record): Longitudinal Patient Record is an EHR that includes all healthcare information from all sources.

[M]

Management information system (MIS): The common term for the computer hardware and software that provides the support of managing the plan.

Master patient/member index: An index or file with a unique identifier for each patient or member that serves as a key to a patient's or member's health record.

Maximum defined data set: All of the required data elements for a particular standard based on a specific implementation specification. An entity creating a transaction is free to include whatever data any receiver might want or need. The recipient is free to ignore any portion of the data that is not needed to conduct their part of the associated business transaction, unless the inessential data is needed for coordination of benefits.

MCI: Medical Council of India

Medical Code Sets: Codes that characterize a medical condition or treatment. These code sets are usually maintained by professional societies and public health organizations. Compare to administrative code sets.

Medical informatics: Medical informatics is the systematic study, or science, of the identification, collection, storage, communication, retrieval, and analysis of data about medical care services to improve decisions made by physicians and managers of healthcare organizations. Medical informatics will be as important to physicians and medical managers as the rules of financial accounting are to auditors.

Medical management information system (MMIS): A data system that allows payers and purchasers to track healthcare expenditure and utilization patterns. It may also be referred to as Health Information System (HIS), Health Information Management (HIM) or Information System (IS). *See* also electronic medical record (EMR).

MIMS: Monthly index of medical specialities

Minimum data set: The minimum set of data elements that must be captured, stored, made available for retrieval, presentation, relay and sharing by an EHR system. It comprises all of the essential data elements required for implementation. An entity creating a transaction must include the mandatory data elements at all times and is free to exclude optional data elements. The entity is free to additionally include whatever other data elements that any receiver might want or need. The recipient is free to ignore any portion of the data that is not mandatory and is further free to ignore any other portion of the data that is not needed to conduct their part of the associated transaction, unless required by sender, intermediaries or receiver. This minimum data set represents the most common data, and system designers are at liberty to add to it as they deem necessary to enrich or enhance their EHR systems.

Modifier: Additional character of a code added to an existing code that is used to help inextending or localization of the existing code.

[N]

NANDA: North American Nursing Diagnosis Association.

National council for prescription drug programs: An ANSI-accredited group that maintains a number of standard formats for use by the retail pharmacy industry.

Non-participating physician (or provider): A provider, doctor or hospital that does not sign acontract to participate in a health plan, usually which requires reduced rates from the provider. In the Medicare Program, this refers to providers who are therefore not obligated to accept assignment on all Medicare claims. In commercial plans, non-participating providers are also called out of network providers or out of plan providers. If a beneficiary receives service from an out of network provider, the health plan (other than medicare) will pay for the service at a reduced rate or will not pay at all.

[O]

Open access: A term describing a member's ability to self-refer for specialty care. Open access arrangements allow a member to see a participating provider without a referral from another doctor. Health plan members' abilities, rights or invitation to self refer for specialty care. Also called Open Panel.

OR: Operating room–synonymous to OT as below.

OT: Operation theatre.

OTC: Over the counter (drugs). Refers to those drugs that are available off the shelf without any prescription or advise from a registered medical practitioner.

Outcome: A clinical outcome is the "change in the health of an individual, group of people or population which is attributable to an intervention or series of interventions". (Taken from: Frommer, Michael; Rubin, George; Lyle, David (1992)."The NSW Health Outcomes program". New South Wales Public Health Bulletin 3: 135. doi:10.1071/NB92067) include the mandatory data elements at all times and is free to exclude optional data elements. The entity is free to additionally include whatever other data elements that any receiver might want or need. The recipient is free to ignore any portion of the data that is not mandatory and is further free to ignore any other portion of the data that is not needed to conduct their part of the associated transaction, unless required by sender, intermediaries or receiver. This minimum data set represents the most common data, and system designers are at liberty to add to it as they deem necessary to enrich or enhance their EHR systems.

Outpatient care: Care given a person who is not bedridden. It is also called ambulatory care. Many surgeries and treatments are now provided on an outpatient basis, while previously they had been considered reason for inpatient hospitalization. Some say this is the fastest growing segment of healthcare.

[P]

Participating physician: A primary care physician in practice in the payer's managed careservice area who has entered into a contract.

Past history: A list of a patient's past health problems, surgeries and specialists.

Patient demographics: All patient's pertinent information such as first and last name, SSN, DOB, insurance, etc.

Patient portal: A secure web-based system that allows a patient to register for an appointment, schedule an appointment, request prescription refills, send and receive secure patient-physician messages, view lab results, pay their bills electronically, access physician directories.

Patient: A person who is under medical care or treatment.

PC based: A program designed to run on an individual PC. This typically means data is notshared in real time among other PCs (users).

PCP: Primary care physician who often acts as the primary gatekeeper in health plans. That is,often the PCP must approval referrals to specialists. Particularly in HMOs and some PPOs, all members must choose or are assigned a PCP.

PHR: A personal health record or PHR is typically a health record that is initiated and maintained by an individual. An ideal PHR would provide a complete and accurate summary of the health and medical history of an individual by gathering data from many sources and making this information accessible online.

Picture archive communication system (PACS): Used by radiology and diagnostic imaging organizations to electronically manage information and images.

Practice parameters, practice guidelines: Systematically developed statements to standardize care and to assist in practitioner and patient decisions about the appropriate healthcare for specific circumstances. Practice guidelines are usually developed through a process that combines scientific evidence of effectiveness with expert opinion. Practice guidelines are also referred to as clinical criteria, protocols, algorithms, review criteria, and guidelines. The American Medical Association defines practice parameters as strategies for patient management, developed to assist physicians in clinical decision-making. Practice parameters may also be referred to as practice options, practice guidelines, practice policies, or practice standards.

Prescription drug: Drug that the law says can only be obtained by prescription.

Primary care: Basic or general healthcare usually rendered by general practitioners, family practitioners, internists, obstetricians and pediatricians who are often referred to as primary care practitioners or PCPs. Professional and related services administered by an internist, family practitioner, obstetrician-gynecologist or pediatrician in an ambulatory setting, with referral to secondary care specialists, as necessary.

Primary care physician: A "generalist" such as a family practitioner, pediatrician, internist, orobstetrician. In a managed care organization, a primary care physician is accountable for the total health services of enrollees including referrals, procedures and hospitalization. Also *see* primary care provider.

Primary care provider: The provider that serves as the initial interface between the memberand the medical care system. The PCP is usually a physician, selected by the member upon enrollment, who is trained in one of the primary care specialties who treats and is responsible for coordinating the treatment of members assigned to his/her plan.

Principal diagnosis: The medical condition that is ultimately determined to have caused a patient's admission to the hospital. The principal diagnosis is used to assign every patient to a diagnosis related group. This diagnosis may differ from the admitting and major diagnoses.

Privacy: Privacy means an individual's interest in limiting who has access to personal healthcare information. Specific patient authorization is required for use and disclosure of clinical notes. As per Fernando and Dawson, 2009, privacy is control of access to private information avoiding certain kinds of embarrassment and can be shared or not shared with others; only authorized (by the patient) people can view the recorded data or part thereof.

Privacy standards: The privacy standards restrict the use and disclosure of individually identifiable health information. Privacy standard applies to all protected health information may it is in physical or electronic form.

Progress note: The documentation of a patient visit or encounter including all or part of the SOAP format.

Protected health information (PHI): Any individually identifiable information whether oral or recorded in any form or medium that is created, or received by a healthcare provider, health plan or healthcare provider and relates to past, present, or future physical or mental health conditions of an individual; the provision of healthcare to the individual; or past, present, or future payment for healthcare to an individual.

[R]

Real time: The instantaneous sharing of data among a user group. It is common to aclient/server database configuration.

Referral: Some insurance companies require that on specific plans a referral must be obtainedfor certain procedures or visits to specialists. The referral is acquired by the primary care physician (PCP) by contacting the insurance company by phone or mail. This is a request for the service. The referral consists of an authorization code, a number of visits allowed (if applicable) and an expiration date.

Referring provider: Referring provider is the provider that referred the patient to a specialist or for a specific procedure.

Relational database: A database program that stores data in a manner similar to excel, with the difference being the data elements are related (linked) to each other.

Remote access: Data travels through a private, protected passage via the internet, allowing healthcare providers to access from home or another practice location and allows EMR vendor to perform system maintenance off-site

Rendering/performing provider: The provider actually treating the patient.

ROS (review of systems): A series of questions related to the system(s) that the patient is having complaints about (i.e. respiratory for cold symptoms).

RxNorm: RxNorm is the name of a US-specific terminology in medicine that contains all medications available on US market; it provides normalized names for clinical drugs and links its names to many of the drug vocabularies commonly used in pharmacy management and drug interaction software.

[S]

Secondary care: Services provided by medical specialists who generally do not have first contact with patients (e.g. cardiologist, urologists, dermatologists). In the US, however, there has been a trend toward self-referral by patients for these services, rather than referral by primary care providers. This is quite different from the practice in England, for example, where all patients must first seek care from primary care providers and are then referred to secondary and/or tertiary providers, as needed.

Security standards: The security standards require measures to protect the confidentiality,integrity and availability of e-PHI while its being stored and exchanged. The security standard applies to all electronic PHI.

Security: This refers to the methods and techniques adopted to protect privacy and are adefense mechanism from any attack (Hong, et al. 2004).

SNOMED (SNOMED CT): Systemized Nomenclature of Medicine Clinical Terms.

SNOMED CT: It is the universal healthcare terminology. It is comprehensive and covers procedures, diseases, and clinical data. SNOMED CT helps to structure and computerize the medical record. It allows for a consistent way of indexing, storing, retrieving and aggregating clinical data across sites of care (i.e. hospitals, doctors offices) and specialties. By standardizing the terminology, the variability in the way data is captured, encoded and used for clinical care of patients and research is reduced. Allows for more accurate reporting of data. It is currently available in English, Spanish and German.

Social history: A description of a patient's social habits and history including marital status, alcohol and drug use and exercise habits.

Solo practice, solo practitioner: A physician who practices alone or with others but does not pool income or expenses. This form of practice is becoming increasingly less common as physicians band together for contracting, overhead costs and risk sharing.

SOP: Standard operating procedures or protocols.

SQL: Structured query language is a computer language aimed to store, manipulate and retrieve data stored in relational databases.

Subjective: Section in a progress note where a patient's account of their current problem is documented. Consists of chief complaint, HPI and ROS.

Sx: Abbreviation for symptoms.

[T]

T1, T3 line: A high-speed internet connection provided via telephone lines often used by businesses needing internet connection speeds greater than DSL/cable.

Therapeutic alternatives: Strong drug products that provide the same pharmacological or chemical effect in equivalent doses. Also *see* drug formulary.

TPA: Third party administrator.

Treatment episode: The period of treatment between admission and discharge from amodality, e.g. inpatient, residential, partial hospitalization, and outpatient, or the period of time between the first procedure and last procedure on an outpatient basis for a given diagnosis. Many healthcare statistics and profiles use this unit as a base for comparisons.

Treatment: The provision of healthcare by one or more healthcare providers. Treatment includes any consultation, referral or other exchanges of information to manage a patient's care.

[V]

Vital statistics: Statistics relating to births (natality), deaths (mortality), marriages, health, and disease (morbidity). Vital statistics for the united states are published by the national center for health statistics. Vital statistics can be obtained from CDC, state health departments, county health departments and other agencies. An individual patient's vital statistics in a healthcare setting may also refer simply to blood pressure, temperature, height and weight, etc.

VPN: Virtual private network—A VPN "tunnel" is a secure connection, typically firewall to firewall that provides for remote access to your data server.

[X]

XML (extensible markup language): Used for defining data elements on a web page and communication between two business systems. Example: Standard messaging system for and EMR to integrate with another software such as a practice management or drug formulary database.

FORMAT FOR MEDICAL RECORDS

(As specified by Medical Council of India)

Name of the patient: ....

Age: ....

Sex: ....

Address: ....

Occupation: ....

Date of 1st visit: ....

Clinical note (summary) of the case: ....

Provisional diagnosis: ....

Investigations advised with reports: ....

Diagnosis after investigation: ....

Advice: ....

Follow up: ....

Observations: ....

Date: ....

Signature in full

....

Name of Treating Physician

MAINTENANCE OF MEDICAL RECORDS

1. Every physician shall maintain the medical records pertaining to his/her indoor patients for a period of 3 years from the date of commencement of the treatment in a standard proforma laid down by the Medical Council of India and available above.
2. If any request is made for medical records either by the patients/authorised attendant or legal authorities involved, the same may be duly acknowledged and documents shall be issued within the period of 72 hours.
3. A registered medical practitioner shall maintain a register of medical certificates giving full details of certificates issued. When issuing a medical certificate he/she shall always enter the identification marks of the patient and keep a copy of the certificate. He/she shall not omit to record the signature and/or thumb mark, address and at least one identification mark of the patient on the medical certificates or report. The medical certificate shall be prepared in the recommended prescribed form.
4. Efforts shall be made to computerize medical records for quick retrieval.

Annexures

ANNEXURE I

Definitions of Medical Specialties

Specialty	*Specialty focus*
Allergy and immunology	Allergic and immunologic diseases and their respirator complications (such as pollen, chemical and food allergies, asthma and AIDS)
Anesthesia	Anesthesia or relief of pain during surgery and childbirth, and control of pain due to various causes.
Bariatric surgery	Weight loss surgery includes a variety of procedures performed on people who are obese, weight loss is achieved by reducing the size of the adjustable gastric band. Gastric bypass surgery-sleeve gastrectomy.
Cardiovascular disease	Diseases of the heart and blood vessels.
Dermatology	Diseases of the skin.
Emergency medicine	Diseases that are acute medical or surgical conditions or injuries that require urgent or immediate care (usually in a hospital emergency room).
Endocrinology and metabolism	Diseases of the internal glands of the body, including diabetes mellitus.
Family practice	All diseases and related total healthcare of an individual and the family
Gastroenterology	Diseases of the digestive tract, including the stomach, bowel, liver and pancreas.
General practice	All diseases and related total healthcare of an individual and the family
Geriatric medicine	Disease of the elderly.
Gynecology	See "Obstetrics and Gynecology.
Gynecology oncology	Cancer diseases of the female reproductive system.
Hematology	Disorders of the blood and blood-forming organs (including cancerous disorders of the blood) such as anemia, leukemia and lymphoma (*see* oncology, medical).
Infectious diseases	Infections of all types.
Internal medicine	All diseases and total healthcare of adults, usually 18 years of age and older.
Neonatology	Diseases of the newborn child.
Nephrology	Diseases of the kidney, including dialysis.
Neurology	Diseases of the brain, spinal cord, nervous system and related *Specialty Specialty focus*structures.
Neurological surgery	Diseases of the brain, spinal cord, nervous system and related structures requiring surgery.

Contd...

Contd…

Specialty	*Specialty focus*
Obstetrics and gynecology	Normal and abnormal pregnancy, diseases of the female reproductive system and fertility disorders.
Oncology, medical	Cancer and disorders of the blood and blood-forming organs (*see* hematology)
Ophthalmology	Diseases of the eye.
Orthopedic surgery	Diseases of the bones, joints, muscles and tendons.
Otorhinolaryngology (ear, nose and throat)	Diseases of the ears, nose, sinuses, throat and upper airway passages.
Pathology	Tissues and specimens removed by biopsy and surgery to diagnose normal from diseased tissues and specimens; supervises and interprets laboratory tests on blood, urine and other body fluids.
Pediatrics	All diseases and total healthcare of newborns, infants, children and adolescents.
Physical medicine and rehabilitation	Diseases with major and minor disabilities requiring restoration of functional ability such as assistance, retaining and recondition of muscles, tendons and extremities for ambulation and other activities of daily living.
Plastic surgery	Diseases and conditions requiring surgical reconstruction for deformity or loss of a body part, or for cosmetic purposes to improve appearance or function.
Podiatric (podiatry) medicine	Diseases of the foot and ankle as they affect the conditions of the feet.
Preventive medicine	Healthcare and other measures to avoid delay or prevent disease or illness from occurring.
Psychiatry	Diseases affecting mental health including diseases of the brain, nervous system and substance abuse of drugs or chemicals.
Pulmonary disease	Diseases of the lung.
Radiology	Diagnostic X-ray, ultrasound and other imaging techniques such as computerized tomography (CT) and magnetic resonance imaging (MRI).
Radiology nuclear	Diseases requiring use of radioactive isotopes or as an aid in diagnosis and/or therapy.
Radiation oncology	Cancer and other diseases with X-ray therapy, radioactive isotopes and linear accelerator particle radiation.
Rheumatology	Diseases of the joints including arthritis and autoimmune diseases.
Sports medicine	Diseases and injuries acquired in sports.
Surgery, general	Diseases that require surgical operation for diagnosis or treatment.
Surgery, hand	Diseases and injuries of the nerves, tendons, muscles, bones or skin of the hand requiring surgery.
Surgery, thoracic	Diseases of the chest, including lungs, heart, blood vessels and chest wall that require surgical operation for diagnosis and or treatment.
Surgery, vascular	Diseases of the blood vessels that require surgical operation for diagnosis or treatment.
Surgery, colon and rectal	Diseases of the large intestine (bowel), rectum and anus that require surgical operation for diagnosis or treatment.
Surgery, urology	Diseases of the kidneys, bladder and male reproductive tract that require surgical operation.

Contd…

ANNEXURE II

Glossary of Terms used in Software Structure for EMR

Addendum	Text that is added to a document after it has been finalized.
Alerts pop-ups or reminders	An automated warning system such as a clinical alerts, preventive health maintenance, medication interactions, etc.
Ambulatory care	Medical care provided on an outpatient basis.
Annotator	A system function that allows and explanatory note or diagram to be added to an image.
ANSI (American National Standard Institute)	Organization that develops industrial standards, in particular recommendations for languages electronic data exchange (EDI) and peripheral devices.
ASP an Application Service Provider (ASP)	ASP is a third party entity that deploys hosts and manages software from a centrally managed host facility (offshore). Applications are delivered over networks (WAN, Internet) on a subscription fee/rental basis. This model is also been referred to as "software-as-a-service".
Audit trail	Security system that tracks a user's access, deletion or modification of data. The term used in healthcare information security refers to a chronological record of system resources usage. This includes user login, file access, other various activities, and whether any actual or attempted security violations occurred, legitimate or unauthorized.
Authentication	The verification of the identity of a person or process.
Bandwidth	A data transmission rate; the maximum amount of information (bits/second) that can be transmitted along a channel.
Bar code	A printed horizontal strip of vertical bars which represent decimal digits use for identification. Bar codes must be read by a bar code reader.
Biometrics	Biometrics are automated methods of recognizing a person based on a physiological characteristic such as fingerprints, retina, voice, etc.
Browser	Short for web browser, a software application used to locate and display web pages.
Case management	A process of identifying individuals at high risk for problems associated with complex healthcare needs and assessing opportunities to coordinate care to optimize the outcome.
Chart of patient/medical record	A document, written by the clinician or healthcare provider, which describes the details of patient's condition including history, physical exam, investigations, progress, diagnosis, treatment including medical and surgical, medication, and the end results.
Client server architecture	Information transmission arrangement, in which a client program sends a request to server. When the server receives the request, it disconnects from the client and processes the request. When the request is processed, the server reconnects to the client program and the information is transferred to the client. This usually implies that the server is located on site as opposed to the ASP (application server provider) architecture.

Contd...

Contd...

Clinical data	A real-time database that consolidates data repository (CDR) from a variety of clinical sources to present a unified rather than to identify a population of patients with common characteristics or to facilitate the management of a specific clinical department.
Clinical decision support system (CDDS)	A clinical decision support system (CDSS) is software designed to aid clinicians in decision making by matching individual patient characteristics to computerized knowledge bases for the purpose of generating patient-specific assessment or recommendations.
Clinical guidelines protocols	Clinical guidelines are recommendations based on the latest available evidence for the appropriate treatment and care of a patient's condition.
Clinical messaging	Communication of clinical information within the electronic medical record to other healthcare personnel.
CPG	Clinical practice guidelines.
CPM	Clinical performance measures.
CPOE	Computerized physician order entry or computerized provider order entry. This order could be investigations, medication or any other orders
CPR	Computer patient record. Electronically maintained information about a patient related to his health history, physical exam, investigations, diagnosis, treatment including medical or surgical, progress, end results, etc.
Current procedural terminology (CPT)	The purpose of CPT codes is to provide a uniform language that accurately describes medical, surgical and diagnosis services.
Data conversion	The conversion of data from one software to another
Data encryption standard (DES)	Data encryption standard (DES) is a widely-used method of data encryption using private (secret) key.
Data integrity	Refers to the validity of data. A condition in which data has not been altered or destroyed in an unauthorized manner.
Data mining	The process of analyzing or extracting data from a database to identify patterns or relationships.
Data set	A group of data element relevant for a particular use.
Data structure	A way to store and organize data in order to facilitate access and modification.
Data base	A collection of information organized in such a way that computer program can quickly select
Data base management system (DBMS)	A set of computer programs for organizing the information in a database. A DBMS supports the structuring of the database in a standard format and provides tools for data input, verification, storage, retrieval, query and manipulation.
DIOCOM	Digital imaging of communications in medicine images such as CT scans, MRI and ultrasound.
Dictation	The process by which a physician records his/her notes about a patient. This recording is intended for reproduction in written word (transcription).

Contd...

Contd...

Digital signature	Digital signature take the traditional hand-written signature and creates a digital image of the signature to eliminate the need to print and sign documents. This is knows as advanced electronic signature.
Discrete data	A set of data is said to be discrete if the values belonging to it are distinct and separate (i.e. they can be counted). Discrete dat is non-discrete or unstructured data.
Document imaging	Converting paper documents into an electronic format usually through a scanning process.
Documentation	The process of recording information.
Document management	Document management's system involving scanning, categorizing and storing vital patient documents.
DOQ-IT doctors office	DOQ-IT is a two-year special study that is designed to improve quality of care, patient safety, and efficiency for services provided to medicare beneficiaries by promoting the adoption of electronic health records.
Quality information	Information technology (IT) in primary care physician offices.
E and M Coding	Documentation guidelines for evaluation and management CPT codes from the Center for Medicare and Medicaid Services (Formerly HCFA).
EDI	Electronic data interchange.
Electronic health record (EHRR)	An electronic repository of information re-generic term for all electronic patient care systems. EHR's simply a level of interoperability beyond the capability of an EMR (electronic medical record).
Electronic super bill	An electronic encounter form used for coding and billing.
Electronic medical record (EMR)	Electronic medical record has a level of sophistication beyond a document management system. An EMR is a provider-based medical record that includes all health documentation for one person covering all services provided within an enterprise.
Electronic order entry (EOE)	The function of this program is to move from hand-written and verbal orders to computer based entry.
Electronic patient record (EPR)	Same as CPR (computerized patient record).
Encryption	Process of converting messages or data into a form that cannot be read without decrypting or deciphering it.
e-prescribing	Prescription medicine through an automated data-entry process and transmitting the information to the participating pharmacies.
Evidence base medicine (EBM0	Evidence based medicine (EBM) is the integration of research evidence with clinical expertise to aid in the diagnosis and management of patients.
Face sheet	Also called summary screen or patient dash-board. This screen includes a summary of patient relevant information on one screen.
Fat client	A fat client is a network computer with a hard disc drive as opposed to a thin client which has no disc drive.

Contd...

Contd...

Firewall	A sytem designed to prevent unauthorized access to or from a private computer network.
Formulary	A listing of prescription drugs established by a particular health plan which includes both brand name and generic drugs. It serves to suggest covered, preferred and lower cost drugs.
FTP	File transfer program.
Graphical user interface (GUI)	Abbreviated GUI. A program interface that takes advantage of the computer's graphics capabilities to make the program easier to use. Well-designed graphical user interfaces can help expedite the software learning process.
HIE	Health information exchange
Health information technology (HIT)	Health information technology
Hot keys	One- or two-keystroke command that switches the user to a different program or function within a software program. Hot keys are useful to expedite movement within a software program.
Informatics	The application of computer technology to the management of information.
Information technology (IT)	The development, installation, and implementation of computer systems and applications.
Interoperability	The capability to provide successful communication between end-users across a mixed environment of different domains, networks, facilities and equipment.
Kiosk	Small computer workstations which allow information to be input. Patient kiosks are used for patients to input information into the system at the medical practice, usually input through a workstation in the waiting room.
Local area network (LAN)	A LAN supplies networking capability to a group of computers in close proximity to each other such as in an office building, a school, or a home.
Longitudinal patient record (LEPR)	Longitudinal Patient Record is an EHR that includes all healthcare information from all sources.
Optical character recognition (OCR)	OCR is recognition of printed or written characters by a computer.
Picture archiving and communication system (PACS)	An information system for the storage and distribution of digital radiology images over a networked environment that allows for instant access to images and reports.
Patient portal	Allow patients and providers to communicate over the Internet in a secure environment.
PHI	Personal health information
Platform	The basic technology of a computer system's hardware and software that defines how a computer is operated and determines what other kinds of software can be used.
Point and click	Allowing the activation of commands by moving the cursor over certain areas or icons and clicking a pointing device.

Contd...

Contd...

Point-of-care	POC refers to the time while with the patient, either bedside or during an encounter.
Portal	A website considered as an entry point to other websites. Examples are a patient portal.
Pull down menu	Also called a drop-down menu. These are a menu of commands or options that appears when you select an item with a mouse.
Query	The primary mechanism for retrieving information from a database and consists of questions presented to the database in a predefined format.
RFID	Radiofrequency identification
Scalable	Refers to how well a hardware or software system can adapt to increased demands.
Security	Is the effort to create a secure computing platform, designed so that agents (users or programs) can only perform actions that have been allowed.
Speech recognition	The ability of a computer to understand the spoken word for the purpose of receiving commands and transforming speech into text.
Structured data	Structured data is managed by technology that allows for querying and reporting against predetermined data types and understood relationships.
Tablet pc	A tablet pc is a computer shaped in the form of a notebook except it has the capabilities of being written on through the use of digitizing tablet technology or a touch screen. A user can use a stylus and operate the computer without having to have a keyboard or mouse.
Template	Often called a library or dictionary. Templates are pre-defined choices of pick-lists designed to stream line the documentation process.
Thin client	A thin client is a network computer without a hard disc drive, as opposed to a fat client which includes a disc drive.
Touch screen	An input device that allows user to interact with the computer by touching the display screen.
Unstructured data	Data which is not structured such as free-text. The computer cannot automatically extract properties and relationships from unstructured data.
Wide area network (WAN)	A computer network that spans a larger geographical area than a LAN (local area network).
Web portal	A website considered as an entry point to other websites.
Wireless	A system employing no connecting wire between the transmitting and receiving stations.
Workflow	The automation of a process, in whole or part, during which documents, information or tasks are passed from one participant to another for action, according to a set of procedural rules.

ANNEXURE III

Electronic Health Records (EHR) Terminology

Addendum	Text that is added to a document after it has been finalized.
Alerts	Pop-ups or reminders. An automated warning system such a clinical alerts, preventive health maintenance, medication interactions, etc.
Ambulatory care	Medical care provided on an outpatient basis.
Annotator	A system function that allows an explanatory note or diagram to be added to an image.
ASP application service provider	An application service provider (ASP) is a third party entity that deploys hosts and manages software from a centrally managed host facility (offsite). Applications are delivered over networks (WAN, Internet) on a subscription fee/rental basis. This model is also been referred to as "software-as-a-service".
Audit trail	Security system that tracks a user's access, deletion or modification of data. The term used in healthcare information security refers to a chronological record of system resource usage. This includes user login, file access, other various activities, and whether any actual or attempted security violations occurred, legitimate or unauthorized.
Authentication	The verification of the identity of a person or process.
Bandwidth	A data transmission rate; the maximum amount of information (bits/second) that can be transmitted along a channel.
Bar code	A printed horizontal strip of vertical bars which represent decimal digits used for identification. Bar codes must be read by a bar code reader.
Biometrics	Biometrics are automated methods of recognizing a person based on a physiological characteristic such as fingerprints, retina, voice, etc.
Browser	Short for web browser, a software application used to locate and display web pages.
Case management	A process of identifying individuals at high risk for problems associated with complex healthcare needs and assessing opportunities to coordinate care to optimize the outcome.
Chart	Medical record
Chart note	A document, written by the clinician or provider, which describes the details of a patient's encounter. Sometimes referred to as a progress note.
Client/Server architecture	An information-transmission arrangement, in which a client program sends a request to a server. When the server receives the request, it disconnects from the client and processes the request. When the request is processed, the server reconnects to the client program and the information is transferred to the client. This usually implies that the server is located on site as opposed to the ASP (application server provider) architecture.

Contd...

Contd...

Clinical data repository (CDR)	A real-time database that consolidates data from a variety of clinical sources to present a unified view of a single patient. It is optimized to allow clinicians to retrieve data for a single patient rather than to identify a population of patients with common characteristics or to facilitate the management of a specific clinical department.
Clinical decision support system (CDSS)	A clinical decision support system (CDSS) is software designed to aid clinicians in decision making by matching individual patient characteristics to computerized knowledge bases for the purpose of generating patient-specific assessments or recommendations.
Clinical guidelines (protocols)	Clinical guidelines are recommendations based on the latest available evidence for the appropriate treatment and care of a patient's condition.
Clinical messaging	Communication of clinical information within the electronic medical record to other healthcare personnel.
CPG	Clinical practice guidelines
CPM	Clinical performance measures
CPOE computerized provider order entry	CPOE refers to the act of a clinician entering an order for patient services into an information system.
CPR computerized patient record, computer-based patient record	Electronically maintained information about an individual's lifetime health status and healthcare from all specialties.
CPT current procedural terminology	The purpose of CPT codes is to provide a uniform language that accurately describes medical, surgical, and diagnostic services.
Data conversion	The conversion of data from one software to another.
Data encryption standard (DES)	Data encryption standard (DES) is a widely-used method of data encryption using a private (secret) key.
Data integrity	Refers to the validity of data. A condition in which data has not been altered or destroyed in an unauthorized manner.
Data mining	The process of analyzing or extracting data from a database to identify patterns or relationships.
Data set	A group of data elements relevant for a particular use.
Data structure	A way to store and organize data in order to facilitate access and modifications.
Data base	A collection of information organized in such a way that a computer program can quickly select desired pieces of data.
Database management system (DBMS)	A set of computer programs for organizing the information in a database. A DBMS supports the structuring of the database in a standard format and provides tools for data input, verification, storage, retrieval, query, and manipulation.
DICOM digital imaging and communications in medicine	Digital Imaging and Communications in Medicine (DICOM) is a standard to aid the distribution and viewing of medical images, such as CT scans, MRIs, and ultrasound.
Dictation	The process by which a physician records his/her notes about a patient. This recording is intended for reproduction in written word (transcription).
Digital signature	Sometimes referred to as advanced electronic signature. Digital signature takes the traditional hand-written signature and creates a digital image of the signature to eliminate the need to print and sign documents.

Contd...

Contd...

Discrete data	A set of data is said to be discrete if the values belonging to it are distinct and separate, (i.e. they can be counted). Discrete data is more easily reportable as opposed to non-discrete or unstructured data.
Document imaging	Converting paper documents into an electronic format usually through a scanning process.
Documentation	The process of recording information.
Document management	It is a system involving scanning, categorizing and storing vital patient documents.
DOQ-IT doctors office	DOQ-IT is a two-year special study that is designed to improve quality of care, patient safety, and efficiency for services provided to medicare beneficiaries by promoting the adoption of EHR's and
Quality information technology	Information technology (IT) in primary care physician offices.
E and M coding evaluation and management	Coding documentation guidelines for evaluation and management CPT codes from the center for medicare and medicaid services (formerly HCFA).
EDI	Electronic data interchange
EHR electronic health record	An electronic repository of information regarding the health of an individual. It is also a generic term for all electronic patient care systems. EHR's imply a level of interoperability beyond the capability of an EMR (electronic medical record).
Electronic super bill	An electronic encounter form used for coding and billing.
EMR electronic medical record	Electronic medical record has a level of sophistication beyond a document management system. An EMR is a provider-based medical record that includes all health documentation for one person covering all services provided within an enterprise.
EOE electronic order entry	The function of this program is to move from hand-written and verbal orders to computer-based entry.
EPR electronic patient record	Same as a CPR—computerized patient record.
Encryption	Process of converting messages or data into a form that cannot be read without decrypting or deciphering it.
e-prescribing	Prescribing medication through an automated data-entry process and transmitting the information to participating pharmacies.
Evidence based medicine	Evidence-based medicine (EBM) is the integration of best research evidence with clinical expertise to aid in the diagnosis and management of patients.
Face sheet	Also called a summary screen or patient dashboard. This screen includes a summary of patient relevant information on one screen.
Fat client	A fat client is a network computer with a hard disc drive, as opposed to a thin client which has no disc drive.
Firewall	A system designed to prevent unauthorized access to or from a private computer network.
Formulary	A listing of prescription drugs established by a particular health plan which includes both Brand name and generic drugs. It serves to suggest covered, preferred and lower cost drugs.
FTP	File transfer program

ANNEXURE IV

Terms and Definitions used in Healthcare Management

The following are some of the important terms and definitions which are required for documenting medical records in general and nursing records in particular.

Accident and emergency record: It is used for emergency (casualty) patients in the A/E department. This term is commonly used as A/E record, or casualty record or emergency room record or emergency file. These records are kept in the casualty department for one year and later transferred to medical record department.

Admission waiting list: A list of names of patients maintained by the admission office waiting for a vacant bed and room for admission to the hospital.

Adult patient: A patient 12–14 years of age or older.

Aetiology: A science dealing with the causation of disease.

Allergy: A condition of unusual or exaggerated specific susceptibility to a substance which is harmless in similar amounts for other members of same species. This term embraces all types of human hypersensitiveness.

Allied health personnel: Those not involved in the direct care of the patient but are vital in providing healthcare (such as dietary, social services, and medical records personnel).

Amalgamation of records: Bringing together of two or more files and numbers of one single patient created at different times under one hospital number and one file.

Anesthesia: Loss of feeling or sensation.

Analysis of hospital service: A gross appraisal of the efficiency of the hospital and medical staff primarily for benefit of, and use by, the patient and hospital. It is intended to give a picture of the type of illnesses cared for by the hospital and their end results.

Anatomy: It is the study of different organs which make up the body, their arrangements, and relationships to each other, and the different types of cells recognizable on microscopic examination.

Anomaly: It is a structure or organ which is irregular in formation (malformation). Examples of congenital anomalies are missing fingers or toes and heart defects.

Angiocardiography: A diagnostic procedure involving an X-ray dye into the blood stream, followed by chest X-rays to show the dimensions of the heart and the large blood vessels.

Arthroscopy: Visual examination of the inside of a joint with an endoscope.

Assembling of records: Arrangement of different forms in a standard prescribed order, e.g. outpatient file and inpatient file as recommended in the work procedures.

Assistant medical record technician (AMRT): It is a trained employee of the medical record department who works under the supervision of a medical record technician (MRT).

Audiometric: An instrument (audiometer) which delivers acoustic stimuli of specific frequencies to determine the patient's hearing for each frequency. The results are plotted on a graph called an audiogram.

Authorized personnel: Employees of the hospital and are directly involved with the medical care of the patient, e.g. medical, nursing, and paramedical staff.

Autopsy: Examination of organs of a dead body (autopsy) to determine the cause of death, is also known as postmortem examination.

Autopsy rate: The ratio during any given period of time of all autopsies to all deaths.

Average daily census: The total number of inpatients days (exclusive of newborn) care rendered for a period is computed and divided by the total number of days in that period.

Average length of stay: The total number of inpatient day's care rendered to discharged patients (exclusive of newborn) in a given fiscal period divided by the total number of patients (exclusive of newborn) who were discharged or who died during the same period. In computing the length of stay, the day of admission should be counted but not the day of discharge.

Bacteriology: The study of bacteria and diseases caused by them.

Bassinet: For the use of infant other than newborns. Bassinets used for newborn infants are not considered to be hospital beds and should not be included in the bed complement of a hospital.

Bed complement: It is the total number of hospital beds, exclusive of newborn bassinets, normally available for 24 hours service to inpatients in the hospital.

Bed occupancy board: This board is maintained by the admission office, is also termed as the "bed control board" or the "bed utilization board" for keeping the account of occupied and vacant beds in different wards of the hospital.

Benign tumor: A benign tumor is a slow growing neoplasm and does not metastasize. Benign tumors are limited in extent and often are surrounded by a capsule.

Biochemistry: The science which deals with the chemistry of life.

Biopsy: Excision of tissue from a living body for microscopic examination to establish a diagnosis.

Birth: Is the acceptance of an infant patient newly born in the hospital for inpatient service. This involves occupancy of a newborn infant bassinet and maintenance of a hospital chart during the period of care.

Birth weight: The first weight of the fetus or newborn obtained after birth. This weight should be measured preferably within the first hour of life before significant postnatal weight has occurred.

Burn: A lesion of the tissues due to chemicals, dry heat, electricity, flame, friction, or radiation. They are usually classified into three types:

- *First degree burns:* No blisters; superficial lesions mainly in the epidermis; hyperesthesia; and erythema.
- *Second degree burns:* Damage to the epidermis and corium; blister; erythema; and hyperesthesia.
- *Third degree burns:* Both the epidermis and corium are destroyed and subcutaneous layer is damaged, leaving charred, white tissue.

Caesarean section: Delivery of the fetus by an incision through the abdominal and uterine wall.

Caesarean section rate: The ratio of caesarean sections performed to viable births.

Carcinomas: The largest group of solid tumors which are derived from epithelial tissue.

Cardiac catheterization: A thin flexible tube (catheter) is introduced into a vein or artery and is guided into the heart for detecting pressure and pattern of blood flow. Dye can also be injected and X-rays taken.

Cardiology: The study of the structure, function, and disease of the heart.

Casualty: This term is synonymous to "accident and emergency" or "emergency".

Causes of death: The causes of death to be entered on the medical certificate of cause of death are all those diseases, morbid conditions, or injuries which either resulted in or contributed to the death and the circumstances of the accident or violence which produced any such injuries.

Cauterization: Burning a part of tissue.

Census: The number of inpatients present in a hospital or healthcare facility at any one time. Ward clerk (AMRT) will prepare a daily ward census report and send it to the medical record department.

Centralized filing system: A system in which all information is filed in one central location. Outpatient and inpatient files are kept in medical record folder and filed in the medical record department.

Central processing unit (CPU): The part of a computer system that contains the circuits which control the interpretation and execution of instructions, including arithmetic, logic, and control functions.

Central registration: This section works around the clock to register new patients for outpatient and inpatient services. This section also maintains patient master index filing to enable verification of previous registration numbers.

Chart (record) analysis: Careful review of the entire record (patient file); identification of specific areas that are incomplete or deficient.

Chemotherapy: It is the administration of a drug which destroys microorganisms, parasites, or malignant cells within the body and is utilized in the treatment of infectious diseases.

Child patient: Any patient less than 12–14 years is called a child patient, excluding newborn infants (born in the hospital).

Coding: A numerical assignment that provides an organized approach to data retrieval. The term coding for disease and operation classification as per international classification of diseases and operations. The medical record staffs are responsible for coding of diseases and operations.

Color coding: It is used in terminal digit filing system, in which ten different color strips or labels are used for numerals 0 to 9 to facilitate and to identify the numbers of records filed by color.

Communicable disease: Causative agents which transfer disease from one person to another directly or indirectly.

Completion of records: Completing the records (patient files) which are deficient in number of forms or content as per the established standards. The medical record staff reviews each case and notes the deficiencies of physician and other documentation.

Complication: A disturbance occurring in the course of a disease and arising wholly or in part separate from the disease itself.

Comprehensive record: It is the one which has all the required forms with detailed and complete clinical and other information in a patient file as per established criteria.

Computer: An electronic device which stores, transmits, and manipulates information according to predetermined instructions known as a program.

Confidential information: A statement made to a physician, an attorney, or a clergyman in confidence with the implicit understanding that it should remain confidential. Patient health records are confidential documents.

Confidentiality: Status accorded to data or information which is sensitive for some reason and therefore must be protected against theft or improper use, and disseminated only to authorized individuals or organizations.

Consent: Concurrence of wills; voluntary yielding of one's will to the proposition of another; acquiescence or compliance. This is obtained in the hospital generally for rendering treatment and performing surgical procedures to patients.

Consultation: A meeting of two or more physicians at the request of the attending physician or other authorized persons or body for study of a problem case, with necessary examinations to arrive at an accurate diagnosis and a written opinion as to prognosis, therapeutic measures, and recommendations proposed.

Contagious disease: One communicable by contact with an individual suffering from it or by contact with an object touched by that person.

Convalescent patient: A patient who is recovering from disease and who is preparing for normal activity.

Cribs: Equipped with sides or guards, for the use of young children (i.e. below 12–14 years of age).

Criteria: Predetermined elements against which aspects of the quality of medical service may be measured; for instance, two criteria for care of urinary tract infection might be the obtaining of a urinalysis and a urine culture.

Cross index: Cross indexing of diseases and operations may be defined as listing on a card for a specific disease or operation entity, according to recognized classification, all essential data of each patient having that particular condition, with a cross reference on other cards to every other entity involved in the particular case.

Cryosurgery: Using cold temperature to destroy tissue. The cold is usually produced by a probe containing liquid nitrogen.

Data bank: Computer term for storage of information.

Death rate: The ratio of total number of deaths in the hospital during any given period of time to the total number of discharges and deaths during that same time.

Deficiency: A non-justifiable variation from expected standards.

Deficiency check: Reviewing of outpatient and inpatient files for deficiencies by the Medical Record Department staff.

Dermatology: The science which deals with the skin, its structure, function, disease, and treatment.

Detrimental: Harmful; damaging; undesirable.

Diagnosis: Is made on the basis of extensive knowledge about the patient such as family history, physical examination, and investigation including X-rays and laboratory tests. The following are some of different kinds:

- *Clinical diagnosis*: Based upon symptoms shown during life, irrespective of the morbid changes producing them.
- *Final diagnosis*: A statement of opinion arrived at after extensive study, which is complete and accurate and is in conformity with the accepted medical terminology.
- *Pathological diagnosis*: Based on gross and microscopic examinations of the structural lesions present.
- *Differential diagnosis*: Based on symptoms and physical signs of two contrasting diseases.
- *Provisional diagnosis*: Based upon the availability of sources of information but subject to change.
- *Tentative diagnosis*: As above (provisional).
- *Preoperative diagnosis*: Made before operation and based on clinical findings.
- *Postoperative diagnosis*: Based upon findings observed during the operation.

Dialysis: Literally means "complete separation". A dialysis machine (artificial kidney) can completely separate out from the blood the harmful waste products of the body which are normally removed in the urine.

Dilatation and curettage: Dilatation (widening) of the cervical opening is accomplished by inserting a series of probes of increasing size. Curettage (scraping) is accomplished by using a curette (metal loop at the end of along, thin handle) to remove the lining of the uterus.

Direct admission: A patient admitted onto a ward and occupying a bed without processing through the admission office. This is permitted in emergency and obstetrics cases.

Discharge analysis: The tabulation of data on discharged hospital patients to reflect the professional services provided in a hospital.

Disease: Any deviation from or interruption of the normal structure and function of any part of the body. It is manifested by a characteristic set of signs and symptoms and in most instances the aetiology, pathology, and prognosis is known.

Disease and operation index: A numerical index of patient problems, diagnoses, and surgical procedures by individual categories. This work is performed by the medical record department.

Dividers: Heavy-weight fabric forms of pressboard, used to designate different sections, e.g. "outpatient", "correspondence", "investigations", and "inpatient" records of the patient folder. Also used to designate alphabetical breaks in the patient master index or numerical divisions of the disease or operation index.

Doctor's conference room: Area in the medical record department allocated exclusively for doctors to periodically complete deficient records.

Doubtful cases: Those in which either hospital number or the name of the patient is recorded wrongly.

Echocardiography: A diagnostic procedure in which pulses of high frequency sound waves (ultrasound) are transmitted into the chest and echoes returning from the surfaces of the heart are electronically plotted and recorded. This can show the structure and movement of the heart over time and may be useful in determining structural defects in the heart.

Elective surgery: A surgical procedure is planned or performed which is subject to the choice or decision of the patient or physician; applied to procedures that are advantageous to the patient but not urgent.

Electrocardiography (ECG or EKG): The record of the electrical activity flows through the heart.

Electrocochleography: A direct recording of the action potential generated following stimulation of the cochlear nerve.

Electroconvulsive therapy (ECT): A form of physical treatment occasionally used by psychiatrists mainly in the management of depression.

Electroencephalography (EEG): Ultrasonic waves are beamed through the head and echoes coming from brain structures are recorded as a image. This procedure is useful in detecting brain tumors, and hydrocephalus.

Electromyography (EMG): The use of an instrument which records electrical current generated by inactive muscle.

Electrooculography (EOG): The use of an instrument which records eye position and movement.

Emergency: Any condition which could result in serious permanent harm to a patient or aggravation of injury or disease, or in which the life of a patient is in immediate danger, and any delay in administering treatment could add to the danger. Casualty or accident and emergency (A/E) or emergency is synonymous terms.

Emergency record: Patient file of an emergency or casualty or A/E patient. If the patient is transferred to outpatient or inpatient care, then the emergency record also becomes part of main patient file.

Emergency treatment: Treatment immediately necessary to save life. *For example*: Treatment of a fracture case is not, whereas the treatment of a shock and hemorrhage case is.

Endemiology: The special study of endemic disease (recurring in an area, e.g. tuberculosis).

Endocrinology: The study of the ductless glands and their internal secretions (hormones).

Endoscopy: An instrument used for visualization of body cavities or organs.

Epidemiology: A branch of medical science that deals with the incidence, distribution, and control of disease in a group of people (population).

Eponym: A name or phrase formed from or including the name of a person such as Brigit's disease or Paget's disease.

Evaluation of medical record service: This evaluation should provide information on how effectively medical record services are being performed; e.g. how accurate is the filing of records or index cards, or how accurate is the disease index, etc.

Fetal death: A death prior to the complete expulsion or extraction of the product of conception from the mother irrespective of the duration of pregnancy. Death is indicated by the fact that, after such separation, the fetus does not breathe or show any other evidence of life such as beating of heart, pulsation of the umbilical cord, or definite movement of voluntary muscle.

Early fetal death or abortion: Completed less than 20 weeks gestation (500 grams or less).

Intermediate death: Completed 20 or more week's gestation but less than 28 weeks gestation (501 to 1000 grams).

Late fetal death or stillbirth: Completed 28 weeks gestation and over 1001 grams.

Filing: Placing a collection of records or cards in a methodical manner so that they may be instantly available.

Alphabetical filing: The method of filing charts or cards in strict alphabetical (dictionary style) sequence.

- **Serial number filing:** The method of filing charts or cards in strict numerical sequence.
- **Centralized serial:** The method of issuing one series of numbers to both the outpatient department and the inpatient department, and storing all records in one place. In addition, a patient is given a new number on each admission either in the outpatient department or in the inpatient department.

Centralized serial unit: Same as centralized serial, but the earlier records of the patient are brought to the folder of the latest admission.

File folders: Solid, two sided binders of Kraft, manila, press-board or patent composition used to store paper records. This term relates to a patient file (folder).

Follow-up: The periodic examination of a patient following disease or injury to determine the progress was being made toward complete recovery and normal health, and to study the end results of treatment.

Follow-up appointment: Giving an appointment for an existing patient to attend the relevant clinic on a particular date and time. All referral hospitals have to observe a follow-up appointment system in collaboration with the related health centers and hospitals.

Forensic medicine: Also called "legal medicine". The application of medical knowledge to legal proceedings.

Format: The arrangement of a form, or an organization of forms in a permanent folder, which directs the type of entries, the way entries are made, and the future use of those entries.

Fracture: The breaking of a bone due to injury or disease; some terms describing fractures and related injuries are:

- *Closed fracture:* A bone is broken but there is no open wound in the skin (simple fracture).
- *Open fracture:* A broken bone with an open wound in the skin (compound fracture).
- *Comminuted fracture:* The bone is splintered or crushed.
- *Impacted fracture:* The bone is broken, and one end is wedged into the anterior portion of the other.
- *Greenstick fracture:* The bone is partially bent and partially broken as when a greenstick breaks.

Gastroenterology: The study of the digestive tract, including the liver, biliary tract, pancreas and the accompanying diseases.

Gerontology: The scientific study of the problems of aging in all their aspects, e.g. clinical, biological, historical, and sociological.

Gestational age: The duration of gestation is measured from the first day of the last normal menstrual period. Gestational age is expressed in completed days or weeks (e.g. events occurring 280 to 286 days after the onset of the last normal menstrual period are considered to have occurred at 40 weeks of gestation).

Gynecology: Study of the female reproductive system (organs, hormones, and diseases).

Health center: Generally provides primary care and, if requiring further special care, refers the patient with a referral letter to an appropriate hospital.

Health information: Any data pertains to the physical, mental, or social well-being of an individual or group of individuals.

Health record: Documentation of direct or indirect healthcare services to patients or clients by providers and users of the data in any type of health-related institution.

Hematology: The science dealing with formation, composition, function, and disease of the blood.

Homonyms: Word of same forms as another word but with different meaning (different spelling but pronounced alike).

Hospital bed: A bed installed for regular 24 hour use by an inpatient (other than newborn infant) during his or her period of hospitalization.

Hospital inpatient: A hospital patient who is provided with a bed, a room, board, medical care, and continuous general nursing service in an area of the hospital where patients generally stay at least overnight.

Hospital number: It is a unit number allocated to a new patient who visits the hospital for outpatient or inpatient service for the first time. This is a permanent number used for all episodes and subsequent admissions. Patient files including relevant forms are represented by this number.

Hospital record: A written account of all the services provided to the patient as an outpatient, emergency, or inpatient from the time of the visit or admission until discharge. This identifies the dates, the ward, the bed, and the room where the patient was physically located, the names of the physicians, the nurses, and the other health professionals who provided care, and the results of that care.

Immature infant: It is a live born infant with a recorded birth weight of 2500 grams or less.

Immunology: The study of the immune system of lymphocytes, inflammatory cells, associated cells, and protein which affect the individuals response to antigens.

Implied consent: That which is given by mutual understanding.

Incident report: In the event of occurrence of an incident in which the patient has suffered during hospitalization that was recorded and intimated to the concerned officials.

Incomplete record: Any hospital record of an outpatient or a discharged patient was lacking essential data.

Index: An organized and condensed list of data selected and recorded on a designed index for easy and quick retrieval of information.

Infectious disease: A disease due to organisms ranging in size from viruses to parasitic worms; it may be contagious in origin, result from nosocomial organisms, or be due to endogenous micro flora from the nose, throat, skin, or bowel.

Information: Knowledge or intelligence; facts and data.

Informed consent: That which is documented to show the following: All procedures and treatment explained (including advantages and disadvantages) signed by a person giving consent as a result of their own decision.

Inpatient: It is defined as a person who occupies a hospital bed, crib, or bassinet while housed in a hospital, for observation, care, diagnosis, or treatment.

Inpatient census: The number of inpatients present at any one time in all of the hospital wards.

Inpatient discharge: The release of a hospitalized inpatient from the hospital by the admitting physician after providing necessary medical care for a period deemed necessary.

Institutional deaths: Those which occur 48 hours or more after admission.

International classification of diseases (ICD): A basic system of three-digit categories with four-and five-digit subcategories in some areas as recommended by the world health organization.

Job description: A document contains information about a position such as required education, training, and experience, as well as lines of authority and designation of supervisor, with a description of general duties and responsibilities and major job functions.

Laparoscopy: Endoscopic examination of the interior of the abdomen by means of a laparoscope.

Legal liability: Accepting responsibility before the court of law for reasonable care of the patients with reasonable maintenance of facilities for that purpose.

Length of stay: The number of days a patient remains in a facility (the day of admission should be counted but not the day of discharge unless the patient was admitted the same day).

Live birth: It is the complete expulsion or extraction from the mother of a product of conception, which, after such separation, breaths or shows any other evidence of life such as beating of heart, pulsation of the umbilical cord, or definite movements of voluntary muscles, whether or not the umbilical cord has been cut or the placenta is attached; each product of such birth is considered a live birth.

Low birth weight: Less than 2500 grams (up to, and including 2499 grams).

Malignant tumor: One that has the properties of invasion and metastasis and that shows a greater degree of anaplasia than do benign tumors.

Malpractice: Improper, careless, or ignorant treatment.

Maternal mortality: The death of a woman while pregnant or within 42 days of termination of pregnancy irrespective of the duration and the site of the pregnancy, from any cause related to or aggravated by the pregnancy or its management but not from accidental or incidental causes.

Medical audit: An evaluation system in which established standards are used to measure performance. Once corrective action has been taken on problems identified through this review process, performance is remeasured after an appropriate time period.

Medical board: A meeting or conference of the medical staff of the hospital held for the purpose of reviewing and analyzing the clinical work of the hospital. This board deals with death cases, unimproved cases, infection, complications, or performance not conforming with the standard. The board also deals with problems concerning organization and management of the various medical services of the hospital.

Medical care evaluation: A structured program to measure the quality of care given to patients. It is a global term that encompasses methods used to carry out such measurement functions as audit, appraisal, peer review, quality assurance, and assessment in various specific forms.

Medical certificate: It is a document containing disease and injury specifications and duration of treatment of a patient in the emergency, outpatient, or inpatient areas of a hospital and attested to by the treating physician.

Medical consultation: The response by one member of the medical staff to a request for consultation by another member of the medical staff, characterized by review of the patient's history, examination of the patient, and completion of a consultation report presenting recommendations and opinions.

Medical file or medical record or patient record or patient file all are synonymous terms. This file contains both outpatient and inpatient records.

Medical record: It is an orderly written report of the patient's history, physical, laboratory findings, treatment, and hospital course. When complete, it should contain sufficient data to justify the diagnosis and also describe the result of the care rendered.

Medical record committee: A committee which ensures that accurate and complete medical records are developed and retained for every patient treated. Also evaluates the work of the Medical Record Department to ensure that the department is functioning efficiently.

Medical record department (MRD): One of the important departments in the hospital responsible for proper custody of the medical records of the patients, for conducting medical audits, for preparing reports necessary to demonstrate the quantity and quality of medical practice, and for assisting in the advancement of medical science through assuring accurately recorded data.

Medical record form: A piece of paper or card, which is a formal arrangement of information (usually with spaces for the entry of additional information). A set of 90 basic medical record forms are recommended for adequate patient care in the hospital.

Medical record officer (MRO): An individual responsible for establishing, organizing, and controlling a medical record department which initiates medical records for patient care. The MRO is also responsible for developing a good information system to compile and distribute patient or client data. He or she is the chief administrator of the medical record department (MRD).

Medical record technician (MRT): A trained person who works under the supervision of a medical record officer. He or she is an intermediate supervisory staff person and performs most of the technical jobs in the department and supervises the work of the assistant medical record technicians.

Medical report: A document containing medical information such as history, physical examination, investigations, diagnosis, and treatment including surgical procedures, end results, duration of treatment, and recommendations about a patient treated in the hospital.

Medical social service: The sociological investigation of a patient and his environment to ascertain any factors which might have a bearing on the diagnosis, treatment, and aftercare of the patient, followed in close collaboration with the physician with respect to the findings.

Medico-legal case (MLC): Case which is accidental, suicidal, or homicidal. The casualty medical officer (CMO) determines a case as medico-legal or not. Except in minor injury cases, all cases of traffic accidents, burns, poisonings, and quarrels have to be treated as medico legal-cases.

Metastasis: Tumor spreading from its primary location to secondary sites throughout the body.

Medicine: (1) The science or art of healing, especially as distinguished from surgery and obstetrics. (2) A therapeutic substance such as a drug.

Microbiology: The science which deals microorganisms.

Microfilming: A process of photographing and reducing a given report to a miniature of the original on film. The medical record department may microfilm certain old records as per the "record retention schedule" as recommended by regulations.

MOH: Ministry of health.

Morbidity: The incidence of disease or proportion of diseases in a given population; statistical data that represents rates or ratios of disease.

Morphology: The science which deals with the structure and form of living things.

Mortality: The incidence of deaths or the proportion of deaths in a given population; statistical data that represents rates or ratios of deaths.

Mounting of investigation (diagnostic) reports: Reports of laboratory, X-ray and other investigations mounted on laboratory mount sheets, and X-ray mount sheets or EKG strips. All inpatient reports are received on the ward and mounted by the ward nurse or clerk (AMRT). Reports of outpatient are received and mounted by the medical record department. The reports of A/E department are received by casualty staff and inserted with the relevant casualty record. If patient is transferred to outpatient or inpatient services, the casualty record along with all associated reports become part of the main patient file.

Necropsy (autopsy): Postmortem examination; see "Autopsy".

Neonatal death: An infant's death occurring less than 28 completed days after delivery.

Neoplasm: New growth; tumor.

Nephrology: The special study of the kidneys and the diseases which affect them.

Neurology: (1) The science and study of the nerves, their structure, function, and pathology. (2) The branch of medicine dealing with diseases of the nervous system.

Newborn: Any infant newly born in the hospital.

New patient: A new patient is one who visits the hospital for the first time, for whom a new hospital number has to be allocated, or an outpatient record has to be created after obtaining accurate and complete identification data.

Non-institutional deaths: Those which occur under 48 hours after admission.

Numbering system: An identifying method that utilizes assigned numbers to label each record for filing in a systematic manner to facilitate easy retention and retrieval.

Obstetrics: A specialty concerned with pregnancy and delivery of the fetus.

Odontology (dentistry): The science which deals with the structure, function, and diseases of the teeth.

Old medical records: Those records which are inactive and kept for a certain duration or period as per the retention schedule for administrative, educational, research, and legal purposes. These include patient files, X-rays, medical registers, reports, index cards, etc.

Old (follow-up) patient: One who has been treated in the hospital either as an outpatient or inpatient for whom a patient file with hospital number exists.

Oncology: The scientific study of tumors.

On-line: A device that currently is an operating part of the computer system. A terminal is on-line if it is logged into the system. An idle service is on-line if it may be activated by the computer.

Operation index: Does a card possess patient information about particular surgical operation undergone by different patients. Operation indexing is performed by the medical record staff.

Ophthalmology: The science which deals with the structure, function, and diseases of the eye.

Oral surgery: Pertaining to structures found in the mouth.

Orthopedics: Branch of study dealing with all conditions affecting the locomotor system.

Otorhinolaryngology (ENT): The science which deals with the structure, function, and diseases of the ear, nose, and throat.

Out guide card: This is also known as the "tracer card" or "locator". This card contains patient identification information which indicates the movement of the patient file.

Outpatient: It is a person who makes use of the diagnostic or therapeutic services of a hospital but does not occupy a regular bed.

Outpatient clinic schedule: The list of patients new and established to be seen in the clinic. Each unit in consultation with the administration and medical record officer decides upon the number of patients (new and established) to be seen in the clinic and the appointments are booked accordingly.

Outpatient record: A patient file created with a hospital number for treatment as an outpatient and generally comprises: The medical record folder, the outpatient form, the history and physical examination report, the outpatient follow-up form, laboratory and X-ray mount sheets, and other special forms added wherever required.

Paramedical: Those personnel who are qualified to render treatment or assist in patient care under the supervision of the medical staff, e.g. occupational therapists, radiographers, laboratory technicians, and so on.

Pathology: The science which deals with the cause and nature of disease.

Patient day: A unit of measure for the service rendered an inpatient between the census-taking hours on two successive days, the day of discharge being counted only if the patient was admitted the same day. Only patients admitted, assigned abed, and having a medical record initiated should be counted in the census. When a patient is admitted and discharged the same day, the length of stay should be considered as one patient day.

Patient file: Medical record.

Patient master index (PMI): A 5″ × 3″ card containing patient identification information with hospital number; this card is filed in the central registration section in strict alphabetical order. This process assists in tracing out whether a patient has registered previously or not. This is also known as "master patient index".

Pediatrics: Any patient less than 12–14 years of age, treated by a pediatrician on a pediatric unit is considered as a pediatric patient or child patient.

Pharmacology: The science that deals with the origin, nature, chemistry, and uses of drugs, as well as their effects on the body.

Physiology: The science which deals with the normal functions of the body.

Policy: A basic guide of action which prescribes the boundaries within which activities are to take place.

Pregnancy: The condition of having a developing embryo or fetus in the body after union of an ovum and a spermatozoon. In normal pregnancy, the embryos develop within the uterus. In an ectopic pregnancy, the embryo is implanted outside the uterus, it is most commonly found in the fallopian tubes, and sometimes in the ovary or in the abdominal cavity.

Premature infant: A live born infant with a period of gestation of less than 37 completed weeks, or specified by the obstetrician as "premature".

Pre-numbered folder: Patient files with required forms numbered well in advance and kept ready for registration of new cases.

Presentation (obstetrical): The relationship of the long axis of the fetus to that of the mother. There are two divisions, the longitudinal, in which the head or breech may be present, and the transverse in which the shoulder is the presenting part and may include shoulder, arm, or any other part of the trunk.

Breech: Presentation of buttocks or feet of the fetus in labor; breech presentation complete mean presentation of the buttocks in labor, with the feet alongside of the buttocks, the feet being in the same position as in vertex presentation, but with polarity reversed.

- *Cephalic (head):* Presentation of any part of the fetal head in labor, including occiput, brow, or face.
- *Transverse:* Shoulder; scapula is the point of direction.

Preservation of records: Patient files and related documents are preserved in a safe location and well protected area for the period recommended in a "record retention schedule" furnished by regulations.

Privacy: A right to declare information confidential and to recognize formally the patient's inherent right to privacy.

Privileged communication: Any information acquired by a physician or surgeon in attending a patient which was necessary to enable him or her to prescribe or act for the patient and which cannot be revealed in a civil action without the consent of the patient.

Procedure: An act or manner of proceeding or method of conducting a business proceeding. A procedure is a series of tasks designed to accomplish work in a given time.

Processing of records: Reviewing of records (files) to determine whether the records are quantitatively and qualitatively complete. This also refers to effective documentation of the details of the patient's history and physical examination, other diagnostic measures, specific treatment procedures, etc.

Prodrome: Symptoms of disease (such as rash or fever) which appear before and signal the onset of an approaching more severe illness.

Prognosis: A prognosis made by a doctor after diagnosis about the nature of the patient's illness. It is a prediction about the disease.

Psychiatry: The branch of medical study devoted to the diagnosis and treatment of mental illness.

Qualitative analysis: Retrospective review program by the organized medical staff. It assesses the quality of care as compared to locally or internally developed standards and verifies that the standards or exceptions are met, that deficiencies are corrected, and that the original problem is reassessed on a planned program basis.

Quality assurance: Activities performed to determine the extent to which a phenomenon fulfills certain values and standards, and to assure changes in practice that fulfill the highest of a predetermined level of values.

Quality assurance program (QAP): A comprehensive and coordinated network of formal mechanisms that provide ongoing objective assessment of patient care services and the correction of identified problems.

Quality control: It is defined as those evaluation procedures that are performed systematically to ensure that established policies and standards are being met.

Quantitative analysis: The responsibility the medical record department to check and analyze the component parts of the medical record to ensure that it is complete, adequate, and accurate, and is available at all times for legitimate needs of the patients, the hospital, and the physician.

Radiology: The study of the diagnosis of disease by using X-rays and other allied imaging techniques.

Record control: The supply of records (patient files) for patient care, administrative, and other reasons and the collection and accounting for that effective control, as well as the safeguarding of the confidentiality of information.

Referral: Two types: From outside, e.g. from health centers and other hospitals or from inside, e.g. within the hospital from one department to another. Any referral of a patient must be on a written prescribed document. Referral forms are in triplicate. When a health center refers a patient, two copies are given to the patient to be forwarded to the hospital, and the third copy is retained by the patient. After treatment, the hospital returns one copy with details as feedback information to the health center and retains one copy in the hospital.

Relapse: A relapse is the reappearance of symptoms of disease.

Remission: A remission is the lessening or disappearance of disease symptoms.

Reports: Relating to statistics: daily, monthly, and yearly. Daily report is the analysis of hospital services which include the work performed by the different departments such as outpatient, accident/emergency, inpatient, and allied departments. Monthly report is a cumulative daily report for calendar months with ratios (or percentage rates) of service facilities used, and other statistical data and rates. Annual report is a compilation of the twelve monthly reports. The figures are cumulated monthly, just as the monthly report figures are cumulated from daily analysis.

Responsibility for medical certificates of cause of death: Medical certification of cause of death should normally be the responsibility of the attending physician. In the case of deaths certified by coroners or other legal authorities, the medical evidence supplied to the certifier should be stated on the certificate in addition to any legal findings.

Retention of records: Keeping information for a specific period so that it may be used in the future. Planning, implementation, and control of a system that safeguards physical and information characteristics of medical or health data for future use. The patient files and other documents are retained in accordance with the "record retention schedule" as suggested per regulations.

Review: Examination of a medical record by a physician to determine if continued hospitalization is medically necessary.

Sarcomas: Rare types of cancer which are derived from supportive and connective tissue, such as bone, fat, muscle, cartilage, bone marrow, lymphatic tissue, or blood cells.

Serial numbering: A system of numbering in which the patient is assigned a new number each time treatment is received.

Sphygmomanometer: Instrument to measure blood pressure.

Stages of labor: The act of giving birth to a child. The following three stages are recognized.

First stage: From beginning of labor to complete dilatation.

Second stage: From complete dilatation to birth of infant.

Third stage: From birth of infant to expulsion of placenta.

Standard: Generally, a measure set by a competent authority as the rule for measuring quantity or quality. Conformity with standards is usually a condition of licensing, accreditation, or payment of service.

Sterilization: The act or process of rendering sterile; the process of freeing from germ life. A procedure by which an individual is made incapable of reproduction by undergoing surgery such as a vasectomy or a tubectomy.

Stethoscope: An instrument used for listening to the various body sounds, especially those of the heart and chest.

Stillbirth: Fetal death

Suit: An action or process in a court of law for the recovery of right or claim.

Summons: A process (document) served on a defendant in civil court action to secure his or her appearance in the action.

Surgery: The branch of medicine which treats diseases, deformities, and injuries wholly or partly, by manual or operative procedures.

Symbiosis: Refers to the living together in close association of two organisms, either for mutual benefit or not. The bacteria which normally lie in the digestive tract of humans are an example of symbiosis.

Syndrome: It is a group of signs or symptoms which commonly occur together and indicate a particular disease or abnormal condition. An example of a syndrome is Homer's syndrome, characterized by ptosis of the eyelid, enophthalmos, and cool, dry face on the affected side due to nerve damage.

System: Related elements that are coordinated to form a unified result, specifically people, activities, equipment, materials, plans, and controls, working together to achieve a unified objective or whole; an array of components that interact to achieve some objective through a network of procedures that are integrated and designed to carry out a major activity.

Terminal digit filing: A method of filing by the last digits of a number instead of by the first digits. The entire number is broken into groups of twos or threes, with the last group being filed first. This system is suggested to all the referral hospitals.

Topography: A description of the regions of the body.

Toxicology: The study of harmful chemicals and their dangerous effects on the body.

Transfer of patient: If a patient is transferred within the hospital (except from casualty) from one unit to another, the same patient file will be continued for the duration of treatment except for change of ward census. In the case of a patient transferred from other hospitals, the case has to be registered and a record has to be created (if he or she is not an established patient).

Traumatology: The branch of surgery dealing with injury caused by accident.

Treating physician: One under whose care, the treatment to the patient is rendered. Physician can be a surgeon, a pediatrician or an obstetrician or gynecologist. This term is synonymous to a medical doctor.

Treatment: The application of any measure to assist in bringing about the cure of disease or relief of symptoms or to correct the disturbances of the function was arising from an infection. Therapeutics or therapy is the general term for all forms of treatment of disease. The kinds of treatment are:

Symptomatic: Directed towards the removal of the cause based on the treatment of symptoms as they are manifested.

- *Prophylactic:* Aimed to prevent the occurrence of disease.
- *Palliative:* Designed to check or to reduce symptoms.
- ***Specific:*** Assigned treatment devised for specific action.

Underlying cause of death: The underlying cause of death is the disease or injury which initiated the chain of events leading directly to death or the circumstances of the accident or violence which produced the fatal injury.

Unit numbering: A system in which only one number is assigned to the patient's record and is retained permanently.

Unit numbering system: Whereby only one serial number is given to the patient irrespective of the number of admissions either in the outpatient department or in the inpatient department and all records of the patient are available in one folder.

Unit record system: A method that compiles all information on a single patient or subject and records it in one document and file folder.

Urology: The branch of medicine which deals with disorders of the female urinary tract and with disorders the male genital urinary tract.

Utilization review: The evaluation of the necessity, appropriateness, and efficiency of the use of medical services, procedures, and facilities. In a hospital, this includes review of the appropriateness of admissions, services ordered and provided, length of stay, and discharge practices on a concurrent and retrospective basis. This can be done by a utilization review committee, by peer review, or by any other assigned committee.

Venereology (sexually transmitted disease): The study and treatment of diseases transmitted during sexual intercourse.

Viable infant: A fetus that has reached a stage of development that has enabled itself to live outside the uterus, usually consider and as 28 completed weeks of gestation or more.

Virology: The study of viruses and the diseases caused by them.

ANNEXURE V

Standardized Medical Abbreviations with Single Meaning

Abbreviations	*Expansion*
A	
A/B	Acid-base ratio
A/G	Albumin-globulin ratio
A2	Aortic second sound
AAA	Abdominal aortic aneurysm
AAR	Antigen anti globulin reaction
AAS	Aortic arch syndrome
AB	Asthmatic bronchitis
ABD HYST	Abdominal hysterectomy
ABE	Acute bacterial endocarditis
ABO	Blood groups (name for agglutinogens)
ABP	Arterial blood pressure
AC	Before meals (ante cibum)
ACC	Adenoid cystic carcinoma
ACE	Adrenocortical extraction
ACH	Adrenal cortical hormone
ACM	Albumin-calcium-magnesium
ACS	Antereticular cytotoxic serum
ACT	Activated coagulation time
ACTH	Adreno cortico tropic hormone
ACVD	Acute cardiovascular disease
AD LIB	As desired (ad libitum)
AD	Right ear (auris dextra)
ADA	Anterior descending artery
ADH	Antidiuretic hormore
ADS	Antibody deficiency syndrome
AEG	Air encephalogram
AFG	Acid fast bacilli
AFT	Acute follicular tonsillitis
AGA	Appropriate for gestational age
AGL	Acute granulocytic leukemia
AGN	Acute glomerulonephritis
AH	Arterial hypertension
AHA	Acquired hemolytic anaemia
AHD	Arteriosclerotic heart disease
AHF	Acute hemophilic factor
AHT	Augumented histamin test
AI	Aortic incompetence
AIDS	Accquired immunme deficiency syndrome
AIHA	Auto-inmune hemolytic anemia
AJ	Ankle jerk
AK	Above knee
AKA	Above knee amputation
ALL	Acute lymphocytic leukemia
Alt. dieb	Every other day (alternis diebus)
Alt. hor	Every other hour (alternis horis)
Alt. noc	Every other night
AM	Auditory meatus
AMA	Against medical advice
AMI	Acute myocardial infarction
AML	Acute myeloblastic leukemia
AMOL	Acute monocytic leukemia
AN	Antenatal
ANA	Antinuclear antibodies
ANT	Anterior
AOM	Acute otitis media
A-P	Anteroposterior
AP	Anterior pituitary
APC	Aspirin, phenacetin, caffeine
APH	Ante-partum hemorrhage
APTT	Activated partial thromboplastin time
AR	Aortic regurgitation
ARD	Acute respiratory disease
ARF	Acute respiratory failure
ARM	Artificial rupture of the membranes
AS	Aortic stenosis
ASD	Arterial septal defect
ASHD	Arteriosclerotic heart disease
ASO	Arteriosclerosis obliteral
ATD	Asphyxiating thoracic dystrophy
ATS	Antitetanic serum
AVF	Arteriovenous fistula
AVH	Acute viral hepatitis
B	
B/K	Bladder kidney (scan ratio)
B12	Vitamin B_{12}
BA	Barium
BB	Blood bank
BBA	Born before arrival
BBB	Bundle branch block
BCG	Bacille calmette guerin (vaccine)
BGTT	Borderline glucose tolerance test
BID	Brought in dead
BID	Twice a day (bis in die)
BIH	Benign intracranial hypertension
BJM	Bones, joints, muscles
BKA	Below knee amputation
BM	Bowel movement
BMR	Basal metabolic rate
BOM	Bilateral otitis media
BP	Blood pressure

Abbreviations	*Expansion*
BPH	Benign prostate hypertrophy
Br Pn.	Bronchopneumonia
BR	Bronchitis
BSOM	Bilateral suppurative otitis media
BSR	Blood sedimentation rate
BT	Bleeding time
BUN	Blood urea nitrogen
BW	Birth weight
Bx.	Biopsy

C

Abbreviations	*Expansion*
C and D	Cystoscopy and dilatation
C	Centigrade (centum gradus)
C1, C2	First, second cervical vertebra
CA (Ca)	Carcinoma
CAD	Coronary artery disease
CAHD	Coronary atherosclerotic heart disease
CAT	Computerized axial tomography
CAV	Congenital absence of vagina
CB	Chronic bronchitis
CBA	Chronic bronchitis with asthma
CBC	Complete blood count
CBC and Diff	Complete blood count and differential
CBD	Common bile duct
CC	Chief complaint
CCF	Congestive cardiac failure
CCU	Coronary care unit
CDH	Congenital dislocation of the hip
CEA	Carcinoembryonic antigen
CHA	Congenital hypoplastic anemia
CHB	Complete heart block
CHD	Congestive heart disease
CHF	Congestive heart failure
CHS	Chédiak-Highshi syndrome
CLBBB	Complete left bundle branch block
CLGL	Correction with glasses
CLL	Chronic lymphocytic leukemia
CM	Costal margin
CML	Chronic myelocytic leukemia
CMR	Cerebral metabolic rate
CNS	Central nervous system
CO2	Carbon dioxide
COAD	Chronic obstructive airways disease
COLD	Chronic obstructive lung disease
COPD	Chronic obstructive pulmonary disease
CPD	Cephalo pelvic disproportion
CPK	Creatinine phosphokinase
CPR	Cardio pulmonary resuscitation
CRBBB	Complete right bundle branch block
CRF	Chronic renal failure
CRH	Corticotrophin releasing hormone
CSF	Cerebro spinal fluid
CSOM	Chronic suppurative otitis media
CSSD	Central sterile supply department
CST	Convulsive shock therapy
CT	Cerebral thrombosis
CV	Cardiovascular
CVA	Cardiovascular accident
CVD	Cardiovascular disease

D

Abbreviations	*Expansion*
D and C	Dilatation and curettage
D and V	Diarrhoea and vomiting
DI	Dibetes insipidus
DIC	Diffuse/disseminated intravascular coagulation
DLE	Discoid lupus erythematous
DM	Diabetic mellitus
DNS	Deflected/deviated nasal septum
DOA	Date of admission
DOB	Date of birth
DOC	Date of confinement
DOD	Date of discharge or death
DTP	Diptheria, tetanus and pertussis
DU	Duodenal ulcer
DUB	Dysfunctional uterine bladder
DVT	Deep vain thrombosis
DX	Diagnosis

E

Abbreviations	*Expansion*
EAM	External auditory meatus
ECG	Electrocardiogram
ECS	Electroconvulsive shock
ECT	Electroconvulsive therapy
EDC	Expected date of confinement
EDD	Expected date of delivery
EEG	Electroencephalogram
EH	Essential hypertension
EMG	Electromyogram
EMI	Eomputed tomography scanner
EN	Emmetropia
ENT	Ear, nose and throat
ER	Emergency room
ERG	Electroretinogram
ESR	Erythrocyte sedimentation rate
EUA	Examination under anesthesia

F

Abbreviations	*Expansion*
F/U	Follow up
FB	Foreign body

Abbreviations	*Expansion*
FBS	Fasting blood sugar
FD	Forceps delivery
FDIU	Fetal death *in utero*
FH	Family history
FHR	Feral heart rate
FHS	Follicle stimulating hormone
FSH	Follicle stimulating hormone
FTM	Fractional test meal
FTND	Full term normal delivery
FUO	Fever of unknown origin
G	
G/S	Glucose and saline
GA	General anesthesia
GB	Gall bladder
GFR	Glomerular filtration rate
GH	Growth hormone
GIT	Gastrointestinal tract
GP	General practitioner
GS	General surgery
GSH	Glomerular-stimulating hormorne
GT	Glucose tolerance
GTT	Glucose tolerance test
GU	Gastric ulcer
H	
HB	Hemoglobin
HBP	High blood pressure
HBW	High birth weight
HCG	Human chorionic gonadotropin
HCT	Hematocrit
HCVD	Hypertensive cardiovascular disease
HD	Heart disease
HDN	Hemolytic disease of the newborn
HF	Heart failure
HHA	Hereditary hemolytic anemia
HHD	Hypertensive heart disease
HIV	Human immuno virus
HPI	History of present illness
HT	Hypertension
HVD	Hypertinsive vascular disease
I	
I and D	Incision and drainage
I and O	Intake and output
ICC	Intensive coronary care
ICCU	Intensive coronary care unit
ICD	International classification of disease
ICM	Intercostal margin
ICU	Intensive care unit
IDK	Internal derangement of knee
IDKJ	Internal derangement of knee joint
IHD	Ishemic heart disease
IMF	Idiopathic myelofibrosis
IMP	Improved
IP	Inpatient
IQ	Intelligence quotient
ITP	Idiopathic thrombocytopenic purpura
IU	Intrauterine
IUD	Intra uterine death
IUFB	Intra uterine foreign body
IV	Intravenously
IVP	Intravenous pyelogram
IVSD	Interventricular septal defect
IVU	Intravenous urography
J	
JBE	Japanese B encephalitis
K	
KJ	Knee jerk
KUB	Kidney, ureter and bladder
L	
L-1, L-2	First, second lumbar vertebrae
L-1, L-2	First, second lumbar vertebrae
LA	Local anesthesia
LA	Local anesthesia
LAG	Lymphangiography
LAG	Lymphangiography
LB	Live birth
LB	Live birth
LBB	Left bundle branch
LBB	Left bundle branch
LBBB	Left bundle branch block
LBBB	Left bundle branch block
LBW	Low birth weight
LBW	Low birth weight
LCM	Left costal margin
LCM	Left costal margin
LE	Left eye
LE	Left eye
LFT	Liver function test
LFT	Liver function test
LHF	Left heart failure
LHF	Left heart failure
LIH	Left inguinal hernia
LK	Left kidney
LL	Left lung
LLE	Left lower extremity

Abbreviations	*Expansion*
LLL	Left lower lobe (lungs)
LMP	Last menstrual period
LP	Lumbar puncture
LSCS	Lower segment cesarean section
LSD	Lysergic acid diethylamide
LTH	Luteotrophic hormone
LUE	Left upper extremity
LUL	Left upper lobe
LV	Left ventricle
LVF	Left ventricular failure
LVH	Left ventricular hypertrophy

M

Abbreviations	*Expansion*
MA	Mental age
MCH	Mean corpuscular hemoglobin
MCT	Mean circulation time
MCV	Mean corpuscular volume
MD	Muscular dystrophy
MFD	Mid forceps delivery
MH	Marital history
MI	Myocardial infarction
MR	Mental retardation
MS	Mitral stenosis
MSW	Medial social worker

N

Abbreviations	*Expansion*
N/C	No complaints
NAD	Nothing abnormal detected
NB	Newborn
NBI	No bone injury
NBM	Nothing by mouth
NBW	Normal birth weight
ND	Normal delivery
NEC	Not elsewhere classified
NED	No evidence of disease
NFTD	Normal full term delivery
NOS	Not otherwise specified
NS	Neurosurgery
NYD	Not yet diagnosed

O

Abbreviations	*Expansion*
O&E	Observation and examination
O/A	On admission
OA	Osteoarthritis
OBG	Obstetrics and gynecology
Od	Once a day
OD	Right eye (ocular dexter)
OE	On examination
OH	Obstetric history
OM	Otitis media
OMI	Old myocardial infarction
OP	Out-patient
OPC	Out-patient clinic
OR	Operating room
OS	Left eye (oculus sinister)
OT	Operation theatre
OU	Each eye (oculi uterque)

P

Abbreviations	*Expansion*
P&A	Percussion and auscultation
P&V	Pyloroplasty and vagotomy
PA	Pernicious anemia
PANT	Posteroanterior
PAP	Primary atypical pneumonia
PAT	Paroxysmal atrial tachycardia
PCV	Packed cell volume
PDA	Patent ductus arterioses
PEG	Pneumo enchephalography
PET	Pre-eclamptic toxemia
PGH	Pituitary growth hormone
PH	Past history
PHT	Pulmonary hypertension
PI	Present illness
PID	Pelvic inflammatory disease
PIVD	Prolapse intervertebral disc
PM	Postmortem
PMA	Progressive muscular atrophy
PMB	Postmenopausal bleeding
PMI	Point of maximum impulse
PMN	Polymorphonuclear neutrophils
PMP	Past menstrual period
PMR	Physical medicine and rehabilitation
PN	Postnatal
PNC	Postnatal clinic
PND	Paroxysmal nocturnal dyspnea
PO	Postoperative
POP	Plaster of Paris
pp	After meals (postprandial)
PP	Postpartum
PPBS	Postprandial blood sugar
PPH	Postpartum hemorrhage
PPU	Perforated peptic ulcer
PRN	As required (pro renata)
PS	Pulmonary stenosis
PT	Pulmonary tuberculosis
PTH	Para thyroid hormone
PTT	Partial thromboplastin time
PU	Peptic ulcer
PUE	Pyrexia of unknown etiology
PUO	Pyrexia of unknown origin

Abbreviations	Expansion
PV	Per vaginum (through the vaginum)
PVC	Premature ventricular contraction
PVP	Portal venous pressure
PVR	Pulmonary vascular resistance
PVT	Paroxysmal ventricular tachycardia
Q	
q.d	Quaque die (every day)
q.d.h	Quaque duo hora (every two hours)
q.h	Quaque horo (every hour)
q.i.d	Quarter in die (four times daily)
q.n	Quaque nocte (every night)
q.n.s	Quantum non-satis (insufficient quantity)
q.q.h	Quaque quator hora (ever)
q.s	Quantum statis (sufficient quantity)
q.t.h	Quaque tres hora (every three hours)
q.v	Quantum vis (as much as desired)
R	
RA	Rhematoid arthritis
RAD	Radiation absorbed dose
RBBB	Right bundle branch block
RBC	Red blood count
RCA	Right coronary artery
RCM	Right costal margin
RCU	Respiratory cardiac unit
RD	Respiratory disease
RDH	Right inguinal hernia
RDS	Respiratory distress syndrome
REM	Rapid eye movement
RF	Rheumatic fever
RFB	Retained foreign body
RFT	Renal function test
Rh. neg	Rhesus factor (negative)
Rh. pos	Rhesus factor (positive)
RHD	Rheumatic heart disease
RHF	Rheumatic heart failure
RIA	Radio immuno assay
RIF	Right iliac fossa
RIH	Right inguinal hernia
RIIH	Right indirect inguinal hernia
RK	Right kidney
RL	Right lobe
RLE	Right lower extremity
RLL	Right lower lobe
RM	Radical mastectomy
RNA	Ribo nucleic acid
ROIH	Right oblique inguinal hernia
ROM	Rupture of membrane
ROP	Right occipito posterior
ROT	Right occipito transverse
RP	Retrograde pyelogram
RPA	Right pulmonary artery
RR	Recovery room
RS	Respiratory system
RT	Radiation therapy
RU	Retrograde urogram
RUE	Right upper extremity
RUL	Right upper lobe
RURTI	Recurrent upper respiratory tract infection
RVF	Right ventricular failure
RVH	Right ventricular hypertrophy
Rx	Recuoe (take)
S	
S-1, S-2	First, second sacral vertebrae
Sa	Sarcoma
SAP	Serum alkaline phosphate
SB	Still birth
SBE	Sub acute bacterial endocarditis
SBP	Systolic blood pressure
SCA	Sickle-cell anemia
SCC	Squamous cell carcinoma
SCI	Spinal cord injury
SD	Spontaneous delivery
SEP	Senile enlarge prostate
SGOT	Serum glutamic oxalic transminase
SGPT	Serum gultamic pyruvic transminase
SH	Serum hepatitis
SLE	Systemic lupus erythematosus
SMR	Sub-mucous resection
SOB	Shortness of breath
SPE	Serum protein electrophoresis
SPP	Suprapubic prostatectomy
SSE	Soapsuds enema
SSG	Split skin graft
STD	Sexually transmitted disease
STOP	Suction termination of pregnancy
SVD	Spontaneous vaginal delivery
SVG	Saphenous vein graft
SVT	Suproventricular tachycardia
Sx.	Symptoms
T	
T&A	Tonsillectomy and adenoidectomy
T-1, T-2	First, second thoracic vertebrae
T-3, T-4	Tri-iodothyronine, thyroxine

Abbreviations	*Expansion*
TAH	Total abdominal hysterectomy
TAL	Tendo Achilles lengthening
TAO	Thromboangiitis obliterans
TB	Tuberculosis
TBM	Tuberculosis meningitis
TEV	Talipes equinovarus
TIA	Transient ischeamic attack
tid	Three times daily (ter in die)
TKR	Total knee replacement
TMJ	Temporomandibular joint
TPR	Temperature, pulse and respiration
TPUR	Transperineal urethral resection
TS	Thoracic surgery
TSH	Thyroid stimulating hormone
TT	Tetanus toxoid
TTH	Thyrotropic hormone
TTP	Thrombotic thrombocytopenic purpura
TUR	Transurethral resection
TURP	Transurethral resection of prostate
TVH	Total vaginal hysterectomy
TVP	Transvesical prostatectomy
TX	Therapy
U	
U/A	Urinalysis
UC	Ulcerative colitis
UD	Urethral discharge
UDT	Undescended testicle
UGI	Upper gastrointestinal
UL	Upper lobe
UNG	Ointment
URI	Upper respiratory infection
URTI	Upper respiratory tract infection
US	Ultrasound
UTI	Urinary tract infection
V	
V&D	Vomiting and diarrhoea
VA	Visual acuity
VD	Veneral disease
VDRL	Veneral disease research laboratory
VE	Visual efficiency
VF	Ventricular fibrillation
VHD	Valvular heart disease
VMR	Vasomotor rhinitis
VRI	Viral respiratory infection
VS	Vital signs
VSD	Ventricular septal defect
VT	Ventricular tachycardia
VV	Varicose veins
W	
WBC	White blood count
WC	Whooping cough
WCC	White cell count
WNL	Within normal limits
WPWS	Wolf-Parkinson-White (syndrome)
WR	Wassermann reaction
X	
XDP	Xeroderma pigmentosum
X-match	Cross-match
XR	X-ray

SYMBOLS

Symbols LS	*Expansion*
´	Foot
#	Fracture
>	Greater than
l	Left
"	Inch
↑	Increase
∞	Infinity
<	Lesser than
♂	Male
ug	Microgram
Y	Year
ul	Microliter
u	Micron
M	Murmur
–	Negative
a	Above
+	Not definite
B	After
oz	Ounce
~	Approximate
/	Per
@	At
+	Positive
*	Birth
:	Ratio
( )	Combined with
√	Right
+	Death
.	Start of operation
<	Decrease
v	Systolic pressure
^	Diastolic pressure
R_x	Take
X	End of operation
c	With
=	Equal
s	Without
♀	Female

Bibliography

1. Abdelhak, M, Grostick, S, and Hanken, MA. (2012). Health information: management of a strategic resource. St. Louis, MO: Elsevier Saunders, 2012.
2. Abrams, K, and Crook, G (2011). The canadian health information management association: health information management in Canada: HIM-Interchange.
3. AHIMA (2008). "Eligibility Requirements". AHIMA. http://www.ahima.org/certification/rhia/requirements.
4. AHIMA (2010). "AHIMA History". AHIMA. Retrieved 2010-01-08.
5. AHIMA (n.d.). New AHIMA Book Addresses PHRs-ADVANCE For Health ... (n.d.).
6. AHIMA. "HIM and Health IT: Discovering Common Ground in an Electronic Healthcare Environment." Journal of AHIMA 79, no. 11 (Nov.-Dec. 2008): 69–74.
7. AHIMA. "Statement on Data Stewardship." December 2008. www.ahima.org/downloads/pdfs/advocacy/AHIMA_PositionStatementDataStewardship_001.pdf.
8. AHIMA. 4/20/2004 HIM Baccalaureate Degree Entry-Level Competencies. AHIMA Education Strategy Committee. Retrieved 1/8/2010.
9. AHIMA. 6/3/2004 HIM Associate Degree Entry-Level Competencies. AHIMA Education Strategy Committee. Accessed 1/8/2010.
10. AHIMA. Eligibility Requirements: Registered Health Information Administrator. Retrieved 1/8/2010.
11. Alberta Occupational Profiles, 2011. Health Information Management Professionalhttp://alis.alberta.ca/occinfo/Content/RequestAction.asp?aspAction=GetHTMLProfile&format=html&OCCPRO_ID= 71002536.
12. Al-Qahtani, MF, Almansour, R, Alharbi, A, Aljasser, M, & Alsunaid, H. (2013). Employer Perceptions of Workforce Preparation of the Graduates of the Health Information Management and Technology Program. Journal of American Science, 9(12).
13. Al-Sawai, A, and Al-Shishtawy, MM (2015). Health Workforce Planning: An overview and suggested approach in Oman. Sultan Qaboos University medical journal, 15(1), e27.
14. Baine, SO, and Kasangaki, A (2014). A scoping study on task shifting; the case of Uganda. BMC Health Services Research, 14, 184. doi: http://dx.doi.org/10.1186/1472-6963-14-184.
15. Bates, David W, and Asaf Bitton. "The Future of Health Information Technology in the Patient-Centered Medical Home." Health Affairs 29, no. 4 (Apr. 2010): 614-21. www.cimit.org/images/events/ciw/IT-in-Patient-Centered-Medical-Home.pdf1.pdf
16. Bennett, V. (2010). Health Information Management Workforce - When Opportunities Abound. Health Information Management Journal, 39(3), 4-6.
17. Bochantin, Felisha, et al. "HIM Expertise Critical for the Advancement of Quality and Patient Safety Initiatives." August 2011, Journal of AHIMA. http://journal.ahima.org
18. CAHIIM. (2005) Interpretation of Standards: Associate Degree section VI.F. Retrieved 1/8/2010.
19. CAHIIM. Interpretation of Standards: Baccalaureate Degree section VI.F. Retrieved 1/8/2010.
20. CAHIIM.org. Retrieved 1/8/2010. Centers for Medicare and Medicaid Services. "Medicare Demonstrations Illustrate Benefits in Paying for Quality Health Care." Press release. December 9, 2010. www.cms.gov/DemoProjectsEvalRpts/downloads/PGP_Press_Release.pdf.

21. Centers for Medicare and Medicaid Services. "Medicare Demonstrations Illustrate Benefits in Paying for Quality Health Care." Press release. December 9, 2010. www.cms.gov/DemoProjectsEvalRpts/downloads/PGP_Press_Release.pdf.
22. Challenges of HIM Professionals with Emerging Technology and Reimbursement Models, by Narendar SampathKurmar, published in the Proceeding of HIM INDIA INFO-2015, 4th-5th December, 2015, pp 47–50.
23. Chicago State University Profession. Retrieved 1/8/2010 CHISP Healthcare IT certification.CHISP Certification Requirement. Retrieved 3/2/2010.
24. Clark, Jill. "Tools for Data Analysis: New Toolkit Provides Resources for Health Data Analysts." Journal of AHIMA 82, no. 2 (Feb. 2011): 40-41.
25. Clausen, David C, et al. "Global Trigger Tool Shows That Adverse Events in Hospitals May Be Ten Times Greater Than Previously Measured." Health Affairs 30, no. 4 (Apr. 2011): 4581–89.
26. Creating HIM Profession in Sultanate of Oman, Journal of AHIMA, Vol. 75, No. 9, October 2004, pp 50–54.
27. Data Retrieval, Analysis, and Reporting Skills are Critical for HIM and Health Information Technology Professionals-UW HIMT BLOG
28. Dentzer, Susan. "Still Crossing the Quality Chasm-Or Suspended over It?" Health Affairs 30, no. 4 (Apr. 2011): 554-55. Eramo, Lisa A. "HIM, Quality, and Safety: Data Collection and Analysis Skills Offer a Natural Role in Patient Safety." Journal of AHIMA 81, no. 4 (Apr. 2010): 48–49.
29. Dyson, SL, Greene, SB, & Fraher, EP (2004). A shortage of health information management professionals: how would we know? Journal of allied health, 33(3), 167–173.
30. EHR Functional Requirements Specifications by Functional Requirements Spcifications by A. Balasubramanian, in the proceedings of HIMA INDIA INFO-2015-4th-5th December, 2015-86:89
31. Eramo, Lisa A. "HIM, Quality, and Safety: Data Collection and Analysis Skills Offer a Natural Role in Patient Safety." Journal of AHIMA 81, no. 4 (Apr. 2010): 48–49.
32. Forster, Alan J, et al. "The Incidence and Severity of Adverse Events Affecting Patients after Discharge from the Hospital." Annals of Internal Medicine 138, no. 3 (2003): 161–67.
33. Giannangelo, Kathy, and Linda Hyde. "Retooling Quality Measures for ICD-10." Journal of AHIMA 81, no. 6 (June 2010): 56–57.
34. Goedert, J (2013). Health information management: WHAT a ride it has been. Health Data Management, 21(10), 22–24, 26–27.
35. Green, MA, and Bowie, MJ (2011). Essentials of Health Information Management: Principles and Practices (Second Edition ed.). USA: Delmar CENGAGE Learning.
36. Green, MA, and Bowie, MJ (2011). Essentials of Health Information Management: Principles and Practices (Second Edition ed). USA: Delmar Cengage Learning.
37. "Health Information as an Aid to Effective Hospital management" published in IHRIM Journal (UK) Vol 45, No. 4, March 2003, 15–19.
38. Health Information Management's Professional Role in Efficient Management of Health Information in USA by Dr Jayachand Pallekonda, BCom. LLM, PhD, RHIM (USA), Retired Health Information Manager (USA, published in the Proceeding of HIM INDIA INFO-2015, 4th - 5th December, 2015: 27–30.
39. "Health Records Paper to Paperless", book published in the year 2015 by Dr G Mogli, JAYPEE Brothers, Medical Publishers (P) Ltd., India, PP 440–445.
40. "Health Records Paper to Paperless", book published in the year 2015 by Dr GD Mogli, JAYPEE Brothers Medical Publishers (P) Ltd., India; PP 440–445.
41. Healthcare Integration and Connectivity: Results of a Survey by the Enterprise Information Systems Steering Committee. Page 4. HIMSS. Retrieved 1/8/2010.
42. Hersh, W, & Wright, A (2008). What workforce is needed to implement the health information technology agenda? Analysis from the HIMSS Analytics™ database. Paper presented at the AMIA Annual Symposium Proceedings.
43. "HIM Leadership Role in Integrating in Healthcare", published in the proceedings of MEDRECON-2012, 12th Annual National Conference on Medical Records, held from 3–4th February, 2012. at Rajiv Gandhi Cancer Institute & Research Centre, Delhi. (PP-107).

44. HIM Professional Current Status and Future Prospects, by Ms RaniyaHumaid M Al-Kiyumi, PhD student, Australia, published in the Proceeding of HIM INDIA INFO-2015, 4th - 5th December, 2015, pp 27–30.
45. HIM Professionals' Endurance in 21st Century, Proceedings of 14th International Health Records Congress, November 2004, held at Washington, DC, USA, by Dr GD Mogli
46. HIMSS (2008). "AHIMA History". HIMSS Legacy Workgroup. Retrieved 2010-01-08.
47. HIMSS. HIMSS.org. Retrieved 1/8/2010.
48. Hurst, K, & Kelley Patterson, D (2014). Health and social care workforce planning and development- an overview. International journal of health care quality assurance, 27(7), 562–572.
49. Information Governance in Healthcare-Benchmarking White Paper-Cohasset Associates-AHIMA International Standard Classification of Occupations, 2008 revision: Unit Group 3252: Medical records and health information technicians. http://www.ilo.org/public/english/bureau/stat/isco/index.htm
50. Information Governance in Healthcare-Benchmarking White Paper-Cohasset Associates-AHIMA. Giannangelo, Kathy, and Linda Hyde. "Retooling Quality Measures for ICD-10." Journal of AHIMA 81, no. 6 (June 2010): 56–57.
51. Jacob, JA (2013). HIM's evolving workforce. Preparing for the electronic age's HIM profession shake-up. Journal of AHIMA / American Health Information Management Association, 84(8), 18–22.
52. LaTour, Kathleen M, and Maki, Shirley Eichenwald. (2010). Health information management concepts, principles, and practice. Chicago, Illinois: American Health Information Management Association.) (LaTour, & Maki, 2010).
53. Ledikwe, JH, Reason, LL, Burnett, SM, Busang, L, Bodika, S, Lebelonyane, R, . . . Mmelesi, M. (2013). Establishing a health information workforce: innovation for low-and middle-income countries. Hum Resour Health, 11(1), 34.
54. Marco, David, and Anne Marie Smith. "Understanding Data Governance and Stewardship, Part 3." Information Management, November 2006. www.information-management.com/issues/20061101/1066745-1.html.
55. Marshall, MN (1996). Sampling for qualitative research. Family practice, 13(6), 522–26.
56. Medical Record Diploma Education Program in Kuwait by Dr Saadpim Faris Al Azmi, MS, PhD (USA), Associate Professor, College of Health Sciences, The Public Authority for Applied Education and Training, Kuwati.
57. Medical Records and Health Information Technicians. Retrieved 1/8/2010.
58. Medical Records Diploma Education Program in Kuwait by Dr. SaadounFarisAlAzmi, MS, PhD, (USA), Associate Professor, College of Health Sciences, The Public Authority for Applied Education and Training, Kuwait, published in the Proceedings of Health Information Management Association (HIMA) India-HIM INDIA INFO-2015, 4th-5th December, 2015 held at Krishna Institute of Medical Sciences Ltd., Hyderabad, India, PP 24–26.
59. "Medical Records in Afghanistan" published in the Medical Record and Health Care Information Journal Vol. 18, No. 2, May 19771, United Kingdom
60. Mervat Abdelhak, et al. "Health Information: Management of a Strategic Resource", Second Edition Occupational Outlook Handbook, 2010-11 Edition. Medical Records and Health Information Technicians. Retrieved 1/8/2010.
61. Moreno, L, D Peikes, and A Krilla. "Strategies to Ensure HITECH Supports the Patient-Centered Medical Home." AHRQ publication no. 11-0013. Agency for Healthcare Research and Quality, February 2011. www.pcmh.ahrq.gov/portal/server.pt/community/pcmh__home/1483/ahrq_commissioned_research.
62. Naylor, Mary D, et al. "The Importance of Transitional Care in Achieving Health Reform." Health Affairs 30, no. 4 (Apr. 2011): 746–54.
63. Partner in the Delivery of Quality Healthcare (nd). Retrieved November 28, 2009, from American Health Information Management Association.
64. "Patient-Centered Medical Homes." Health Affairs. September 14, 2010. www.healthaffairs.org/healthpolicybriefs/brief.php?brief_id=25.

65. Price Waterhouse Coopers. "Transforming Healthcare through Secondary Use of Health Data." 2009. www.pwc.com/us/en/healthcare/publications/secondary-health-data.jhtml
66. Pronovost, Peter J, and Richard Lilford. "A Road Map for Improving the Performance of Performance Measures." Health Affairs 30, no. 4 (Apr. 2011): 569–73.
67. Riyami, AA (2012). Health Vision 2050 Oman: A Committed Step towards Reforms. Oman Medical Journal, 27(3), 190–191. doi: 10.5001/omj.2012.43
68. Role of Associate of Health Information for Care, Cost and Quality Assurance in the Millennium by Dr Mogli & Mogli SK Presented in 13th International Health Record Congress, 2nd to 6th October, 2000, Melbourne, Australia
69. Safian, SC (2012). Factors Influencing Students to Enroll in Health Information Management Programs. Longwook, FL: Capella University.
70. Safian, SC (2012). Factors Influencing Students to Enroll in Health Information Management Programs. Longwook, FL: Capella University.
71. Sandefer, R, DeAlmeda, D, Dougherty, M, Mancilla, D, and Marc, D (2014). Keeping Current in the Electronic Era. Journal of AHIMA, 39–44.
72. Sandelowski, M (2000). Focus on research methods combining qualitative and quantitative sampling, data collection, and analysis techniques. Research in nursing and health, 23, 246–255.
73. Shepheard, J (2010). Health Information Management and Clinical Coding Workforce Issues. Health Information Management Journal, 39(3), 37–41.
74. Sheridan, PT, and Smith, LB (2009). Redefining HIM Leadership: Toward an HIM Leadership Framework: A Commentary on HIM Leadership. Perspectives in Health Information Management / AHIMA, American Health Information Management Association, 6(Summer), 1c.
75. "Standards for Medical Record Services" published in IHRIM Journal (UK), vol. 41, No. 2, March 2000 pp. 24–27
76. Stansfield S (2005). "Structuring information and incentives to improve health". Bulletin of the World Health Organization, 83(8):562.
77. Street, T (2012). Creating change in the health information management profession. Health Information Management Journal, 41(1), A20-A20.
78. Tips for Evaluating the Pre-implementation of Electronic Health Records Software by Vikky (ND Vikram) published in the Proceeding of HIM INDIA INFO-2015, 4th-5th December, 2015, pp 65–68.
79. Van Den Bos, Jill, et al. "The $17.1 Billion Problem: The Annual Cost of Measurable Medical Errors." Health Affairs 30, no. 4 (Apr. 2011): 4596–603.
80. Wall Street Journal. "Benefits of Electronic Health Records Seen as Outweighing Privacy Risks". Retrieved 1/8/2010.
81. Watson, PJ (2008). Health information management in Australia: a brief history of the profession and the association. Health Information Management Journal, 37(2), 40.
82. Watzlaf, VJ, Rudman, WJ, Hart-Hester, S, and Ren, P (2009). The Progression of the Roles and Functions of HIM Professionals: A Look into the Past, Present, and Future. Perspectives in Health Information Management/AHIMA, American Health Information Management Association, 6 (Summer).
83. White, Susan, Crystal Kallem, Allison Viola, and June Bronnert. "An ACO Primer." Journal of AHIMA 82, no. 6 (June 2011): 48–50.
84. White, Susan, Crystal Kallem, Allison Viola, and June Bronnert. "An ACO Primer." Journal of AHIMA 82, no. 6 (June 2011): 48–50.
85. World Health Organization. (2010). Classifying health workers. Geneva: WHO.
86. Zeng, X, Reynolds, R, and Sharp, M (2009). Redefining the roles of health information management professionals in health information technology. Perspectives in Health Information Management/ AHIMA, American Health Information Management Association, 6 (Summer).

Index